OXFORD MEDICAL PUBLICATIONS

Health care for Asians

OXFORD GENERAL PRACTICE SERIES

1. Paediatric problems in general practice
   M. Modell and R. H. Boyd
2. Geriatric problems in general practice
   G. Wilcock, J. A. M. Gray, and P. M. M. Pritchard
3. Preventive medicine in general practice
   edited by J. A. M. Gray and G. H. Fowler
5. Locomotor disability in general practice
   edited by M. I. V. Jayson and R. Million
6. The consultation: an approach to learning and teaching
   D. Pendleton, P. Tate, P. Havelock, and T. Schofield
8. Management in general practice
   P. M. M. Pritchard, K. B. Low, and M. Whalen
9. Modern obstetrics in general practice
   edited by G. N. Marsh
10. Terminal care at home
    edited by R. Spilling
11. Rheumatology for general practitioners
    H. L. F. Currey and S. Hull
12. Women's problems in general practice
    (Second edition)
    edited by Ann McPherson
13. Paediatric problems in general practice
    (Second edition)
    M. Modell and R. H. Boyd
14. Epidemiology in general practice
    edited by D. Morrell
15. Psychological problems in general practice
    A. C. Markus, C. Murray Parkes, P. Tomson, and M. Johnston
16. Research methods for general practitioners
    D. Armstrong, M. Calnan, and J. Grace
17. Family problems
    Peter R. Williams
18. Health care for Asians
    edited by Brian R. McAvoy and Liam J. Donaldson
19. Continuing care: the management of chronic disease
    (Second edition)
    edited by J. C. Hasler and T. P. C. Schofield

Health Care for Asians

Oxford General Practice Series 18

Edited by

BRIAN R. McAVOY

Department of General Practice,
University of Auckland, New Zealand

and

LIAM J. DONALDSON

Northern Regional Health Authority,
Newcastle-upon-Tyne

OXFORD   NEW YORK   TOKYO

OXFORD UNIVERSITY PRESS

1990

Oxford University Press, Walton Street, Oxford OX2 6DP

Oxford   New York   Toronto
Delhi   Bombay   Calcutta   Madras   Karachi
Petaling Jaya   Singapore   Hong Kong   Tokyo
Nairobi   Dar es Salaam   Cape Town
Melbourne   Auckland

and associated companies in
Berlin   Ibadan

Oxford is a trade mark of Oxford University Press

Published in the United States
by Oxford University Press, New York

British Library Cataloguing in Publication Data
Health care for Asians. – (Oxford general practice series; 18)
1. Great Britain. Health services. Requirements of Asian immigrants
I. McAvoy, Brian R.   II. Donaldson, Liam J.
362.8'4
ISBN 0–19–261733–8

Library of Congress Cataloging in Publication Data
Health care for Asians/edited by Brian R. McAvoy, Liam J. Donaldson.
p. cm. – (Oxford general practice series; 18)
1. Asians – Health and hygiene – Great Britain.   2. Asians – Medical
care – Great Britain.   3. Asians – Great Britain – Social life and
Oxford general practice series ; no. 18.
RA485.H34   1990   362.1'089'95041 – dc20
89-22973
ISBN 0–19–261733–8

Set by
BP Integraphics, Bath
Printed in Great Britain
by Courier International,
Tiptree, Essex

Foreword

Sir Robert Kilpatrick
President of the General Medical Council

The public has always expected, and indeed received, a high standard of medical care from doctors in the United Kingdom. This public expectation, while a source of pride for the medical profession, imposes a heavy obligation on practitioners to maintain, and where necessary improve, those standards. The emphasis which we naturally place on undergraduate and postgraduate training should not obscure the need to pay proper attention to the continuing education needs of independent practitioners, both in hospital and general practice. The care of patients from ethnic minority backgrounds is an excellent case in point. Given the overcrowded state of undergraduate curricula and the heavy demands of postgraduate training programmes, doctors may have received little or no guidance on ethnic minority health issues, in spite of its importance for those practising in urban areas.

This book addresses these matters directly and comprehensively. Its scope is wide and the approach is consciously interdisciplinary. The contributors write from first-hand experience, as practitioners and researchers, of the problems—medical, social, or cultural—faced by Asians and those responsible for their care. It deserves the widest circulation, and I commend it most warmly to all those who have a professional interest in the delivery of health care to ethnic minorities and in the continuing improvement in standards of medical practice in the United Kingdom and elsewhere.

Acknowledgements

We are indebted to the following people who have helped us enormously by their critical comments, suggestions and support: Dr Azhar Farooqi, Dr Salim Khan, Terjinder Manku, Dr Joseph Owusu-Bempah, and Rabia Raza. We would also like to thank all the authors for their efforts and support, Drs Kevin Browne and Pauline McAvoy for their contributions to Chapters 13 and 10 respectively, Chris Shaw of OPCS for advice during the preparation of Chapter 6, and Dr Raj Bhopal for advice during the preparation of Chapter 14. Thanks to Ishbel Rans for secretarial help and Bernadette Hayes for repeated typing, checking, and general assembly of the book. We are grateful to the Health Education Authority and the National Extension College for permission to use material from their publications in Chapter 5, and to OPCS for their permission to quote statistical data in Chapters 6 and 14.

Finally we are indebted to our wives and children for tolerating our preoccupations during this time.

B.R.M.
L.J.D.

Colour plate section

The editors and publisher are grateful to E. Merck Ltd for the company's contribution towards the production costs of the colour plate section.

Contents

List of contributors   ix

Cultural and religious aspects

1 Asians in Britain—
origins and lifestyles   3
Colette Taylor
2 Cultural factors in health and   17
illness
Cecil Helman

Organizational aspects

3 Organization and delivery of care   31
Allan McNaught
4 Asian doctors and nurses in the NHS   40
Aly Rashid
5 Communication   57
Brian McAvoy
Akram Sayeed
6 Asians in Britain: the population   72
and its characteristics
Liam Donaldson
Luise Parsons

Clinical aspects

7 Alternative/complementary medicine   93
Bashir Qureshi
8 Diet and nutrition   117
Bashir Qureshi
9 General medical problems   130
Stephen Sturman
D. G. Beevers
10 Women's health   150
Brian McAvoy
11 Obstetrics   172
John MacVicar
12 Hereditary disorders   192
Ian Young

viii *Contents*

13 Paediatrics   210
    John Black
14 Elderly Asians   237
    Liam Donaldson
    Marie Johnson
15 Infectious diseases   250
    Karl Nicholson
16 Skin diseases   272
    Derek Barker
17 Psychological/psychiatric disorders   290
    Philip Rack
18 Terminal care and bereavement   304
    Dewi Rees

Index   321

Plates fall between pp 276 and 277 in the text

Contributors

Derek John Barker, MA, MB, MRCP
Consultant Dermatologist, Bradford Royal Infirmary.

He has been a Consultant Dermatologist in Bradford for nearly ten years. The majority of Bradford's Asian citizens originated in Pakistan but there are also Sikhs and Indians. Bradford also has substantial West Indian, Polish, and Ukrainian communities. Among the Department's other interests are contact dermatitis and the use of remedial camouflage techniques.

D. G. Beevers, MD, FRCP
Reader in Medicine, Department of Medicine, University of Birmingham and Honorary Consultant, Dudley Road Hospital, Birmingham.

Prior to the present appointment he was a clinical scientist in the MRC Blood Pressure Unit at the Western Infirmary, Glasgow. Dr Beevers' research interests are mainly in the field of the epidemiology of high blood-pressure, but he has a subsidiary interest in racial differences in common diseases. He is the Editor of the *Journal of Human Hypertension*.

John Angus Black, MD, FRCP
Late: Consultant Paediatrician, Children's Hospital and Jessop Hospital for Women (1963–1981)—Sheffield. Honorary Consultant Paediatrician, King's College Hospital, London (1982–).

His special interests are in paediatric aspects of ethnic minorities in Britain, metabolic disorders and diabetes mellitus in children. He is also Chairman of the Eritrean Medical Association (UK).

Liam J. Donaldson, MSc, MD, FRCS(Ed), FFCM
Regional Medical Officer/Head of Clinical Policy Northern Regional Health Authority.

Prior to taking up his present post he was Senior Lecturer at the University of Leicester. His research interests include the health of ethnic minorities and the application of epidemiology to health service problems. Dr Donaldson is Editor of the *Journal of Public Health Medicine* and co-author of *Essential community medicine*.

Cecil G. Helman, MB ChB, Dip Soc Anthrop
Lecturer, Department of Primary Health Care, University College and Middlesex Medical School, and Research Fellow, Department of Anthropology, University College London.

He is a Fellow of the Royal Anthropological Institute and author of *Culture, health and illness: an introduction for health professionals*.

Marie Johnson, BA (Hons) Anthropology, PhD
Senior Clinical Policy Officer, Northern Regional Health Authority.

She has carried out research in Iceland and Britain and her particular interest is in people's perception of illness and health and the quality of service they receive from the NHS.

John MacVicar, MD, FRCS, FRCOG
Foundation Professor of Obstetrics and Gynaecology at the University of Leicester School of Medicine.

He has a special interest in perinatal and maternal mortality, nutrition in pregnancy, and, in particular, obstetric problems of the Asian community.

Brian R. McAvoy, MB, ChB, BSc, MRCP, FRCGP
Elaine Gurr Professor of General Practice at the University of Auckland, New Zealand.

He qualified at Glasgow in 1972 and spent a year as a Teaching Fellow in the Department of Family Medicine at McMaster University, Hamilton, Ontario. He was a Lecturer, then Senior Lecturer in the General Practice Unit at Leicester University. He has a special interest in Asian health care, the application of roleplay and simulated patients in the teaching of clinical and communication skills, and health-care delivery.

Allan McNaught, BSc, MPhil
A former health administrator.

For the past seven years he has been involved in health-management training, development, and consultancy. He is currently Programme Director: Health Administration with the Overseas Development Administration, London. He was on loan to the Government of Zimbabwe until the end of 1989 and is now undertaking similar work at the Medical School of Punjab University.

Karl Nicholson, MB, FRCP, MRC Path.
Senior Lecturer and Honorary Consultant in Infectious Diseases at the University of Leicester and Groby Road Hospital, Leicester.

His particular interests include rabies, viral respiratory infections, and antiviral agents.

Luise Parsons, MB BS, MFCM
Consultant Epidemiologist/Specialist in Community Medicine to the Northern Regional Health Authority.

Prior to her present post she worked in City and Hackney in Community Medicine where she was closely involved with a project which provided advocates for non-English speaking women in the maternity department. She has also worked in Peru, and Papua New Guinea. Her special interests are ethnic health care, womens and childrens health care, and inequalities in health.

Bashir Qureshi, FRCGP, DCH, AFOM (RCP), FRSH, MICGP, FRIPHH
General Practitioner and Community Medical Officer, Hounslow, London.

Writer, lecturer, and broadcaster in transcultural medicine, Dr Qureshi was formerly a member of the Communication Executive of the RCGP. Currently he is a member of the Council of Section of General Practice of the RSM and Chairman of the South Middlesex Division of the BMA.

Philip H. Rack, MA, MB, BChir, FRCPsych, DPM
Consultant Psychiatrist from 1967–1987 in Bradford, Yorkshire.

He developed a multidisciplinary transcultural team to cater for the psychiatric and social problems of the ethnic minority population of Bradford. He retired from clinical practice in 1987, but continues lecturing and writing. He has published over 40 articles and a book *Race, culture and mental disorder*. He is a Visiting Lecturer at the Department of Psychiatry, University of Leeds; Consultant to Fountain House, Lahore; and Honorary Life Member of the Pakistan Psychiatric Society.

Aly Rashid, MB, ChB, MRCGP, DRCOG
General Practitioner, Leicester
Honorary Research Associate, Leicester University.

His interests are in research and teaching in general practice facilitating improvement in communication skills of health care professions, resulting in better communication between patients and their carers.

(Abul Fatah) Akram Sayeed, OBE, MB BS
Leicester inner-city General Practitioner.

Has done pioneering Community Relations work and remains actively involved in transcultural health care and ethnic minority health problems.

William Dewi Rees, MD, FRCGP
Former rural general practitioner; now Medical Director, St Mary's Hospice, Birmingham, and Honorary Senior Clinical Lecturer, University of Birmingham.

Stephen George Sturman, MB, ChB, MRCP
Sheldon Clinical Research Fellow, Department of Neurology, University of Birmingham. Formerly Registrar, University Department of Medicine, Dudley Road Hospital, Birmingham.

Colette Taylor, BSc
Medical anthropologist

Currently completing postgraduate research at University College, London, on the adaptation of Asian (Ayurvedic) medicine in London and the implications for health policy and planning.

Ian D. Young, MSc, MD, FRCP, DCH
Senior Lecturer/Honorary Consultant in Child Health (Clinical Genetics), University of Leicester.
Research interests include: the aetiology, delineation, and epidemiology of multiple malformation syndromes, inherited connective tissue disorders, and the skeletal dysplasias; and, the delivery of genetic services to the community and the likely impact of new developments in molecular genetics.

Cultural and religious aspects

1 Asians in Britain— origins and lifestyles

Colette Taylor

Introduction

The phrase 'Asians in Britain' somehow suggests a cohesive group, a single community; whereas 'Asian' people in Britain represent a variety of communities and individuals, with fundamental differences in terms of country of origin, language, religion, social class, politics, and many other factors. Just as Europe can be divided into separate countries, languages, cultures, and subcultures, so too can Asia, or, to be more specific in the context of this book, South Asia. But such a breakdown, particularly in one chapter, is of limited use (the risk of stereotyping being all too obvious), and should only be taken as an impression of the range and complexity of the Asian communities in Britain. Information, for example, about beliefs, languages, and lifestyles is not enough to improve health-care delivery, but it can help to create awareness of the range of factors to be taken into account in planning and providing an appropriate and equitable service. Regarding everyone in the same way does not constitute an equal opportunities policy, nor does special provision have to be separate provision; rather, it should be an integral part of a comprehensive health service.

The term 'immigrant' tends to stereotype communities and individuals as 'new', and outside the mainstream of society or of service provision. Asian communities in Britain vary from those newly arrived (largely limited since 1971 to certain dependants) to individuals of the third or even some later generation to become settled here. Lifestyles are constantly changing, and although culture, the effects of migration, and the added dimensions of racism, discrimination, and prejudice are factors determining health-care needs, 'Asian' people are also subject to all the common socio-economic factors affecting health—for example, occupation, housing, and unemployment.

This chapter will provide an overview of the origins of the main Asian communities and of why people came to Britain, and a brief outline of the main languages, religions and naming systems among them, and of some aspects of their lifestyles. This information is not definitive, and local resources such as Community Relations Councils and voluntary groups should be contacted for more specific information.

Origins

Since partition in 1947, and the war of independence in East Pakistan (now Bangladesh), the Indian subcontinent consists politically of Pakistan, India, Bangladesh, and Sri Lanka. People who have come from the subcontinent have tended to come from a few main areas (Fig. 1.1).

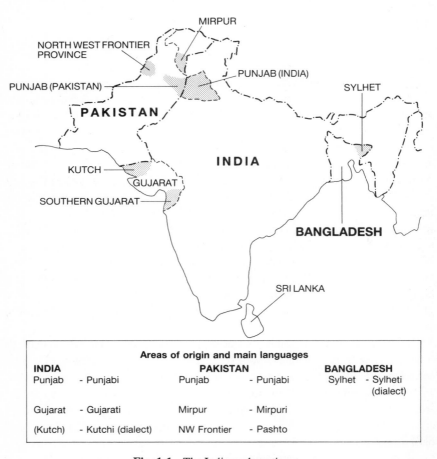

Areas of origin and main languages					
INDIA		**PAKISTAN**		**BANGLADESH**	
Punjab	- Punjabi	Punjab	- Punjabi	Sylhet	- Sylheti (dialect)
Gujarat	- Gujarati	Mirpur	- Mirpuri		
(Kutch)	- Kutchi (dialect)	NW Frontier	- Pashto		

Fig. 1.1   The Indian subcontinent.

In India the main areas from which people have come to Britain are the Punjab and the state of Gujarat. Since partition in 1947 the Punjab has been divided into two parts—the Indian Punjab and the Pakistani Punjab. Punjabis from the Indian Punjab are predominantly Sikh; and predominantly Muslim from the Pakistani Punjab. The state of Gujarat on the west coast of Indian has had a tradition of migration (particularly to East Africa) for hundreds of years. Gujaratis from Gujarat state constitute the largest group of 'Asians' in Britain, and are mainly settled in the South East and the Midlands. They have tended to come from two areas of Gujarat; the northern area—Kutch—and southern Gujarat. The majority of Gujaratis in Britain are Hindu, although there are communities of Gujarati Muslims—for example, in the West Midlands. There are Tamil communities in Britain from the state of Tamil Nadu in South India, and from Sri Lanka; these are predominantly Hindu. There are also communities of Christian Asians, particularly from Goa on the east coast of India.

People from Pakistan tend to have come either from the Pakistani Punjab—Punjabis; from the North-West Frontier province—Pathans; or from Mirpur District—Mirpuris. They are predominantly Muslim, and have settled mainly in the West Midlands, Yorkshire, and the North West. People from Bangladesh have usually come from one main area in the north-east of the country—the district of Sylhet; and Bengalis (predominantly Muslim), have settled mainly in the South East, the largest community being in the London borough of Tower Hamlets.

A proportion of the Asian communities in Britain originate from East Africa—mainly from Uganda, Kenya, Tanzania, Malawi, and Zambia (see Fig. 1.2). The main areas in the Indian subcontinent from which migration to East Africa occurred were Gujarat and the Punjab. East African Asians are largely settled in the South East and West Midlands; those of Gujarati origins are mainly Hindus (some Muslims), and those of Punjabi origins are Hindu, Sikh, and Muslim. There are some Asian communities in Britain originating from the Caribbean, mainly from Trinidad and Guyana. These consist mainly of Hindus and Muslims.

Reasons for migration

The main migration from the Indian subcontinent occurred after the Second World War, largely in response to post-war labour shortages in Britain. Migration from the main 'sending' areas of the Indian subcontinent and East Africa occurred for a variety of social, economic, and political reasons.

In considering the main factors which affect migration it is helpful to conceptualize them broadly as 'push' or 'pull' factors. The 'pull' factors, in Britain, of gaps in the labour market, particularly in manual jobs and shift work, influenced migration and patterns of settlement. Positive recruitment and 'chain migration' based on kin-networks also influenced patterns of settlement. Southall, for instance, became a focus of settlement for Punjabi Sikhs partly as a result of a rubber vulcanizing plant's operating a positive recruitment drive among members of the Indian Army after the Second World War. The settlement pattern of Pakistanis, largely concentrated in the West Midlands, Yorkshire and Humberside, and the North West, is a reflection of post-war job vacancies in the textile industries, as well as of kin-networks.

In contrast, the 'push' factors from the Indian subcontinent were mainly lack

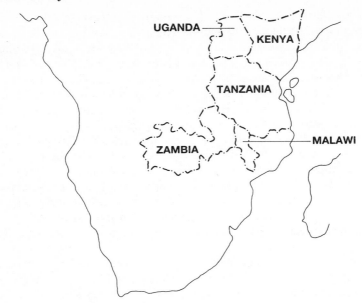

Fig. 1.2   East Africa.

of employment in rural areas, a tradition of emigration from certain areas, and the aftermath of political reorganization—such as the unsettlement caused by partition in 1947. For example in Mirpur the construction of the Mangla Dam in the early 1960s resulted in high levels of migration of people who had only recently resettled after partition. Mirpuris were given priority for immigration at that time, and whole communities from that area migrated to Britain, and resettled particularly in the West Midlands and Yorkshire.

The main factors influencing migration to Britain from East Africa were political. By 1960, longterm migration from the Indian subcontinent to East Africa had resulted in many Asian families, mainly Gujarati and Punjabi in origin, settling in the main towns and cities, usually either as self-employed persons or working in the professions and civil service.

From the early 1960s, East African governments started to implement a policy of 'Africanization' which, among other things, gave preference in employment to Africans. Employment and life-style became increasingly restricted for the East African Asians, particularly those who retained British citizenship; and eventually, in the most extreme case, Uganda, in 1972, all Ugandan Asians holding British passports were expelled in the space of three months. East African Asians migrating as a result of these policies settled in England mainly in the South East and in the East and West Midlands.

The pattern of migration from the Indian subcontinent of men arriving initially in response to labour shortages and with the intention of returning, but followed later by the gradual arrival of relatives and dependants, contrasts with the pattern of refugee migration from East Africa. Migration from the Caribbean was influenced by economic and political factors. Since independence, the Asian communities there have been in a marginal position, though not as unstable as that which the Asians in East Africa experienced.

Tamils from the state of Tamil Nadu in South India settled in Britain mainly after the Second World War, largely in response to labour shortages; while the migration of Tamils from Sri Lanka has been influenced by the unstable political and religious position of the Tamil minority in relation to the Sinhalese majority.

Since 1968 immigration into Britain has been increasingly restricted, particularly since the 1971 Immigration Act. Primary immigration (people coming mainly for work and accepted for settlement after the expiry of a time limit) peaked in 1972, and has been falling since then. Secondary immigration (of relatives and dependants) was restricted by the 1971 Immigration Act and has been steadily declining since 1972.

The analysis of the main 'sending' areas of the Indian subcontinent described above is not always applicable to the various professional groups who migrated to Britain: doctors and other professionals have tended to come from all over the subcontinent, mainly from the urban areas, and will not necessarily be familiar with the majority community languages used by South Asians in Britain.

Language

There are many different languages and dialects in the Indian subcontinent. The main languages spoken in Britain—Gujarati, Punjabi, Bengali, Pashto, Hindi, and Urdu—belong to the Northern Indian group of languages. Some people may speak a dialect of these languages: for example, Gujaratis from the northern area of Gujarat (Kutch) may speak Kutchi, a dialect of Gujarati. Mirpuris from Mirpur may speak Mirpuri, a dialect of Punjabi. Bengalis from the Sylhet district of Bangladesh may speak Sylheti, which is a dialect of Bengali. East African Asians will usually speak the language of the area of the Indian subcontinent from which their families originated—mainly Gujarati and Punjabi; and most of them speak English, which was the administrative language of East Africa.

The languages mentioned above are spoken by the majority Asian communities in Britain, but there are smaller communities from other areas: for example, the Tamil speakers from the Southern Indian state of Tamil Nadu and from Sri Lanka, and the Kokni Muslims from the state of Maharashtra, who speak Kokni. Many people speak more than one Asian language. Hindi (from India) and Urdu (from Pakistan) spoken colloquially are virtually the same language, with only some small variations in vocabulary and pronunciation. Formal Hindi and Urdu have more differences from each other, and may not be understood by a colloquial speaker.

In a written form, the Asian languages referred to above use three alphabets. The Indian languages (Punjabi, Gujarati, Hindi) use two alphabets: Punjabi is written in 'Gurmukhi' script, and Gujarati and Hindi are written in 'Devanagri' script. The Pakistani languages (Urdu, Punjabi, Pashto) are all written in 'Arabic' script, which is read from left to right. Bengali is written in 'Devanagri' script, but in a very different form of it from that used for Gujarati and Hindi.

Examples of different Asian languages and scripts are shown in Fig. 10.1. In these alphabets a word can only be written in one form, which is not the case with their transliterations into the Roman alphabet, in which the same word can sometimes be spelt in more than one way: for instance a name which may appear in English as Choudrey, Choudhury, Chowdry, or Choudri can only be spelt one way in Arabic script. Transliteration of names from Asian scripts into the Roman alphabet has sometimes caused confusion, because of the various forms that may be used in the latter.

The variety and complexity of Asian languages should be taken into account in any situation requiring an interpreter. Professional interpreters should be used rather than *ad hoc* interpreters, as the role demands skill and sensitivity to facilitate communication. In particular it is often inappropriate and unsuccessful to use relatives, friends, and children. Professional staff are often used as interpreters, but may not adequately speak or understand the language needed in the situation if it is not their first language, or they do not possess adequate interpreting skills. Further discussions on this will be found in Chapter 5.

Religion

There are three major religions practised by the majority Asian communities in Britain: Hinduism, Islam, and Sikhism. Like Christianity, each of these religions is interpreted and practised by various groups in different ways, and will vary in its influence on communities and individuals. Trying to define a major religion in a few brief paragraphs tends to result in a resume of the main tenets, historical developments, and sect divisions. General information about religions provides a basic background, but just as there is no such person as a 'typical Christian', the same applies to Hindu, Sikhs, and Muslims. The implications of adherence to a particular religion should always be worked out on an individual basis.

Hinduism

Hinduism is based on a belief in one God, who can be worshipped in many different forms, of which the most important are Brahma (the creator), Vishnu (the preserver), and Shiva (the destroyer). There are many other manifestations, which represent the various qualities of God worshipped by different groups and sects. One of the main Gujarati sects in Britain is the Swami Narayan sect, with communities in the South East and North West. Common to all groups is a belief in non-violence and the idea of a never-ending cycle of creation and destruction—reincarnation. Reincarnation is the cycle of birth and rebirth, based on the belief that all persons are responsible for their actions in each life, and will be reborn again and again until their lifestyles raise them above the cycle of rebirth and unite them with God. Status and condition in each life is determined by behaviour in the last life.

The caste system is linked to the belief in reincarnation. Hindu society is divided into four major castes—the Brahmins (priests); the Kshatriyas (warriors); the Vaisyas (farmers, merchants), and the Sudras (labourers and servants). There is a fifth group of outcastes (untouchables). The caste system resulted in a rigid form of social structure amongst Hindus in Indian society, and although the Indian government has outlawed caste discrimination, the system is deep-rooted, with strong religious connotations. The effect of migration has in some instances reinforced the system, maintaining its social and political implications, and in other instances has contributed to a reduction in its influence. Each caste group contains many subcaste groups, composed of people from a particular social and occupational group and geographical origin. People from the same subcaste group will share a common subcaste name (see section on Names, p. 11).

Jainism is an offshoot of Hinduism founded in the sixth century BC, but Jains are not Hindus, although their beliefs are influenced by Hinduism and they may attend Hindu temples. Most of the Jains in Britain are Gujarati in origin.

Sikhism

Sikhism developed as a reformist movement from Hinduism in the sixteenth century. Sikhism was founded by Guru Nanak, and is based on the teachings of ten Gurus. The Sikh holy book is the *Guru Granth Sahab*, which is a collection of the writings of the ten Gurus. Sikhism is based on belief in one God, with the emphasis on a personal relationship with, and worship of, God. Reincarnation, the cycles of birth and rebirth, is a belief included in Sikhism; but theoretically Sikhism is opposed to the caste system, because of a belief in equality for all, although caste is still reflected in social divisions, particularly in marriage patterns and, for example, in the selection of a *gurdwara* (temple). This provides a centre for communal worship, as well as providing a meeting place for the community; and each *gurdwara* has a kitchen which provides communal food. There are five signs of Sikhism:

Kara — a metal bangle which is usually not removed, worn by men and women;
Kesh — uncut hair;
Kangha — the comb used to secure long hair under a turban;
Kirpan — a small symbolic dagger; and
Kaccha — a sacred under-garment.

There is a special devotion in Sikhism—'taking *Amrit*'—and Sikhs who undertake this are known as *'Amrit Dari'*, and promise to wear the five signs of Sikhism, say special prayers, not eat meat, and attend the *gurdwara* every day. The last Sikh Guru ordered all Sikhs not to use a subcaste name (see section on Names, p. 12), but to use the titles *Singh* (for males), and *Kaur* (for females), in an attempt to alter the caste system and promote equality.

Islam

Islam was founded in the Middle East at the beginning of the seventh century by the prophet Muhammad. Muslims believe in one God—Allah—and believe that Muhammad was the last and most important in a long line of prophets including Jesus Christ. Muhammad was God's messenger, an instrument to proclaim the will of God. According to Muhammad, he was instructed by God to lay down specific rules about the spiritual, physical, and community life of Muslims in the form of a holy book—the Quran.

Islam is a major world religion, and although there is a great deal of similarity in the practices and beliefs of all Muslims, different sects have developed because of differing interpretations and explanations of the Quran. These differences have resulted in two main sects in Islam—the Sunni Muslims and the Shia Muslims. Most Muslims from Pakistan and Bangladesh belong to the Sunni sect, and most Muslims from India, particularly from Gujarat, belong to the Shia sect.

Decisions on matters not discussed in the Quran, or which have new implications—for example, because of developments in technology—are agreed upon mutually by discussion between the Imams (religious leaders) based on the principles in the Quran. Muslims are encouraged to learn Arabic to read the Quran in its Arabic form, and many children go to mosque school in the evenings and at weekends to read and study the Quran. Mosques provide a community centre, as well as holding services and classes. The local community mosque can be approached for information about and for contact with the local community.

The pillars of Islam are the five main duties which devout Muslims should follow:

Faith   —   in God and in the prophet Muhammad; only God is to be worshipped.

Prayer   —   all Muslims should pray formally five times a day—before sunrise; in the early and in the late afternoon; just after sunset; and during the night. Ritual washing should take place before prayers, which should be said with the head towards Mecca. Friday is a holy day; and prayer, especially congregational prayer, is very important.

Charity	—	every Muslim is expected to give money, where possible and appropriate, to the poor.
Fasting	—	Adult Muslims are expected to fast throughout the day during the period known as Ramadan. The date for Ramadan changes each year, as it is based (as are all Muslim festivals) on the lunar calendar—twelve months of 28 days each. Ramadan lasts for approximately one month, and fasting should take place from dawn to dusk. Because the date of Ramadan is not fixed, the daily period of fasting can be very long in Britain when it occurs in the summer months. The rules for fasting are not inflexible, and there are exceptions to the requirement for fasting—for example, in case of illness or travelling—which may be compensated for at other times. Children may or may not be expected to fast, depending on their age and health.
Pilgrimage—		A pilgrimage to Mecca—the holy city—should be aimed for by every Muslim, and should be made in the twelfth month of the Islamic year. Anyone who completes a pilgrimage may add the title '*Hajji*' ('*Al hajj*' or '*Hadji*') to their name.

Asian naming systems

Asian names, like European names, involve a variety of systems based on different patterns and usages. The majority of Asian names from the Indian subcontinent are based on Hindu or Sikh or Muslim naming systems. This section briefly describes these three systems, because confusion has arisen in the process of 'fitting' these names to British records. The spelling convention of the alphabets used in the subcontinent, which means that a name can only be spelt one way, is lost when an Asian name is transliterated into a Roman alphabet in which it can be spelt in a variety of ways. Many adaptions have been made to the 'traditional' usage of names in order to 'fit' the British system of records and usage. This section outlines the three systems, and points to common areas of confusion and adaptation; but, to state the obvious, names belong to individuals, and no guide can be definitive.

Hindu names

Hindu names are based on a three-part system: first name—middle name—family name, thus:

First name	*Middle name*	*Family name*
Usha	behn	Patel
Vijay	lal	Sharma.

First name: personal, used by family and friends; male and female names are usually different.

Middle name: used to complement the first name, for example, Lakshmi (goddess); Rani (princess).

Common middle names:
Men: Bhai, Chand, Das, Dev, Lal, Kant, Kumar, Nath, Pal.
Women: Behn, Devi, Gowri, Kumari, Lakshmi, Rani.

Surname: usually a subcaste name; as most of the Hindus in Britain come from a few subcaste groups there are a limited number of 'surnames' in use, some very common—for example, 'Patel', from the Patidar subcaste in Gujarat.

Gujarati Hindus may use a father's or husband's first and middle names after their own as an extra means of identification, meaning 'son of' or 'daughter/wife of', for example:

Jayantilal	(son of) Mohandas	Patel
Ushabehn	(daughter of/wife of) Rajkumar	Sharma

Gujarati Hindus often use the middle name Bhai (brother) or Behn (sister). This does not necessarily denote relationship, and may be used as a courtesy title, particularly to older people.

As a result of the 'traditional' usage of first and middle name, one of the main confusions in the recording of Hindu names in British records has been the recording (usually in error) of the middle name as the family name, and the creation of a duplicate record if the subcaste name is subsequently recorded as the family name.

Sikh names

Sikh names, like Hindu names, are derived from a three-part system: first name—middle name—family (subcaste) name. However, the Sikh religion discourged the use of the subcaste name in order to promote equality, and encouraged the use of the titles *Singh* ('lion') for men and *Kaur* ('princess') for women. These names are of religious significance. Subcaste or family names have been retained by most families, and, though rarely used in the subcontinent, are used by many Sikhs in Britain, often as the result of an effort to comply with the British records system.

First name: not usually related to sex; for example, 'Baljit' or 'Ravinder' can be male or female.
Middle name: 'Singh' (male), or 'Kaur' (female)—may also be used as individual's 'surname'.

Many Sikhs may only use their first name with 'Singh' or 'Kaur'. 'Singh' (never 'Kaur') may be used as a family name, usually as the result of an adaptation to the British records system. Records in the subcontinent tend to be filed under the initial of the first name.

Subcaste name   Sikh family (subcaste) names are Punjabi in origin, and, as most of the Sikhs in Britain have come from a few main groups, there are al limited number of family names in use in Britain—for example, Dhillon, Sahota, Gill. The main confusion in British records is the misrecording of the 'surname', resulting in duplicate records—one with Singh/Kaur, and one with the family name as surname. Children's names have been confused where no family name is used; for example, Amarjit Kaur's son—Rajinder Singh—may have been misrecorded at birth as Rajinder 'Kaur'. The whole name should be used when addressing someone, unless they indicate otherwise—for instance, Baljit Kaur Siddhu may only be using 'Siddhu' for records purposes.

Muslim names

In common with all Hindu and Sikh names, the Muslim naming system is derived from a religious source; however that is all that Muslim names have in common with Hindu and Sikh names. Muslim names are derived from Islam, a major world religion, and the outline of Muslim naming systems described here is appropriate to the Indian subcontinent, and not necessarily to Muslim names throughout the rest of the world. Muslim names are entirely different for males and females. Traditionaly, women do not take their husband's name on marriage and, therefore, would not share either their husband's or their father's name; but as with all naming systems, there are adaptations to the standard conventions, and many women in Britain do use a family name.

Male Muslim names   Asian Muslim men usually have two or more names—order and usage are flexible, so the first name is not necessarily the 'personal' name. For example, 'Muhammad Anwar' (personal name: 'Anwar'). Many men have a religious name (for example, Allah (Ullah)—God; Muhammad—the prophet), which, when used with the personal name, may have a religious meaning—for example, 'Habib Ullah'—'Friend of God'. Some men may use an hereditary 'clan' name—for example, Qureshi, Choudrey, Khan. Traditionally this is a male name, but it is now sometimes used as a family name; there are a limited number of these hereditary names. The title 'Mia' (Mian) is sometimes used as a 'Surname' or family name in Britain by Bengalis. In Bangladesh it does not represent a name, but is a male title similar to 'Mr', and is used to indicate respect. The use of the hereditary name and the title 'Mia' are usually adaptations to recording systems; another adaptation is the use of a male personal name as a family name—for example, where the father is 'Muhammad Ali Anwar', 'Anwar' (the personal name) may be adopted as the family name. Most of the confusion in records in Britain has resulted from the flexible pattern and order of these names. Addressing someone by their whole name (unless they indicate otherwise) will avoid misusing the name.

Female names   Asian Muslim women do not have a religious name, and traditionally have a two-part name: a personal name, and a title or second personal name, for example, 'Amina Bibi' or 'Fatma Jan'. The common female titles are: Bano, Bibi, Begum, Khanam, Khatoon, Sultana. There are a few common second personal names: Akhtar ('the chosen one'); Jan ('soul'); Kausar ('heavenly drink'); Nissa/Nessa ('amongst women'). Many complex two-part names have a meaning, and should not be broken up, for example, 'Mehrun Nessa'— 'Blessing amongst women'. Many women have adapted to using a 'family name' from the male naming system. This is usually the husband's or father's last name, particularly one of the hereditary names, such as Khan, Choudrey, or Salimi; but they may only be using this for records purposes, and should be addressed by their whole name unless they indicate otherwise.

Lifestyles

A general description of 'Asian lifestyles' usually includes images of the extended family, arranged marriages, and the role of women.

Asian family patterns are undergoing constant change and pressure in British society. Social and economic factors effect constant changes in lifestyle. The 'tradition' of the extended family is maintained to a certain extent, but is also breaking down for a variety of reasons. The extended family has tended, for example, to have been stereotyped as an infallible support system, providing, among other things, support for the handicapped and elderly. The extended family is in transition; and this 'vision' of it, where it exists, should not be seen as an alternative to service provision.

Prior to the 1981 census, the proportion of ethnic minority elderly was low in proportion to the whole ethnic minority population. By 1981, there were some 87 000 people of pensionable age or over. Of the Asian elderly, people who came in the 1950s and 1960s did not always expect to remain and grow old in Britain, and others have arrived as dependants of people settled here, or as members of refugee families. The 'grief' attached to separation from a home country experienced by many people after migration may particularly affect the elderly. They may experience feelings of isolation, perhaps due to language barriers and loss of status in the changing structure of family lifestyles.

The 'tradition' of arranged marriages is also in transition, the conflicts arising from this often widening a generation gap, and causing stress both within families and in the community.

The role of women is also undergoing constant change, with an increasing shift from 'domestic power' to roles outside the home; yet some women experience isolation because of a language barrier, and that isolation is increased where that barrier does not exist for other family members, particularly if they are partners and/or children.

Conclusion

Background information on lifestyles, beliefs, languages, etc. in itself does not always create greater understanding, but may help to indicate some of the factors to be taken into account in providing an adequate and equitable service.

'Culture' is not static, and neither are communities or individuals. Clients may belong to different 'cultural' groups, but they are individuals within those groups, and culture may only be one of the many elements influencing their health-care needs. 'Cultural' aspects should not be seen in isolation, but as an integral part of community health-care and service-delivery.

Further Reading

Anwar, M. (1979). *The myth of return: Pakistanis in Britain.* Heinemann, London.

Anwar, M. (1985). *Pakistanis in Britain: a sociological study.* New Century, Durham.

Bhachu, P. (1985). *Twice migrants. East African settlers in Britain.* Tavistock, London.

Brown, C. (1984). *Black and white Britain*, Policy Studies Institute. Heinemann, London.

Burghart, R. (ed.) (1987). *Hinduism in Great Britain.* Tavistock, London.

Commission for Racial Equality (1985). *Ethnic minorities in Britain: statistical information on the pattern of settlement.* C.R.E., London.

Fenton, S. (1987). *Ageing minorities: black people as they grow old in Britain.* Commission for Racial Equality, London.

Helman, C. F. (1984). *Culture, health and illness: an introduction for health professionals.* Wright, Bristol.

Henley, A. (1979). *Asian patients in hospital and at home.* King's Fund, London.

Henley, A. (1982). *Asians in Britain. Caring for Muslims and their families: religious aspects of care.* National Extension College, Cambridge.

Henley, A. (1983a). *Asians in Britain. Caring for Hindus and their families: religious aspects of care.* National Extension College, Cambridge.

Henley, A. (1983b). *Asians in Britain. Caring for Sikhs and their families: religious aspects of care.* National Extension College, Cambridge.

Henley, A. and Taylor, C. (1981). *Asian names and records*, King's Fund/DHSS Training Pack. National Extension College, Cambridge.

Igbal, M., Vohra, K. D., and Singh, S. A. (1981). *East meets West: a background to some Asian faiths.* Commission for Racial Equality, London.

Joly, D. and Nielsen, J. (ed.) (1984). *Muslims in Britain an annotated bibliography (1960–1984).* Bibliographies in ethnic relations. Centre for Research in Ethnic Relations, University of Warwick.

Littlewood, R. and Lipsedge, K. (1982). *Aliens and alienists.* Penguin, Harmondsworth.

Mares, P., Henley, A., and Baxter, C. (1985). *Health care in multiracial Britain.* Health Education Council/National Extension College, Cambridge.

Nelson Swinerton, E., Kuepper, W. G., and Lynne Lacket, G. (1985). *Ugandan Asians in Great Britain.* Croom Helm, London.

Radwell, T. (ed.) (1986). *Health, race and ethnicity*. Croom Helm, London.
Saifullan Khan, V. (ed.) (1979). *Minority families in Britain*. Macmillan, Basingstoke.
Schackle, C. (1984). *The Sikhs*. Minority Rights Group, London.
Schwarz, V. (1986). *The Tamils of Sri Lanka*. Minority Rights Group, London.
Singh, R. (1980). *The Sikh community in Bradford*. Bradford College.
Tambs-Lyche, H. (1980). *London Patidars*. Routledge and Kegan Paul, London.
Tandon, Y. (1978). *Problems of a displaced minority: the new position of East African Asians*. Minority Rights Group, London.
Townsend, P. and Tibbs, N. (1984). *Inequalities in health in Bristol*. Dept of Social Administration, University of Bristol.
Wilson, A. (1978). *Finding a voice: Asian women in Britain*. Virago, London.

2 Cultural factors in health and illness

Cecil Helman

Introduction

In modern Britain, general practitioners are increasingly likely to encounter patients from backgrounds different to their own. In urban areas, particularly, they may have among their patients: foreign tourists, businessmen, students, migrant workers, or au pair girls; as well as émigrés and refugees from many countries, and immigrants from both the Commonwealth and Europe. The patient population may also now include members of different religions, cults, or life-styles. Finally, the patients may be further divided from the GP—and from each other—by barriers of social class, gender, and education. This means that the average urban practice may well include many groups of patients whose experiences of life, beliefs about illness, and expectations of treatment, differ widely from that of their doctor.

In order to provide health care which is efficient, humane, and appropriate to the needs of this heterogeneous population, the modern GP may have to become an applied *social* scientist—as well as an applied medical scientist: in addition to considering the physical signs and symptoms of illness, the GP will also have to consider the role of social or cultural factors in its origin, presentation, and treatment. These factors are many, and complex: they include patients' cultural and religious backgrounds, their social class and gender, and their beliefs and behaviours in relation to health and illness. But to complete the picture, the GP will also have to consider the role of his or her own background and beliefs, and how they may influence the ways that illness is interpreted, and how it is treated.

The concept of 'culture'

This chapter outlines some of the basic concepts and research findings of medical anthropology, which may be useful to those health professionals dealing with patients from different backgrounds from their own—whether from South Asia, or from elsewhere. Medical anthropology—a branch of social anthropology—is about how people of different social and cultural groups explain the causes of ill-health, the meanings they given to their ill-health, the types of treatment they believe in, and to whom they turn if they do get ill. It is also the study of how these beliefs and behaviours relate to biological changes in the human organism, in both health and disease (Helman 1984).

The reasons why one group of people have a particular set of health beliefs, and not another, are many and various. In general, it can be said that an individual's health beliefs are usually a unique blend of a number of influences. These include a variety of factors encompassing:

- individual factors (such as age, gender, size, appearance, personality, and experience of life);
- educational aspects (both formal and informal, including education into a religious, professional, or ethnic sub-culture);
- social aspects (such as social class, economic status, and social pressures or support from other people); and
- cultural aspects (including the culture into which he was born, and that which now surrounds him).

As well as being unique to each individual, health beliefs are often complex and multicausal, and tend to change over time, depending on circumstances (Helman 1987). They are important since they help determine how patients interpret their ill-health, and what they think should be done about it. Cultural background is—as noted above—only one of the many factors that influence patients' health beliefs, as well as those of their health professionals. The notion of 'culture' derived from social anthropology, was defined by E. B. Taylor in 1871 as:

> That complex whole which includes knowledge, belief, art, morals, law, custom and any other capabilities and habits acquired by man as a member of society. (Leach 1982).

Culture can also be understood as an inherited 'lens' of shared concepts and rules of meaning, through which the members of a group or society perceive the world they live in, and which guides their behaviour in their daily lives, and influences their emotional reactions to it. Culture is a set of guidelines—both implicit and explicit—which an individual inherits as a member of a particular group, and which tells him how to view the world, and how to behave in it in relation to other people, to the natural environment, and to supernatural forces or gods. Culture is transmitted from generation to generation by the use of language, symbols, and ritual. Without a shared cultural 'lens' both the cohesion and the continuity of any human group would be impossible. An interesting feature of culture, noted by Hall (1984), is that many of our cultural influences are unconscious, and hidden from the individual's awareness. We may not, therefore, know what hidden cultural 'grammars' or 'paradigms' we carry round with us (for example, certain types of prejudice), or how they play an important role in our daily lives.

Culture is thus one of the factors which influences individuals' beliefs, behaviours, perceptions, affects, language, religion, family structure, diet, dress, body-image, and attitudes to ill-health, pain, and other forms of misfortune—and all of these may have important implications for health and health care.

Sub-cultures

A sub-culture is a group of people whose view of the world, while developed from the larger culture in which they live, and sharing many of its values and concepts, also has certain unique, distinctive features of its own. Sub-cultures can include religious, ethnic, or social minorities, as well as the members of certain cults or lifestyles. The term can also be used to describe certain professional groups—such as the medical, legal, or military professions. Each sub-culture has its own particular world-view, its patterns of social organization into different roles and ranks, its specific view of its own history and *raison d'être*, and its own private rituals and language. Sub-cultures vary in the degree to which they try to blend in with the majority culture, from either doing so in all but a few aspects of their lives, to trying to live in a wholly distinctive way, with their own dress and public behaviour. Schools, universities, hospitals, clubs, regiments, and other institutions (such as the House of Commons, or the House of Lords), all have their own specific sub-cultures—often developed over many years—which mark off their members from the rest of society. Ethnic minorities can generally not be regarded as a single sub-culture, since they are so diverse and heterogeneous. The Asian population of Britain, for example, includes many social, religious, and regional sub-cultures within it—a point that will be discussed later in this chapter, and which is emphasized in many other chapters of this book.

At the interface between different cultures—or between members of different sub-cultures—a *culture clash* can occur. In this situation, one set of (often hidden) assumptions and concepts encounters a different set of assumptions and concepts. This may not only result in poor communications between the two parties (see Chapter 5), but also in feelings of bafflement, irritation, or even hostility in one or both parties. To some extent, the relation between doctor and patient may provide opportunities for such a 'culture clash'. This is partly due to the sub-culture of the medical school and the hospital acquired by one of the parties; but it is also due to differences in social class, economic status, legal power, gender, and ethnic or religious background between doctor and patient.

The medical sub-culture tends to inculcate into its members a respect for the principles of scientific rationality, and an emphasis on the objective, numerical measurement of physical and psychological states (Helman 1984). Furthermore, as Kleinman *et al.* (1978) point out, modern medicine has become increasingly dualistic in its approach to ill-health, splitting 'mind' from 'body', and emphasizing the latter at the expense of the former. Physical and chemical data are seen as intrinsically more 'real' and clinically significant—especially when they can be measured with the aid of diagnostic technology—than the patient's psychological state, cultural background, or social class. Thus reducing the complexity of ill-health to merely physiological phenomena may lead to the doctor's missing many of the factors which influence the origin, presentation, and prognosis of that ill-health. It may also lead to 'culture clash' between doctor and patient which can be hard to avoid.

'Disease' versus 'illness'

There is an ever-growing literature on the meaning of and on perceptions of the phenomena of health, illness, and disease. From the perspective of medical anthropology (Cassell 1976; Eisenberg 1977) two main interpretations of ill-health can be identified. The *disease* or *medical* perspective tends to emphasize physiological data and measurement, and sees individual diseases as abstract entities (such as 'pneumonia' or 'diabetes') which have specific properties and a recurring identity in whatever setting they occur. Diseases can be assumed to be universal in their form, progress, and content. By contrast, the *illness* or *lay* perspective refers to the subjective response of the patient to being unwell; how he—and his family and friends—perceive the origin and significance of this event; how it affects his behaviour or relationships with other people; and the steps he takes to remedy the situation. Thus it includes not only his subjective experience of ill-health, but the types of meaning that he gives to that experience.

In understanding 'illness' it is useful to consider the types of questions that people ask themselves when they feel unwell, or when they experience any sudden, unexpected event in their daily lives. These questions include: What has happened? Why has it happened? Why to me? What would happen to me if nothing were done about it? What are its likely effects on other people (such as family, friends, or employers)? And what should I do about it—or to whom should I turn for further help? (Helman 1981). The answers to these questions, include references to individual factors, education, cultural background, and economic status, and all of these combine in a unique blend in each individual patient, and determine how 'illness' is constructed for him or her.

Although most 'disease' is also accompanied by 'illness', it is possible to have illness without disease (a subjective feeling of being unwell, or unhappy, but without any physiological abnormality), or disease without illness (as in asymptomatic hypertension, or carcinoma-in-situ). Thus medical and lay beliefs about ill-health may differ widely, and this may influence the types of conditions that people bring to doctors, and how they present them to the doctor, and the type and quality of treatment that they are given.

Misuse of the concept of 'culture'

Although the anthropological concept of culture is a useful one in explaining both health beliefs and health behaviours, it can be misused in a number of ways. Health professionals should be aware of the dangers of this misuse, and take the following points into account in evaluating patients from different backgrounds to their own:

Both cultures and sub-cultures do not exist in a vacuum

They are always part of a particular context, which is made up of historical, geographical, economic, social, and political elements. This means that the culture of any group of people, at a particular point in time, is always influenced by many other factors. Thus it may not be possible to isolate 'pure' cultural beliefs and behaviours from the social and material background where they occur. For example, people may act or think in a particular way, not because of their inherited 'culture', but because they are rich or poor, employed or unemployed, able or disabled, educated or uneducated, powerful or powerless. The material circumstances of people's lives, and the situations in which they find themselves, are therefore just as important as their cultural background. One should avoid the dangers of 'culturalism'—reducing all aspects of a group's life down to its 'culture', while ignoring such important factors as its members' social class or economic status.

Cultural background may therefore be a misleading explanation of the inequalities of health in a society (Mares *et al.* 1985)

Social and economic factors may both lead to the development and to the perpetuation of ill-health in a particular community. For example, low incomes, unemployment, sub-standard housing, poor diet, limited educational opportunities, and exposure to crime or the fear of crime may all contribute to the development of physical or mental ill-health. Furthermore, discrimination or persecution—whether this is based on class, ethnicity, religion, or gender—may also seriously undermine the health of a particular group. As an example, Artley (1987) has described the effect of racialist attacks and harassment on the mental and physical health of Bengalis living in Tower Hamlets and other parts of inner London.

In understanding the culture of minority groups in society it is also important to consider the culture of the majority community

In the case of a recent immigrant group the culture of the 'host' community, who hold the reins of political and numerical power, is just as relevant to the health status of the immigrants as the culture they have brought with them. For example, the degree of xenophobia on the one hand, or tolerance on the other in the 'host' community, may affect whether the immigrants are able to get a job, and to afford decent housing, a nutritious diet, and adequate clothing. On another level, societies whose culture defines its members and citizens by the depth of their ancestral roots in the country may be less accepting of immigrants than more recently created societies with a 'melting pot' ideology. In both cases, however, the culture of the 'host' community—as well as that of the immigrants—is an important determinant of health and illness.

In dealing with health issues, the culture of the doctor is just as important as that of the patient

On one level this refers to the medical sub-culture that doctors acquire as part of their training; on another level, however, doctors also express the culture of the wider society in which they live—including its prejudices and social assumptions. For example, Littlewood and Lipsedge (1982) have suggested that in Britain psychiatry can sometimes be used as an agent of social control, by misinterpreting the religious and cultural behaviours of some ethnic minority patients as evidence of mental illness, and thus 'disguising disadvantage as disease'. In dealing with patients from social classes or cultural backgrounds different from their own, some members of the medical profession may see these people as 'difficult', 'odd', 'resistant to treatment', or 'hypochondriacal', instead of understanding the nature of the hidden 'culture clash'.

Cultures are usually not homogeneous

In other chapters of this book, the point has been made that the Asian population itself is made up of many communities, differing in, for example, religion or migration-history. Even within groups, however, it is important to be aware of variation. It is therefore not possible to make broad generalizations about the members of a cultural group without taking into account that differences among the group's members may be just as striking as those between the members of different cultural groups. One cannot necessarily predict the beliefs or behaviours of a group of people by basing onself simply on knowledge of a small number of them. That is, one must always avoid cultural stereotypes in understanding, for example, how patients respond to ill-health, or the types of treatment they believe in. Broad genralizations, such as 'No Muslim will eat pork, pork products, or anything that contains pork or pig derivatives; if there is any doubt about the origin or content of a food they will refuse it,' (Black 1985) can provide a useful introduction and background for those who have no knowledge, but may *not* apply literally and practically to all individual members of that group, all the time—whatever their belief system. One should differentiate, therefore, between the rules that govern how people ought to act in certain situations, and how they actually behave in their daily lives. There is thus no such thing as 'the typical Asian patient', no more than there is a 'typical European patient' or a 'typical British patient'.

Culture is not static

It is continually in a process of change and adaptation to new conditions. In the modern industrialized world, no cultural groups are completely isolated from those around them. Much of this is due to the influence of the media, education, and travel on all members of a society. Even small sub-cultural groups tend to be syncretic in their world-view and behaviour—that is, they combine their own cultural elements with some of those of the majority culture. It follows from this point that immigrant groups, for example, often differ culturally from those of their compatriots that have remained behind in their countries of origin, as they assimilate more and more of the cultural elements of their new home. Similarly, there are changes within immigrant communities over time, as each generation becomes progressively more encultured into the new society than the previous one. It is thus inaccurate to refer to many of the members of ethnic minority groups in Britain as 'immigrants', since many were born here, or at least educated in this country.

Cultural beliefs and behaviours can be used as a form of 'victim-blaming'

Responsibility for ill-health can be shifted on to the patient's 'culture', rather than being ascribed to wider social problems, such as unemployment, discrimination, or pollution (Crawford 1977). Culture alone is often not a sufficient explanation for the types of lives that people lead, and should not be used as a basis for condemnation. No one culture is necessarily 'healthier', for its members, than another. As La Fontaine (1986) points out, 'Modern anthropology takes as axiomatic that differences of culture cannot be used to judge individuals, categories of individuals, or groups.'

In interpreting patients' behaviour and symptomatology, the cultural aspects of the clinical picture may be over-emphasized

That is, the clinician may mistakenly ascribe most of the patients' behaviour to their 'culture', and thus miss or underestimate an underlying physical or mental disorder (Lopez and Hernandez 1986).

For these reasons, the anthropological concept of 'culture' is a useful one, but it should always be modified with reference to the unique circumstances of each patient's life.

Immigration and cultural bereavement

Migration from one country to another is almost always a stressful experience for the immigrant and his or her family (Helman 1984). There is considerable evidence that immigration is often accompanied by an increase in mental and physical illness among immigrants (Littlewood and Lipsedge 1982), as manifested by higher rates of hypertension (Cassell 1975), paranoid reactions and schizophrenia (Carpenter and Brockington 1980), admissions to psychiatric hospitals (Hitch and Rack 1980), and attempted suicide (Burke 1976).

The reasons for the stress of migration are many and varied. One useful way of looking at the problem is Parkes' (1971) concept of *psycho-social transitions—*

of which migration is an important example. He points out that changes in an individual's life that are likely to be most stressful are those that take place in those parts of his world that impinge on his 'life space'. This consists of 'those parts of the environment with which the self interacts and in relation to which behaviour is organized; other persons, material possessions, the familiar world of home and place of work, and the individual's body and mind in so far as he can view these as separate from his self.'

Changes in this 'life space' also involve changes in the basic assumptions that people have made about their world—that is, their 'assumptive world'; and then they can sometimes no longer take some, or even any, of these assumptions for granted any longer.

In Parkes' view, those psycho-social transitions that are likely to be most stressful are those which are lasting in their effects, take place over a relatively short period of time, and affect many of the basic assumptions that people make about their world. Migration is thus a clear example of a stressful 'psycho-social transition'—especially if the cultural and social distance between old and new countries is very marked. A further useful way of viewing migration is Eisenbruch's (1984) concept of *cultural bereavement*, in which he compares the psychological effects of migration to those of a grief reaction after the death of a loved one. This reaction is likely to be most serious when the change in country has been very rapid (as in refugees in wartime), and the individual is removed from the supportive social networks of friends and family. The whole 'structure of meaning' of people's assumptive world is shattered, and the old cultural 'lens' is no longer adequate as a guide to daily life. The individual experiences grief, therefore, not only for the country he has left behind, but also for the culture (or sub-culture) into which he was born.

In addition to the experience of migration itself, the social, cultural and economic features of the new 'host' community are also relevant to the degree of stress that immigrants experience, as mentioned earlier. Discrimination and prejudice—whether individual or institutionalized—all make the process of adaptation to a new country more difficult for the immigrant. A further point, to complete the picture, is that some aspects of the immigrant's culture—such as rigid gender roles and expectations (Schofield 1981)—may, at least in the first generation, contribute to ill-health within that community. The reasons why people migrate are also relevant to how stressful their migration will be. This has been termed the 'push-pull' model of migration (see also Chapter 1). That is, whether people are pushed out of their home country, or pulled towards a new country, is something which it is important to know in understanding their migration experiences. In practice, migration usually contains elements of both 'push' and 'pull'. In the former case, migrants are unwillingly pushed out of their home country by famine, unemployment, war, or persecution, and arrive in another country as refugees, exiles, or émigrés. Many of them will harbour a deep wish to return home, once their life has improved and events have settled down at home. This may make adaptation to the new country more difficult. By contrast, migrants who are 'pulled' towards a new country by the promise of a better standard of living, better education, more security, and freedom of worship, may also experience adaptation problems if their ambitions are not fulfilled. They may cling to a 'myth of return' which never becomes reality, and not return home for fear of being branded a failure.

A further model which seeks to explain increased rates of mental illness among immigrants has been summarized by Cox (1977). He describes three hypotheses:

1. Certain mental disorders incite their victims to migrate (the selection hypothesis).
2. The process of migration itself creates mental stress, which may precipitate mental illness in susceptible individuals (the stress hypothesis).
3. There is a non-essential association between migration and certain other variables such as age and class.

Whatever the explanation, the process of being an immigrant is a stressful one, and the individual may only be protected from this by his or her social support networks: religious organizations, community groups, extended family, circle of friends, and traditional healers. The degree of assimilation of the immigrant may lessen his stress in some situations, but increase it in others—and there may be no way of predicting how any particular individual (or family) may cope with assimilation and the processes of 'cultural bereavement'.

Conclusion

This chapter has outlined some of the anthropological concepts of 'culture' and 'sub-culture'. Both of these are important influences on the ways that people perceive their world, and how they act in it in relation to other people, and to the natural and supernatural environments. The pervasive influence of our cultural premises is hidden from awareness. However, it has also been stressed that culture is only one explanation for the ways that people think and act. Other factors—such as personality, experience, education, social class, and economic status—are all relevant, and influence the role that culture plays in any particular situation.

Some of the misuses of the term 'culture' have also been described—especially the erroneous view that cultural groups are isolated, static, and homogeneous. The dangers of stereotyping and 'victim-blaming' have been pointed out, as well as those of misinterpreting symptoms as 'cultural', when they are actually evidence of underlying physical or mental disorder. In the case of immigrants, the importance of the social and cultural attributes of the 'host' community has also been stressed.

In understanding intrinsic differences between medical and lay perspectives on ill-health, the medical anthropological concepts of 'disease' versus 'illness' have been described, and the possibility this raises of a 'cultural clash' between doctor and patient.

Some of the hypotheses about the reasons for increased rates of mental and physical ill-health among migrants have been reviewed. They point to the importance of certain types of 'psycho-social transitions' and 'cultural bereavement' in the origin, and perpetuation, of ill-health.

As a result of the complexity of social and cultural factors, it is essential that the health professional should treat each patient—from whatever background—as an individual, the unique blend of many influences and circumstances. To understand the patient's perspective on health and illness, the clinician should ask about his or her health beliefs and practices, and respect them even if they are different from his own. It is also important not to make broad generalizations or assumptions about individual patients, based on a superficial knowledge of their social or cultural background.

References

Artley, A. (1987). Out of sight, out of mind. *Spectator*, **258**, 8–10.

Black, J. (1985). Asian families 1: cultures. *British Medical Journal*, **290**, 762–4.

Burke, A. W. (1976). Attempted suicide among Asian immigrants in Birmingham. *British Journal of Psychiatry*, **128**, 528–33.

Carpenter, L. and Brockington, I. F. (1980). A study of mental illness in Asians, West Indians and Africans living in Manchester. *British Journal of Psychiatry*, **137**, 201–5.

Cassell, J. (1975). Studies of hypertension in migrants. In *Epidemiology and control of hypertension* (ed. O. Paul), pp. 41–61. Stratton, New York.

Cassell, E. J. (1976). *The healer's art: a new approach to the doctor-patient relationship*. Lippincott, New York.

Cox, J. L. (1977). Aspects of transcultural psychiatry. *British Journal of Psychiatry*, **130**, 211–21.

Crawford, R. (1977). You are dangerous to your health: the ideology and politics of victim blaming. *International Journal of Health Services*, **7**, 663–80.

Eisenberg, L. (1977). Disease and illness: distinctions between professional and popular ideas of sickness. *Culture, Medicine and Psychiatry*, **1**, 9–23.

Eisenbruch, M. (1984). Cross-cultural aspects of bereavement. 1: A conceptual framework for comparative analysis. *Culture, Medicine and Psychiatry*, **8**, 283–309.

Hall, E. T. (1977). *Beyond culture*. Anchor Books, New York.

Helman, C. G. (1981). Disease versus illness in general practice. *Journal of the Royal College of General Practitioners*, **31**, 548–52.

Helman, C. G. (1984). *Culture, health and illness: an introduction for health professionals*. John Wright, Bristol.

Helman, C. G. (1987). General practice and the hidden health care system. *Journal of the Royal Society of Medicine*, **80**, 738–40.

Hitch, P. J. and Rack, P. H. (1980). Mental illness among Polish and Russian refugees in Bradford. *British Journal of Psychiatry*, **137**, 206–11.

Kleinman, A., Eisenberg, L. and Good, B. (1978). Culture, illness and care: clinical lessons from anthropological and cross-cultural research. *Annals of Internal Medicine*, **88**, 251–8.

La Fontaine, J. (1986). Countering racial prejudice: a better starting point. *Anthropology Today*, **2**(6), 1–2.

Leach, E. (1982). *Social anthropology*. Fontaine, Glasgow.

Littlewood, R. and Lipsedge, M. (1982). *Aliens and alienists*. Penguin, Harmondsworth.

Lopez, S. and Hernandez, P. (1986). How culture is considered in evaluations of psychopathology. *Journal of Nervous and Mental Disease*, **176**, 598–606.

Mares, P., Henley, A., and Baxter, C. (1985). *Health care in multiracial Britain*. Health Education Council/National Extension College, Cambridge.

Parkes, C. M. (1971). Psycho-social transitions: a field for study. *Social Science and Medicine*, **5**, 101–15.

Schofield, J. (1981). Behind the veil: the mental health of Asian women in Britain. *Health Visitor*, **54**, 138–41.

Further reading

Foster, G. M. and Anderson, B. G. (1978). *Medical anthropology*. Wiley, New York.

Helman, C. G. (1984). *Culture, health and illness: an introduction for health professionals*. Wright, Bristol.

Kessing, R. M. (1981). *Cultural anthropology*. Holt, Rinehart, and Winston, New York.

Kleinman, A. (1980). *Patients and healers in the context of culture*. University of California Press, New York.

Landy, D. (ed.) (1977). *Culture, disease and healing*. Macmillan, New York.

Littlewood, R. and Lipsedge, M. (1982). *Aliens and alienists*. Penguin, Harmondsworth.

Organizational aspects

3 Organization and delivery of care

Allan McNaught

Introduction

How to deliver relevant and high-quality health care in a multi-racial or multi-cultural setting is a perennial problem for health systems throughout the world, whether in developed or developing countries. The attempt by one inner London health authority to develop a multi-racial approach to health service provision has been described (McNaught 1988). While there had been considerable developments in relevant policies, in West Lambeth there was a lack of a robust strategy to achieve practical improvements. Racial prejudice and insensitivity to the socio-cultural features of the local population were found to pervade the whole organization, even among staff in senior management and professional roles. The West Lambeth case-study clearly showed that, despite the existence of policy statements, there was an inability or reluctance to implement the clinical and organizational measures which it was known would lead to an improvement in services to local ethnic minorities. It was clear that fairly intense personal, social, and organizational factors in part accounted for this situation; but the predominant influences seemed to have been a combination of poor management, insensitivity to ethnic minorities and their needs, and racial prejudice.

In trying to explore the extent to which general practice has responded to the needs of minority patients, there is the immediate difficulty that the service is much less open to scrutiny than, for example, a health authority. General practice is also, of course, intensely personal: it is a setting in which difficulties can very easily be attributed to the personality, ability, and opinions of individuals. Thus it is difficult to generalize from the experience of an individual practice or doctor. However, there is sufficient social and professional homogeneity among GPs to make it worthwhile to attempt to draw conclusions on the issues of Asian health care, and on other matters. While recognizing these problems, this chapter will attempt to do two things. Firstly, it will briefly summarize and discuss the findings of some existing studies concerned with Asians and general practice. Secondly, it will identify and discuss the main practical implications of these findings for the organization and delivery of services at practice level.

Background

The literature on Asian people's use of general medical services is very scanty—somewhat surprisingly, given that most individuals from minority communities seem to be registered with and make use of their GP. The absence of an extensive literature should not lead to the assumptions either that all is well from the point of view of such patients and their GPs, or that there are no problems which merit serious attention in their own right rather than being considered as part of the wider problems which are said to afflict general practice, particularly in 'inner cities'. An example of the view often taken of ethnic minorities and general practice is reflected in the assumptions in Smith and Stiff's report on general practice in north-west London (1985). In this report ethnic minorities are categorized as one of the 'main problem(s) for general practice in their area'. The exact nature of the problems posed for general practice by ethnic minorities is not stated, but it is widely assumed that ethnic minorities place some sort of 'burden' on GPs.

Viewed from the perspective of ethnic minority communities themselves, general practice is often seen to be inappropriate and of poor quality. This dissatisfaction is noted in Weightman's (1977) article, which records West Indian use and perception of GPs, and also in a later study of the health experiences and perceptions of Asian and Afro-Caribbean patients in the general practice setting (Donovan 1986).

There is, however, a growing body of literature on ethnic minorities and the NHS; and the aspect which deals with Asians and general practice tends to address one of three questions: firstly, the extent to which Asians register with and use GPs; secondly, the identification of experiences or difficulties which GPs have in providing a service to Asians; and thirdly, the patient's perspective of the extent to which general practitioner services are sensitive to the socio-cultural features and health needs of the Asian community.

(a) Asians' use of general medical services

A large-scale household survey carried out in the West Midlands in 1981 found that 99 per cent of all groups (white, Asian, and Afro-Caribbean) were registered with a GP. Only 10 per cent were not registered with GPs practising in their immediate area of residence. Over 60 per cent of Asians had a GP of Asian origin, and a further 10 per cent were registered with practices containing a doctor of Asian origin. Asian households were also more likely to have visited their GP in the preceding year, and were more likely to have had a domiciliary visit. The latter finding the researchers attributed to the higher number of children in Asian households (Johnson 1986).

Blakemore (1982) found that a high proportion of elderly Asians (70 per cent) had visited their GP within the previous year, while a study of younger people found that only 8 per cent of young Asians had not visited their GP in the previous twelve months. This compared with 27 per cent of white respondents and 18 per cent of Afro-Caribbean respondents (Norman 1985).

Many studies have been concerned to assess the extent to which Asians use traditional medical practitioners (*hakims*). Davies and Aslam (1980) maintained that *hakims* were at work in all the main Asian communities in Britain; but no other researchers have reported significant use of *hakims* by Asians. Indeed several investigators have remarked on how little use Asians made of these practitioners (Johnson 1986; Jain *et al.* 1985). The extent to which Asians use private GPs has rarely been addressed, and it is often assumed that this is more characteristic of Afro-Caribbean people. Donovan's (1986) methodology did not assess use of private doctors or *hakims*. Jain *et al.* (1985), on the other hand, were concerned with this phenomenon, and found that a small number of Asian patients from two practices said that they had consulted an alternative private doctor. Further details on alternative/complementary medicine are contained in Chapter 7.

(b) General practitioners and Asian patients

Wright's (1983) questionnaire-based survey of thirty-nine GPs' contact with the Asian community in Newcastle upon Tyne showed that the commonest comments volunteered by the GPs did not concern language or modesty, but their view that their Asian patients tended to complain of trivial ailments, while on the other hand they presented less often with psychosocial problems than the average patient. Thirty of the GPs who responded reported reluctance on the part of Asian women to be examined. More than half also felt that Asians consulted more often and took up more time than English patients. Four of the doctors, two of them Asians themselves, who responded saw, between them, nearly half the Asian population concerned. Another was an English woman doctor who had learned Hindi. The fourth doctor spoke no Asian languages at all, and Asians comprised 5–10 per cent of his list. Twenty-nine of the doctors in the sample (74 per cent) were dependent upon patients' relatives for interpreting, and few seemed to have been aware of the presence of two Asian liaison health-visitors in the study area. Wright concluded that his overwhelming impression was of GPs puzzled by the influx of Asians to their practices, aware of considerable problems of management, and yet unable or unwilling to make appropriate adjustments. He observed that each doctor seemed to see his Asian families as his private problem, and did not look for, or expect, aid from elsewhere.

Quite a contrary conclusion is arrived at by Jain *et al.* (1985) in their study of the attitudes of Asian patients in two general practices in Birmingham. While observing some of the same issues as Wright (that is, communications, female modesty, etc.) they concluded that many of the difficulties encountered by Asian patients are those which are inherent in the National Health Service system of primary care, and which are experienced by the population in general. This is not a view which is widely shared: Lobo's work (1978, 1985) suggests fairly elementary gaps in medical practitioners' knowledge of the health and social features of ethnic minorities in the UK. My own examination of the responsiveness of community health services within a small patch in the community health unit of an outer London district encompassed three general practices. It was found, as has been shown in other studies, that Asian patients tended to be registered with doctors of Asian origin. However, when referrals for secondary care arose, particularly for psychiatric treatment, language differences posed enormous problems in a number of individual cases. Another factor which was found to be important was social class. Although the assignment of social class categories in the Asian community is difficult, as a broad observation it seemed that GPs and community nurses noted fewer problems with Asians with 'middle class' or westernized backgrounds. This could suggest that education or economic achievement resulted in a loosening of traditional patterns of behaviour, and thus meant that language and communication were less likely to be problematic in the relationship between the health worker and Asian patients.

It must not be forgotten, of course, that a significant number of GPs are from the Indian subcontinent themselves: in 1986, 26 per cent of all doctors in general practice in England and Wales were born outside Great Britain, the majority coming from the Indian subcontinent (DHSS 1987). Their presence, and the considerable use made of them by Asian people, must have shielded many GPs from the necessity to address the issue of improving their standards in the treatment and care of Asian people. Despite their contribution towards primary health-care, Asian doctors tend to be regarded as second-class doctors. At a common sense level this assumption was reinforced by the change in General Medical Council (GMC) regulations in 1975 which required overseas doctors to take a language test. This concern was not extended to consider the professional implications of the situation where many British-born doctors could not understand the culture or language of non-English-speaking patients.

(c) Asians' experience of general practice

The literature on the Asian experience of the NHS often portrays the service as insensitive to their health, social, and cultural needs, as well as being characterized by racism (see for example Baxter *et al.* 1985). In a somewhat different vein, Donovan's study looks at the health experience of fourteen Asian women, which included their views of and use of GPs. The majority were registered with GPs of Asian origin. Their ability to communicate was the main reason given for this preference. All had seen their GP within the past year, and at least six respondents reported being dissatisfied with their doctor. Many of these latter were also less keen than the average patient about seeing their GP even when they were unwell (Donovan 1986). The work on the attitudes of Asian patients by Jain *et al.* (1985) was carried out mainly by GPs, and they failed to capture the largely critical attitude that most ethnic minorities now share about the performance and sensitivity of the NHS. Clearly, though, neither party in this debate is wholly right. It seems that considerable insensitivity to the health and related needs of ethnic minorities, and racism, exist alongside a situation of high usage and considerable satisfaction with general-practice services. Whether this satisfaction is merely a reflection of good personal relationships (between patients and their doctors), or is a feature of social-class aspects of the relationship, is difficult to discern.

Implications for the organization and delivery of care

While the literature on Asians and general-practice services is to a degree contradictory, it is possible to identify the core issues that would need to be considered and acted upon by any practitioner concerned to improve the quality and relevance of the care he or she provides. These issues include: language and communication, knowledge of relevant aspects of Asian culture, female modesty, racial discrimination, familiarity, and up-to-date knowledge of relevant clinical issues. These issues can be considered under two headings:

    (a) human resources management; and
    (b) practice organization and facilities.

(a) Human resources management

Language and communication The key resource in every general practice is the people within it. In trying to improve the quality and relevance of services to ethnic minorities, we have to start with the character, performance, and quality of our human resources. From the literature it is clear that language and communication problems are common. Practices with no Asian partner or who are unable to speak Asian languages rely on the willingness of relatives to act as interpreters. This practice is increasingly being perceived as unprofessional (see Chapter 5). Reliance on family members tends to reduce the ability of the practitioner to act in his patient's best interest on issues where there is family conflict or misunderstanding. The practitioner cannot be sure of the competence or accuracy of the translation. It also means that the content of advice, and guidance on critical matters such as compliance with drug regimes, may also be ineffective. The other problem with lack of effective communication between patients and GPs is that it distorts their relationship. Wright (1983), for example, postulates that what the GP perceives as trivial complaints may in fact be ailments that the language barrier prevents from being explained adequately by the patients, and thus from being diagnosed and managed appropriately by the doctor.

Staff mix and training Practices which seek to improve services to Asian patients or to attract Asian patients, will need to improve on their language and communications capabilities. This could be achieved through a recruitment policy which brings in Asian partners or ancillary staff, or by making more active use of such resources as may exist within voluntary organizations, the local authority, or the health authority. The training of staff in Asian languages or culture is another innovation which could take place either alongside or separate from attempts to develop a staff group which contains Asian members.

In terms of the practice as a whole, it seems that a more effective strategy is to combine staff development and language and cultural training with an explicit recruitment policy. Apart from looking at language and culture, practice members should be encouraged to examine and discuss the quality of the clinical and non-clinical services provided to patients. This would help individuals to learn how to improve their performance; it would also promote professional development and standard-setting for the whole practice, to the benefit of patients and practitioners alike. The danger with one-off initiatives is that they do not become integrated with the culture and operational expectations of the practice, and hence have no lasting impact on performance.

It must also be remembered that training and development must be for the whole staff group. There really is little point in the clinical members enhancing their capacity to help Asian patients when all is undone by patient-contacts with receptionists or secretaries who may not have had such training. It must also be recognized, however, that this is an immensely sensitive area of staff development and training, which must be handled with considerable diplomacy and tact if the desired results are to be achieved in practice. Concerned practitioners would do well to study the experience of other agencies or professional groups who have attempted to improve services to ethnic minorities. The publications *Social Work Today* and *Community Care* are rich sources of initiatives and development in statutory and voluntary social services, and may be of particular interest to GPs. Examples here include articles by Bhaduri (1984) and Fogarthy (1984). The pitfalls are many, but it is clear that professionally and socially such training and development have considerable benefits.

(b) Practice organization and facilities

Accommodation   Practitioners frequently overlook the need to consider the administration and organization of their practice as they affect or promote services to ethnic minorities. For example, in situations when interpreters are frequently used the number of persons in a consulting room can increase from two or three to four or more. Female modesty, too, might require the presence of a chaperon in the consulting room. For practices with poor or cramped accommodation these demands put an undeniable pressure on both patients and practitioners and can have wider effects on the practice, as they reduce the effective waiting area and put additional pressure on receptionists. While there may be no short-term solutions, the problem should be taken into account when designing new or altered practice premises, and may be eased by a closer examination of the use of space in existing practice premises.

Medical records   With non-European names there is often confusion and mis-spelling in medical records. Practitioners should anticipate such practical difficulties and assist their staff to resolve them, while at the same time maintaining the quality of service to patients. In the case of medical records, guidance may be required on Asian naming systems; and considerable care needs to be given to the completion and pulling of records, in order to minimize confusion and promote the maintenance of accurate records. Further details on Asian naming systems are given in Chapter 1.

Appointment systems Wright (1983) and other investigators have found that Asian patients require longer consultations than English patients. Language and communication difficulties are one obvious reason for this. Whatever the actual appointment system being followed in a practice, this need is bound to cause problems unless it is explicitly taken into account. In the Jain *et al.* study (1985) a large proportion of Asian patients felt that there was a need to improve the appointment system in one location because they had to wait two or three days to see the doctor; but at another location (where there was no appointment system) some complained because of long delays in seeing the doctor after arrival at the surgery.

The future

The White Paper *Promoting better health. The Government's programme for improving primary health care* (1987) devotes a complete chapter to inner cities. Proposals include:

- encouraging the development of primary health-care teams;
- introducing a 'deprived area allowance';
- improving standards of practice premises;
- encouraging more women to enter and remain in general practice; and
- providing incentives for the employment of link workers as members of primary health-care teams.

If implemented these changes should facilitate improvements in the quality of primary health care to all residents in inner cities and deprived areas.

A further incentive to improved services is the recent announcement by the Health Minister that Regional Health Authorities will be required to report on progress towards improving care for ethnic minority groups as part of their annual performance review.

Conclusion

Very little attention has been given in general practice literature to the care or management of Asian patients. The studies explored in this chapter have shown that a number of problems crop up in the interaction between Asians and GPs, including: language and communication; the gravity of the complaints which Asians bring to their GPs; and female modesty. The large number of

Asian doctors practising in the UK, and the fact that they have many Asian patients on their lists, has meant that the majority of British-born, white GPs never have to think seriously about the quality of the service they provide to Asian patients. Although levels of registration with GPs by Asians are high, it is also clear that levels of satisfaction with the general-practitioner service are not particularly high.

Attempts to improve the quality of service to Asians have to include the human resources of the practice, as well as its organization and facilities. This chapter has suggested that improvements in human resources management could be fruitfully pursued through a strategy which combined the deliberate ethnic mixing of practice staff with training and development for all practice workers. The overall objective would be the improvement of the clinical and non-clinical services available to patients regardless of their ethnic background.

There are limitations to what individual practices can do. However, there are a tremendous range of people and resources available in health and local authorities and the voluntary sector. Contact addresses of a sample of organizations which might provide guidance are included at the end of this chapter. Currently GPs make little and ineffective use of those resources that are available, to the detriment of their patients.

Tackling problems of practice organization and facilities, by contrast, are rather easier to conceptualize. The need for interpreters and the possible need for chaperons for some female Asian patients results in a need for more operational space in some practices. How this can be achieved is very much about the resources and building opportunities available to individual practices. In comparison, improving appointment systems, reception arrangements, and medical records seems cheap and easy to do. However, we should not underestimate the difficulties in trying to improve standards in general practice. If a GP does not see the benefit or advantage in providing a better service for his whole practice population, it seems unlikely that the needs of Asians will motivate him to do better!

References

Baxter, C., Henley, A., and Mares, P. (1985). *Health care in multi-racial Britain*. Health Education Council/National Extension College, Cambridge.

Blakemore, K. (1982). Health and illness among the elderly of minority ethnic groups living in Birmingham: some new findings. *Health Trends*, **14**, (3), 69–72.

Bhaduri, R. (1984). Patient minority: immigrants in hospital. *Social Work Today*, **15**, 18–19 (27.2.84).

Davies, S. and Aslam, M. (1980). *The Hakim and his role*. Department of Health and Social Security, London.

DHSS (Department of Health and Social Security). (1987). *Health and Personal Social Services statistics for England*, 1987 ed. HMSO, London.

DHSS (Department of Health and Social Security). (1987). *Promoting better health*.

The Government's programme for improving primary health care, **CM 249**. HMSO, London.

Donovan, J. (1986). *We don't buy sickness, it just comes: health and illness and health care in the lives of black people in London*. Gower, Aldershot.

Fogarthy, M. (1984). Psychiatry and race: uncomfortable questions. *Social Work Today*, **15**, 8 (25.6.84).

Jain, C., Narayan, N., Narayan, K., Pike, L. A., Clarkson, M. E., Cox, I. G. and Chatterjee, J. (1985). Attitudes of Asian patients in Birmingham to general practitioner services. *Journal of the Royal College of General Practitioners*, **35**, 416–18.

Johnson, M. (1986). Inner city residents, ethnic minorities and primary health care in the West Midlands. In *Health, race and ethnicity*. (ed. T. Rathwell and D. Phillips), pp. 192–212. Croom Helm, London.

Lobo, E. de H. (1978). *Children of immigrants to Britain: their health and social problems*. Hodder and Stoughton, London.

Lobo, E. de H. (1985). Health problems in immigrant mothers and children. *Update*, **30**, 429–37.

McNaught, A. (1988). *Race and health policy*. Croom Helm, London.

Norman, A. (1985). *Triple jeopardy: growing old in a second homeland*. Centre for Policy on Ageing, London.

Smith, C., and Stiff, J. (1985). Problems of inner city general practice in North-East London. *Journal of the Royal College of General Practitioners*, **35**, 71–6.

Weightman, C. (1977). Poor man's Harley Street. *New Society*, **42**, 118–19.

Wright, C. (1983). Language and communication problems in an Asian community. *Journal of the Royal College of General Practitioners*, **33**, 101–4.

Possible sources of guidance

Standing Conference of Ethnic Minority Senior Citizens (SCEMSC), 5 Westminster Bridge Road, London SE1 7XW. Tel: 01-928-0095.

National Association of Health Authorities (NAHA), Garth House, 47 Edgbaston Park Road, Birmingham B15 2RS.

Afro-Caribbean Mental Health Association (ACMHA), 35–7 Electric Avenue, London SW9. Tel: 01-737-3603.

Local Authorities Race Relations Information Exchange (LARRIE), 100 Park Village East, London NW1. Tel: 01-828-7055.

4 Asian doctors and nurses in the NHS

Aly Rashid

Introduction

As the recruitment (both historically and today), training, and career structure experienced by Asian doctors are completely different from those experienced by Asian nurses in the National Health Service, the two groups are considered separately in this chapter.

Asian doctors in the NHS

From the late 1950s onwards, Asian doctors have formed a substantial proportion of the medical manpower in the National Health Service. DHSS figures (DHSS 1986a) show that 24 per cent of all doctors in the NHS are from overseas, and that approximately 80 per cent of these are of Asian origin (Table 4.1). By far the largest contingent of Asian doctors in the NHS is from the Indian subcontinent, and in particular, from India itself. Other countries from which Asian doctors have emigrated include: Pakistan, Bangladesh, Sri Lanka, Kenya, Uganda, Zimbabwe, Tanzania, and Malawi.

Table 4.1 *Number of NHS doctors in Great Britain (DHSS census survey of Medical Manpower 1986)*

Workplace	All doctors	Overseas doctors	Overseas %
Hospital	52 790	13 790	26
Community Health	7000	1760	25
General Practice	31 870	6700	21
Total	91 660	22 250	24

There is some duplication in that some GPs work in hospitals as clinical assistants and hospital practitioners.
Figures are rounded to the nearest 10.
Source: DHSS 1986a

With few immigration restrictions in the 1950s, 1960s, and 1970s, Asian doctors migrated in large numbers to the United Kingdom, at a time when the demand for doctors in the NHS could not be met by British medical schools. This migration of foreign graduates, particularly of Asian origin, was essential to the NHS at a time when it was rapidly expanding.

The majority of these Asian doctors came to the UK with the intention of obtaining some postgraduate medical training or postgraduate medical qualifications, such as Membership or Fellowship of the Royal Colleges. However, this significant input of overseas doctors into the NHS has had important and far-reaching implications for their training and career structure within the NHS.

As most of the Asian doctors had initially come for a limited period early in their careers, they were mainly concentrated in the lower hospital grades (junior house officer (JHO), senior house officer (SHO), and registrar). Many of the Asian doctors were to be found working in the least popular hospital specialties, such as geriatrics or psychiatry, where language and communication are of prime importance. The NHS, therefore, had a pool of Asian doctors who filled a large proportion of junior hospital posts, particularly in peripheral hospitals where training and teaching prospects are often said to be poor.

Asian doctors, therefore, found themselves in an unenviable position. As very little postgraduate teaching takes place in peripheral hospitals, the doctors working within them often found it difficult to obtain postgraduate qualifications, and this resulted in them flitting from one poor job to another. These doctors then faced the prospect of either returning to their country of origin with no postgraduate qualifications, and therefore to low-paid posts, or continuing to stay in this country.

In real terms, the NHS did not benefit either, as Asian doctors were often forced to take jobs which were inappropriate to their career aims, with little of the job-satisfaction which is such an essential ingredient in providing good-quality patient-care. As the majority of overseas doctors left before becoming general practitioners or consultants, a 'pool' of Asian doctors at JHO and SHO level in hospitals was maintained. Today that pool has gradually diminished, particularly since 1985, when it became mandatory for overseas doctors to take the Professional and Linguistic Assessment Board (PLAB) examination. This examination (which has a low pass-rate) enables overseas doctors to apply for limited registration for the purposes of postgraduate training in a hospital for up to four years. The second factor in diminishing the pool of Asian doctors in the lower grades in hospitals is the increased output of graduates from British medical schools.

Categories of Asian doctors

There are three categories of Asian doctors in the NHS: those who were born and graduated overseas; those who were born and graduated in the UK; and those who were born overseas, but graduated in the UK. Expectations, attitudes, and hopes for achievement are different for each category. To some extent their ambitions are determined by the influence of their own culture and identity, and to some by the experience of adaptation to a new 'western' culture.

Currently, by far the largest group is that comprising Asian doctors who graduated abroad, came here to obtain further qualifications or experience, but decided to stay. This category is discussed in detail below. Of the other two groups mentioned above, very little is written, perhaps because they are a relatively new phenomenon. These latter two groups are discussed in the light of the author's personal experiences, those of his colleagues, and those of students from medical schools whom he has taught over the last five years.

Characteristics of Asian doctors

Language spoken   Many Asian doctors speak more than one language (see Table 4.2). There are considerable advantages to patients as consumers and to the NHS of having Asian doctors who speak a second language as well as English (Baxter 1987). This is particularly important in areas of high Asian populations, such as Leicester, Manchester, Bradford, Rochdale, London, Birmingham, and Coventry. Firstly, it obviates the need for an interpreter. Secondly, in such areas, whether working in hospitals or in general practice, Asian doctors are more likely to be able to understand the community's social conventions, and its expectations of the health service. Thirdly, there is some anecdotal evidence (Mares *et al.* 1985) that individuals and families are likely to be more receptive to health care and advice given by someone from their own community whom they respect and trust. Finally, colleagues of non-Asian origin working with patients from Asian communities can gain valuable understanding and practical expertise by drawing on the insight and experience of Asian doctors working in these communities.

Table 4.2.   *Main languages spoken by overseas doctors with their families*

Language	No.	Percentage
English	134	49
Hindi	26	10
Bengali	23	8
Urdu	20	7
Punjabi	12	4
Gujarati	7	3
Others	51	19
Total	273	100

Some doctors spoke more than one language.
Source: Anwar and Ali 1987

Age   Asian doctors are mainly concentrated in the 30–44 age-group (although this statistic is rapidly changing with the output of Asian graduates from British medical schools), so that relatively few have reached the age at which they may be expected to occupy senior posts. Despite possessing relevant medical postgraduate qualifications many Asian doctors feel that they have experienced discrimination on the part of selection committees for consultant posts in hospitals, and also in general practice, with the result that these doctors are concentrated in the lower hospital grades (Smith 1980; Smith 1987) and less desirable practices.

Geographical distribution   It is interesting, with the recent focus of attention on the North–South divide, that the lowest percentage of Asian doctors are to be found in the prosperous South East, and the highest in the North Western region. The latter region is continually in the news as an underfunded area with respect to both health and social-service resources. Asian doctors in general practice are often found to be working in inner-city deprived areas, and not necessarily those with large ethnic minority populations. It is well-known and acknowledged that practices within these communities are less attractive, and more demanding in terms of workload. Asian doctors in these areas are often subjected to racial abuse, which may be both verbal and physical. It may be that Asian doctors take such practices not from choice, but because they find it impossible to obtain anything better. Family Practitioner Committees and Health Boards ought to be aware that the Asian population in many cities is rapidly becoming more prosperous, and moving out of the inner-city areas, creating a need for Asian doctors in more prosperous areas of the country. Medical school curricula will need to adapt to include teaching on health care for ethnic minorities.

Career paths for Asian general practitioners

A great deal of evidence has accumulated (Smith 1980; CRE 1983; Mares *et al.* 1985; McNaught 1985; Anwar and Ali 1987; Smith 1987) that Asian doctors who became GPs did so reluctantly in the 1960s, when general practice was regarded as 'less prestigious' than it is today, and morale in the profession was low. Doctors were at that time able to 'opt out' into general practice after having failed to pursue a successful career in the hospital service, despite possessing relevant higher medical qualifications, such as MRCP or FRCS. It is interesting that many Asian doctors from that era possess these qualifications, and yet had to become GPs.

This is in contrast to British graduates, who usually chose general practice as a career from the outset. General practice does, of course, offer a good income and status at a comparatively early stage after qualification. It could be that Asian doctors who decided to stay in Britain found general practice the most appropriate career in the British context, as its organization is less hierarchical, and perhaps therefore less open to the practice of discrimination than that of the hospital service.

Career paths for Asian hospital doctors

British and Asian doctors are agreed (Smith 1980; CRE 1983; Mares *et al.* 1985; McNaught 1985; Smith 1987) that an Asian doctor with a basic degree from a recognized overseas medical school and with postgraduate qualifications is likely to be rejected when in competitition with a white applicant with similar or identical qualifications and experience. As Smith (1987) pointed out recently, what is more disturbing is that this also appears to be true of Asian graduates from this country. British doctors in one survey (CRE 1983) felt that rejection of Asian doctors when applying for jobs was either likely to be based on the supposition that their qualifications were inferior, or came about because Asian overseas graduates were thought to be less competent to practise within the UK. However, they also believed that these views are based on stereotyping, and that these beliefs and judgements are misguided.

This notion of rejection is strongly confirmed by data on the number of applications made for jobs by Asians, which is much higher than the number made by their white British counterparts (Smith 1987).

Achieving a balance

The NHS has left within it, therefore, a group of doctors (contained in the 'pool' described above) who have decided to stay in the UK, but who graduated from overseas, and who have, for the reasons previously explained, few or no career prospects in the NHS. This group of doctors, some approaching middle age, move between the least desirable posts in the NHS to make a living.

In 1987 the Government published *Hospital medical staffing: achieving a balance: plan for action* (DHSS 1987a). This document plans a ten-year improvement in training arrangements and career prospects for hospital doctors. In addition to increasing the number of consultants and reducing the number of senior registrars, it proposes to divide registrar posts into those for overseas graduates who are limited to four years' training in their country, and posts for those graduates who will be making a career in the NHS hospital service. A further proposal concerns mechanisms to identify doctors unlikely to make further progress ('stuck doctors'), and to provide counselling and help in obtaining secure employment for them. In the first instance this may be by means of a single four-year extension of the contract, followed by retraining for another specialty or for general practice, appointment to a staff-grade post, regrading as an associate specialist, or, exceptionally, the granting of a five-year rolling contract. These proposals will be of particular interest to many Asian doctors within the hospital service, especially those who are 'stuck'.

Problems experienced by Asian doctors entering general practice

Previously those Asian doctors who were unsuccessful in pursuing a successful hospital career went into general practice. However, since the introduction of compulsory vocational training programmes, and the rise in popularity of general practice as a career, Asian doctors have again become disadvantaged when applying for jobs in this field. Today, there can be as many as one hundred applicants for a principal's post in general practice, and competition is naturally very fierce. Existing and established practices often express the view that they are unwilling to accept hospital 'dropouts', or those not choosing general practice as a primary career choice. As a result of these attitudes many Asian doctors who qualified abroad are unable to compete on equal terms with British graduates in the general practice market, despite being vocationally trained. These doctors for whom there is no place in the hospital career structure either man general-practitioner deputizing services, do locums, or, in desperation, set up as single-handed practitioners. Their conditions of work, especially their unsocial hours, would be totally unacceptable to many white British graduates. Paradoxically, if Asian doctors did not man deputizing services during unsocial hours, one wonders how many general practice vacancies would occur through the early retirement of elderly GPs or through resignations by female GPs unwilling to do night visits in dangerous areas. Would those practices then be willing to take on partners from the pool who work for deputizing services? Just as there is a pool of Asian hospital doctors destined to go nowhere by the end of this decade, it is likely that, unless remedial steps are taken, a similar pool will exist in general practice.

The Government still officially encourages group practices within the inner city with incentive allowances. There is a marked tendency for Asian doctors to belong to the smaller single-handed or two-doctor practices, which are generally less desirable and popular. As Smith (1980) correctly pointed out 'this contrast is particularly strong when account is taken of the fact that most Asian doctors entered general practice at a time when small practices were on the decrease'.

At least in its recently published White Paper on primary care the Government has recognized the excessive workload inner-city practices are exposed to by the proposed provision of an 'inner-city allowance' (DHSS 1987*b*).

Attitudes towards Asian doctors

There is considerable evidence of racial discrimination against Asian doctors (Smith 1980; Mares *et al.* 1985; McNaught 1985) both from patients and colleagues. Recently, there have been several reports in the press of racial attacks on Asian doctors and their surgeries. Of course, many of them are particularly vulnerable, as they practise in the inner cities amongst a deprived population. Asian doctors who work for deputizing services are reported to be terrified of visiting high-rise flats; and yet Family Practitioner Committees allow the situation to continue, with patients' own GPs often unwilling to do night calls in these areas. Police escorts are not always available; and, as the proportion of female practitioners increases, one can envisage a situation in the future when night visits to patients' homes will not take place, as in the United States of America.

Asian doctors from overseas but who grad*u*ted from British medical schools

This group of doctors came to Britain at an early age, had most of their schooling here, and then graduated from a British medical school. In common with white British graduates, their parents are often from professional backgrounds. Parental guidance in children's education in an Asian household is very important; and from that perspective here was a profession of high status and salary, with a career structure and a secure future, in which discrimination was unlikely to occur. The motivation for this second generation to go to medical school was therefore very substantial. Reality, however, fell far short of this ideal. The first-generation migrants came to establish a foothold, and the second generation was expected to build on that, so that they could be treated as equals in a multiracial society. Despite the high aims of their parents and their own expectations, this second generation have also experienced discrimination at each stage in their careers. The evidence for this is considerable (Smith 1987). A recent investigation at St George's Medical School in London discovered a computer program which gave negative weighting to ethnic minority candidates. Furthermore, a study from St Mary's Hospital Medical School showed that only 11.2 per cent of applicants with non-European names were interviewed, compared to 30 per cent of those with European names. This despite the health and academic suitability of applicants being the same. What differed, however, was the nebulous concept of their 'non-academic suitability' (Collier and Burke 1986)!

A recently published report on disadvantage experienced by ethnic minority groups applying to medical schools revealed that twenty-four variables ranked in order of importance could be used for predicting successful applications to medical schools (McManus *et al.* 1989).

From these 'predictors' of 301 Asian applicants to medical schools in 1986, 101 (33.4 per cent) were predicted to be accepted, but only 76 (25.2 per cent) were actually accepted. For white Europeans, out of 1406 applicants 672 (47.8 per cent) were predicted to be accepted whereas the actual number accepted was 697 (49.6 per cent). Applicants from ethnic minority groups were less likely to be accepted than their white European counterparts at all grades of 'A' level achievements. It could be said that this is not conclusive evidence of discrimination by medical schools against non-white candidates, as entry to medical school should be judged on other criteria such as interest, initiative, enthusiasm, and ability to communicate and empathize. While these factors are undoubtedly important, and the public has a right to expect such qualities in future doctors, the fact remains that many medical schools still do not interview candidates prior to entry. What is also questionable is the ability and skills of admission officers to medical schools to evaluate the qualities stated above on the basis of application forms and a single interview. Indeed candidates are often subjected to different interviewers, whose personal attitudes may affect any objective qualitative criteria for admission, leading to a non-uniform selection policy.

Adaptations in practice made by Asian doctors treating Asian patients

Treatment of female Asian patients by male doctors poses particular problems in an Asian culture, and paradoxically more so if the doctors are of Asian origin. Asian women, especially Muslim and Sikh women, will often not allow Asian male doctors to examine their chests or perform vaginal examinations. Some Asian doctors in general practice have adapted to the needs of such patients. Some practices employ female practice nurses to carry out vaginal examinations, do cervical smears, and advise on breast examinations. Such 'in house' facilities play a vital role in the delivery of anticipatory care amongst the Asian community.

Future policies and recommendations

The NHS needs to effect some fundamental changes if discriminatory practices are to be eliminated from its structure. The following recommendations have been suggested by the Commission for Racial Equality, and supplemented by the author:

1. There is a paucity of data on doctors of different ethnic origins in the NHS. If problems of racial discrimination exist it is essential to gather a large and accurate database to monitor the career development of the second generation of ethnic minority doctors (that is, of those who are British graduates.)
2. Interviewers on selection committees should be given appropriate guidance and training to ensure that decisions taken in appointing medical staff are not based on stereotyped assumptions about cultural backgrounds and places of qualification.
3. Royal Colleges have been accused of passing fewer Asian candidates as against white British graduates, at examinations for Membership or Fellowship. The reasons for these differences should be urgently investigated, and a programme instituted to remedy the situation. It is both unfair and unethical to keep on collecting examination fees from candidates who have little chance of passing.
4. Medical schools need to critically evaluate their entry criteria to ensure that discriminatory practices are eliminated.

5. The DHSS, District Health Authorities, and Regional Health Authorities should make certain that action is taken to ensure that all specialties are accessible to Asian doctors working in hospitals.

6. Family Practitioner Committees and Health Boards should ensure that similar action is taken in appointing practitioners to single-handed or new-practice vacancies.

7. There should be greater representation of Asian doctors on selection committees, merit award committees, hospital committees, and District Management Boards.

8. The Government, the British Medical Association, Family Practitioner Committees, and Health Boards should investigate who mans deputizing services, and the proportion of locums of Asian origin. Remedial action should be taken where necessary.

9. Family Practitioner Committees and Health Boards should ensure that Asian doctors are not just concentrated in inner-city areas, and act in anticipation of Asian populations moving away from deprived areas as they become more affluent.

10. Medical schools should be sensitive to the needs of a multiracial society, and teach students how to deal with patients from different cultures and backgrounds.

Finally, the National Association of Health Authorities has recently published a report (NAHA 1988) which states 'The NHS must acknowledge the existence of institutional and individual racism, and realise that widespread racial discrimination occurs in both employment practices and service provision'. Among the proposals made in the report is a call for more ethnic minority appointments to Health Authorities, Family Practitioner Committees, and Community Health Councils.

Conclusion

The NHS, over the last three decades, has received a substantial contribution in the form of medical manpower from doctors of Asian origin. While this relationship may have been beneficial to the NHS, it has not, in many cases, been beneficial to the career and promotion propects of those Asian doctors who decided to stay permanently in the UK.

Today, the number of Asian doctors entering the NHS having qualified overseas is gradually decreasing. This situation has occurred because of three fundamental changes.

Firstly, the Medical Act of 1978 drastically reduced the number of overseas medical schools whose degrees could be recognized for the purposes of full registration. Secondly, Asian doctors are now required to be successful in the Professional and Linguistic Assessment Board (PLAB) examination, which has a particularly low pass-rate. Thirdly, the higher output from British medical schools has increased the pool of home graduates competing for jobs.

While the majority of overseas doctors came to the UK to obtain higher qualifications and enhance their career prospects in their country of origin few intended to stay permanently. Those who stayed on in the UK did so either because of their success in the medical profession, for example as consultants or general practitioners, or because they had failed to achieve their career aims. Others married local women and wished to have their children educated and brought up in the UK.

Whether successful or not, many Asian doctors who graduated from overseas feel they have experienced discrimination within the NHS. This sinister experience unfortunately appears to be extending to affect the second generation of Asian graduates from British medical schools. These feelings and experiences are backed up by statistical and anecdotal evidence (Smith 1987).

There is thus an urgent need for the NHS to renew its recruitment, training, and selection procedures to ensure that there is equality of opportunity, both at junior and senior levels, for Asian doctors within its structure.

Asian nurses in the NHS

Very little has been written on Asian nurses in the NHS. They are nearly always discussed as part of a larger group of ethnic minority nurses. While the experiences of ethnic minority nurses may on the whole be similar, cultural and religious differences pose particular problems for Asian nurses, who have experienced difficulties in adaptation, integration, and promotion within the Health Service. These factors have played an important role in influencing nurse recruitment from the Asian community, which is currently running at very low levels even in areas with large Asian populations.

As the DHSS, District Health Authorities, and Royal Colleges of Nurses and Midwives claim not to identify the ethnic origin of nurses, it is not possible to deduce what proportion of the 465 000 nurses working in the UK (DHSS 1986*b*) are of Asian origin. However, in 1972 a survey by the Policy Studies Institute found 9 per cent of all NHS hospital nurses were from overseas (Thomas and Williams 1972).

Historical perspective

During the 1960s and 1970s a significant proportion of nurses were recruited from overseas, specifically from the West Indies, Africa, and Malaysia. These nurses were mainly channelled into state enrolled nurse (SEN) training, which is both less well-paid and less prestigious than state registered nurse (SRN) training. SEN is not recognized as a qualification in most countries outside the UK, and, consequently, was of no value to overseas nurses if they wanted to return home and continue nursing.

During this period very few nurses of Asian origin other than from Malaysia were recruited into the NHS. The reasons for this recruitment policy remain unclear, despite the obvious need for Asian nurses in areas with large Asian populations where knowledge of Asian languages and Asian culture would be of great advantage both to patients and to the NHS.

Of those ethnic minority nurses recruited in the 1970s many, it appears, were positively encouraged to specialize in low-status disciplines such as geriatrics and mental subnormality. Indeed, current General Nursing Council figures show that, even today, up to one-third of overseas nurse trainees are in psychiatric and mental-handicap nursing (Mares *et al.* 1985).

Promotion prospects

A review of the ethnic minority composition of nursing staff in South Derbyshire (Pearson 1987) reveals some startling statistics (Table 4.3).

Table 4.3   *Ethnic origins of nursing staff in South Derbyshire*

Ethnic origin	No.	% of nurses	% of population
White	1193	82.7	(85.2)
Afro-Caribbean	198	13.8	(4.2)
Asian	28	2.0	(9.7)
Other European	22	1.5	(0.7)
Total	1441	100.0	(100.0)

Figures in brackets represent estimated percentage of population in Derby City, the home of over 80 per cent of Derbyshire's Asians.
Sources: Pearson 1987 and Derbyshire FPC 1988

In this district, of 29 clinical nurse managers 1 (3 per cent) was of Asian origin and 1 (3 per cent) of Afro-Caribbean origin. Eighty-nine per cent of 227 ward sisters were white and British, 15 (7 per cent) Afro-Caribbean, 4 (2 per cent) were European and 1 (0.4 per cent) was of Asian origin. Similarly, 291 (92 per cent) of 382 staff nurses were white and British, 20 (5 per cent) were Afro-Caribbean, and 3 (0.8 per cent) were of Asian origin.

The situation for SENs was different: here overseas Asian and Afro-Caribbean nurses take more responsibility, but with no real prospects for promotion into management. Of 352 SENs 54 (15 per cent) were Afro-Caribbeans and 11 (3 per cent) Asian. Ethnic minority nurses were also over-represented among 427 nursing auxiliaries, of whom 97 (23 per cent) were Afro-Caribbean and 12 (3 per cent) were Asian.

Nurse training

The policy of non-identification of ethnic origin pursued by nursing institutions and their hierarchy has posed considerable problems, and is a source of embarrassment to the nurse managers, particularly in areas with large ethnic minority populations.

In these areas it is increasingly recognized that inequalities in the delivery of health care may be partially remedied by the provision of health-care workers who have a culture and a language in common with the local populations.

A recent survey by the Commission for Racial Equality (CRE 1987) identified under-representation of ethnic minority students in nurse training. Only 3 per cent of existing trainees in general nursing courses are black, while the ethnic minority proportion of the economically active population in the UK is 5 per cent. However, the national figure of 3 per cent for general nurse trainees conceals substantial differences between individual nursing schools. In Leicester, for example, where the city's ethnic minority population is 25 per cent (22 per cent Asian, 3 per cent West Indian), only 4 per cent of the nursing-school intakes are of Asian extraction.

The CRE has challenged advertising procedures, selection procedures, and the stereotype of 'white, middle-class nurses', which they say may be applied informally by selectors. Schools of nursing suggest that the imbalance in recruitment between Asian and West Indian minorities may have cultural causes. Within the Asian communities nursing may be seen as a low-status occupation for youngsters with five or more 'O' levels; or the 'hands-on' intimate touching nature of many nursing practices may be a deterrent.

Figures collated by the CRE show the ethnic origins of existing trainees in nursing at 22 schools of nursing throughout the UK (Table 4.4).

This table highlights the low intake of Asian nurse trainees nationally. The

Table 4.4 *Ethnic origins of Registered General Nursing (RGN) and Registered Mental Nursing (RMN) trainees at 14 schools of nursing in the United Kingdom*

	No.	%
Total white	7765	96.9
Total black	245	3.1
Afro-Caribbean	97	1.2
African	26	0.3
Asian	104	1.3
Other	18	0.2

Source: CRE 1987

CRE points to certain differences between individual nursing schools, some of which have no Asian recruits at all.

According to the 1981 census the proportion of persons of Asian origin resident in households in Greater London was 14.6 per cent. Three schools in Greater London had only 15 black trainees out of a total of 1365 (just over 1 per cent). At one school of nursing in Leeds there were only two black trainees out of a total of 425. At another school in the same city, there were 14 trainees out of a total of 335. The Asian population in Leeds is about 4 per cent (CRE 1985).

Nursing and cultural conventions

While it is recognized that there is a clear need for Asian nurses in areas with large Asian populations, national nursing bodies and most District Health Authorities have not actively pursued an equal opportunities policy in nursing. Nor have these institutions looked at ways of surmounting factors which may deter students from Asian families taking up a career in nursing.

Factors which may deter Asian students from taking up nursing as a career

Different cultural conventions and practices are often difficult to integrate into an established system. Much is dependent on the family and socio-religious background of the individual, and on the ability and willingness of nursing institutions to recognize these differences.

These factors influence the differing needs of Asian nursing students, who may experience particular difficulties in adjusting and adapting in the unfamiliar environment of a hospital or working in the community. Nurse teachers and managers need to be aware of these cultural differences, which may lead to a sense of disharmony and isolation amongst Asian recruits to the nursing profession. The nursing profession needs to be aware of the fact that working in a different culture may lead to compulsory involvement in practices totally forbidden by various Asian cultures and religions. The profession needs to devise strategies to overcome these problems in nurse training (Wong and Wong 1982).

Punjabi women (Muslim and Sikh) prefer not to show their legs, for cultural and religious reasons. However, until 1981 nurses of Asian origin were not permitted to wear trousers instead of skirts. Rochdale Health Authority was the first to allow the wearing of trouser suits as part of nurses' uniform, to encourage women of Asian origin to apply for nursing posts.

Some Asian females may be embarrassed or apprehensive at the thought of touching male patients while giving them baths or helping them change or dressing wounds. Close contact with strange men is thought to be socially unacceptable in many Asian households. Some women from an Asian background are deterred by catering arrangements in living-in accommodation, especially during training, when it is often impossible to self-cater. As hospital canteens do not cater for

Asian staff, for example by providing halal meat for Muslims, Muslim nurses in such situations would be forced to eat a very restricted diet.

Certain Asian cultures, for example, the Malaysian, forbid women going near the dead whilst menstruating.

Asian nurses may be ostracized by their English counterparts if they do not conform to traditional hospital social activities such as parties and nights out. This cultural difference may be further aggravated if Asians are resident in nurses' homes. Traditionally Asian females are not encouraged to 'go out' late at night; but the dilemma facing many Asian nurse students is that if they do not conform to 'accepted social practices' then they may be rejected by their peers.

Some career guidance advisers, who are aware of the difficulties mentioned above, actively discourage ethnic minority students (Asian females in particular) from considering nursing as a career (Mares *et al.* 1985). This attitude has obviously been unhelpful in the recruitment of Asian nurses. Nurse training needs to be made more sensitive to the attitudes, beliefs, and experiences of Asian applicants if schools of nursing are to improve their recruitment record. Finally, the past experience of many Asian nurse recruits has not been good, and may play an important role in deterring Asians from the nursing profession. Promotion prospects for Asian nurses have been poor, and many trained nurses are working in unpopular specialties such as geriatrics and mental health (Hicks 1982*a*, 1982*b*), which parallels the experience of Asian doctors. Asian nurses have an important role to play in the delivery of effective health care, and should be represented at all grades in the nursing profession, not just the lowest.

Health visitors

Ethnic minority communities, particularly Asians, are under-represented in the health-visiting profession. Until recently, there had been very little effort to recruit people from an Asian background. Slowly, however, District Health Authorities have begun to ask for health visitors who are able to converse in Asian languages, to try and improve the service provided to the Asian community and increase the number of health visitors. This kind of positive discrimination is not yet the norm.

One of the reasons why there are few Asian health visitors is because community nursing is lagging behind social service departments in recognizing that appropriate experience and the ability to understand a culture and speak a patient's language is a more relevant qualification than high academic achievement.

The curriculum for nurse education and its implications for Asian nurse learners

There has been a tendency for nursing curricula to reflect the values of the indigenous British population, despite the fact that we live in a multiracial society. Nurse training should have a multicultural approach, to benefit students by increasing their understanding of the impact of cultural diversities in health care.

Such curricula would be far more attractive to potential recruits from the Asian community, and would contribute to some extent to alleviate the social and cultural isolation Asian student nurses have experienced in the past (Wong and Wong 1982). The Asian community too would benefit if white British nurses understood Asian illness and health behaviour, as this knowledge would improve communication and help to eliminate some of the misunderstandings that occur between health-care staff from the indigenous population and Asian patients.

Conclusion

New developments in the structure and scope of nursing with respect to Asian students present an opportunity to which nursing management must respond with vision (Baxter 1987). They could recruit, retrain, and redeploy Asian nurses to care for patients in the community where they are currently grossly under-represented. From 1987, many schools of nursing started recording information about the ethnic origins of nursing applicants to ensure that an appropriate ethnic mix is achieved, and, where necessary, to identify where positive discrimination policies need to be deployed.

Because of the present low number of Asian nurses and the current national shortage of qualified nurses, prospects for future employment and promotion within the National Health Service are excellent for Asian men and women who choose nursing as a career.

A final word

Over the last two decades, Asian doctors and nurses appear to have experienced considerable disadvantage in their career-development within the National Health Service. Whether this is due to discrimination on grounds of race is often very difficult to determine. There is no disputing, however, that a large majority of Asian doctors and nurses are to be found practising in the less popular special-ties in medicine, particularly in geriatrics and psychiatry. Paradoxically, these are the branches of medicine in which a good understanding of English culture and language are probably most important. There is clear evidence that Asian doctors with similar experience and qualifications to their white Anglo-Saxon counterparts find it more difficult to obtain consultant posts in hospital in the more popular specialties.

Asian doctors and nurses are under-represented on selection committees and in management. In general practice, most Asian doctors are to be found working in underprivileged and deprived inner-city areas. These practices are thought to be unattractive to white British graduates. Lack of Asian nurses in the community is recognized as a problem, especially in areas with large Asian populations.

With new policies on recruitment and training being adopted by many schools of nursing, this situation should gradually change over the next few years. The situation for Asian medical students and graduates from British medical schools remains somewhat worrying, however. Recent evidence has emerged of dubious selection procedures in certain London medical schools, which may discriminate against ethnic minority candidates. Most irksome, however, is the fact that Asian graduates from British medical schools are beginning to experience some of the difficulties their first-generation predecessors did in finding jobs of their choice with good promotion prospects. It is for the General Medical Council and the British Medical Association to ensure that the numbers of Asians represented in all specialties in medicine and in management are appropriate to their numbers in the medical profession as a whole.

For general practice some way must be found to ensure that Asian GPs are not just concentrated in the inner-city areas. As the Asian population expands and acquires wealth, many are moving to more prestigious areas. There is also clear evidence that Asian people retain their culture through many generations as migrants. In the future, more Asian GPs and nurses will be needed in suburban areas, especially if medical and nursing schools continue not to train doctors and nurses with a multicultural approach to health care.

References

Anwar, M. and Ali, A. (1987). *Overseas doctors: experience and expectations.* Commission for Racial Equality, London.

Baxter, C. (1987). Steps to sensitising the service. *The Health Service Journal,* **97,** 642–3.

Collier, J. and Burke, A. (1986). Racial and sexual discrimination of students applying for London medical schools. *Medical Education,* **20,** 86–90.

CRE (Commission for Racial Equality) (1983). *Ethnic minority hospital staff.* CRE, London.

CRE (Commission for Racial Equality) (1985). *Ethnic minorities in Britain.* CRE, London.

CRE (Commission for Racial Equality) (1987). *Ethnic origins of nurses applying for and in training.* CRE, London.

DHSS (Department of Health and Social Security) (1986*a*). Statistics and research division. *Census survey of NHS medical manpower in the United Kingdom.* DHSS, London.

DHSS (Department of Health and Social Security) (1986*b*). *Statistics and research division. Annual census of NHS non-medical manpower.* DHSS, London.

DHSS (Department of Health and Social Security) (1987*a*). *Hospital medical staffing: achieving a balance: plan for action.* DHSS, London.

DHSS (Department of Health and Social Security) (1987*b*). *Promoting better health—the Government's programme for improving primary health care.* CM **249.** HMSO, London.

...shire Family Practitioner Committee (1988). *Raising the issues. A review of social provision for the ethnic minorities.* Derbyshire FPC, Derby.

Hicks, C. (1982*a*). Racism in nursing. *Nursing Times*, **78**, 743–8.

Hicks, C. (1982*b*). Racism in nursing. *Nursing Times*, **78**, 789–91.

Mares, P., Henley, A. and Baxter, C. (1985). *Health care in multiracial Britain.* Health Education Council/National Extension College, Cambridge.

McManus, I. C., Richards, P. and Maitlis, S. L. (1989). Prospective study of the disadvantage of people from ethnic minority groups applying to medical schools in the United Kingdom. *British Medical Journal.* **298**: 723–6.

McNaught, A. (1985). *Race and health care in the United Kingdom*, Occasional paper no. 2. Health Education Council, London.

NAHA (National Association of Health Authorities) (1988). *Action not words.* NAHA, Birmingham.

Pearson, M. (1987). Racism the great divide. Discrepancies between promotion prospects of black and white nurses. *Nursing Times*, **83**, 24–6.

Smith, D. J. (1980). *Overseas doctors in the NHS.* Heinemann for the Policy Studies Institute, London.

Smith, R. (1987). Prejudice against doctors and students from ethnic minorities. *British Medical Journal*, **294**, 328–9.

Thomas, M. and Williams, J. M. (1972). *Overseas nurses in Britain: a PEP survey for the United Kingdom Council for Overseas Student Affairs.* Broadsheet No. 539 of the former Political and Economic Planning (now Policy Studies) Institute, London.

Wong, S. and Wong, J. (1982). Problems in teaching ethnic minority students. *Journal of Advanced Nursing*, **7**, 255–9.

Further reading

Baxter, C. (1988). *The black nurse—An endangered species.* National Extension College for Training in Health and Race, Cambridge.

Office of Health Economics (1987). *Compendium of Health Statistics*, 6th edn. OHE, London.

5 Communication

Brian McAvoy and Akram Sayeed

Introduction

Good communication is central to clinical competence. In hospital consultations, the diagnosis is established from the history alone in 56–82 per cent of cases (Hampton *et al*. 1975; Sandler 1979); the figures are probably higher in general practice. Communication skills exert a major influence on the adequacy of the consultation, on patients' satisfaction, and consequently on the quality of the doctor–patient relationship. Good communication is also sensitive to the needs of relatives and other health professionals, and is a pivotal factor in effective health education.

Surveys in Great Britain and the United States have shown that the commonest source of dissatisfaction with medical care is poor communication, mentioned by up to 51 per cent of general practice patients and up to 65 per cent of hospital patients (Ley 1983). These findings hold good in the context of a single language and culture. Their import and significance is even greater when there is no common language or culture. The variety of Asian languages and dialects, and the differences in the written word, are described in Chapter 1.

Cross-cultural communication

Communication is the process whereby individuals impart or exchange information, experiences, or feelings. The process is complex, and involves verbal and non-verbal components, including paralinguistics (how things are being said). The potential for confusion and misunderstanding is considerable in the context of a single language and culture, but is compounded when different cultures and languages are involved.

Several general factors underlie communication difficulties and misunderstandings. These factors, which very often operate in combination, are applicable to consultations as much as to any other settings. In clinical settings Bochner (1982) has identified four sources of error:

(a) Role uncertainty.
(b) Role non-correspondence.
(c) Definition disparity.
(d) Goal disparity.

(a) *Role uncertainty* arises when the doctor or patient is unclear about mutual expectations and obligations. For example, if a parent uncertain of the workings of the NHS believes that calling out her general practitioner would incur a fee, she may delay seeking help for her sick child. The difficulties may be compounded if, when the general practitioner is eventually called, he scolds the parent for not seeking help earlier, unaware of her misconception. If such difficulties arise it is helpful to discuss mutual expectations with the patient, and 'clear the air'.

(b) *Role non-correspondence* occurs when the doctor and patient have clear views on what they want and expect from the consultation, but these views conflict. For example, a patient with chest pain which the doctor believes is musculoskeletal in origin may expect to have a chest X-ray or electrocardiograph done, fearing a more serious cause. Unless the doctor allows the patient to express these anxieties and explains why such investigations are unnecessary, the patient may leave the consultation disgruntled and dissatisfied. Cultural factors play a major part in influencing patients' health beliefs and treatment expectations (see Chapter 2).

(c) *Definition disparity* arises when the doctor and patient use different terms to describe the same situation. There is some evidence (Hussain and Gommersall 1978) that depressed immigrant Asians show a strong tendency to present with somatic symptoms. Unless the doctor is aware of this, considerable time and effort may be wasted pursuing elusive organic causes for the symptoms, or worse still, the patient may be labelled as a 'neurotic' or 'hypochondriac'. Similarly, it is well-recognized that individuals from different cultures respond in different ways to pain, coping with it in a variety of ways (Zborowski 1952; Zola 1966). The 'stoical' British doctor should never assume that patients from a more 'emotional' culture are over-reacting to pain—they still need sympathy and support. Further discussion on this is contained in Chapter 17.

(d) *Goal disparity* occurs when the aims of the doctor and patient are totally different—a potent source of conflict. Difficulties may arise when a patient who just wishes for relief from the symptoms of his acute bronchitis consults with a doctor who is also concerned with the longer-term implications of the patient's continuing to smoke heavily. The doctor's main aim may be to stop the patient smoking, the patient's to obtain a prescription for an antibictic. Cultural factors can compound such difficulties, and careful negotiation is often required to avoid overt conflict.

A further source of communication difficulties is distancing between the participants, related to differences in social class, age, education, religion, and culture. Indeed, communication difficulties between sexes, as between generations, demonstrate that cultural differences are not the only barriers to successful communication between participants from different cultural or ethnic backgrounds. In general, the closer the cultural, social, and linguistic backgrounds of the doctor and patient, the less likely they are to be confused about roles or to have communication problems. Unfortunately, stereotyping of individuals from other cultures or backgrounds tends to reinforce distancing, and thereby increases the potential for misunderstanding.

A person's culture exercises a far greater influence on his behaviour than is generally recognized. Indeed, an individual's cultural background, which is inseparable from his psychological processes, determines what he perceives—what he sees, hears, feels, or believes. That is to say we perceive our physical as well as social environment according to the cultural map we carry in our minds. Often, however, this map, which represents our beliefs, deceives us; it leads us to perceive things that are not there, and vice versa (Owusu-Bempah 1988). For example, to Western eyes white clothes symbolize purity, brightness, and clinical efficiency, making the hospital doctor's white coat and the nurse's uniform reassuring. However, they may not be perceived in the same way by Asian patients, for whom white is the traditional colour worn by widows.

While generalizations about the attitudes, customs, or behaviours of Asians or different subgroups within the Asian community can provide a useful introduction and background for those who have no knowledge, it is critical that this information is interpreted in the context of the enormous variability between individuals (see Chapter 2). These who have ventured North of the border realize the inaccuracy of the steretyped image of the Scotsman—mean, whisky-sodden, haggis-eating, and wrapped in a kilt. It is important not to fall into similar traps when dealing with Hindus, Muslims, or Sikhs. In other words, the doctor's attitude to, and cultural assumptions about, the patient significantly affect the relationship between them. Similarly patients' attitudes to the NHS and to health professionals can have a major influence on communication.

Attitudes to the N.H.S.

In the Indian subcontinent the idea of a National Health Service is not universal. A system of regular health care by a particular doctor is well beyond the economic reach of many people. Consequently the Western-style medical practitioner is called only after initial 'home remedies' and other cheaper systems have failed; dramatic results are expected. Moreover, the costly, often sole, consultation is expected to be comprehensive, and to include a full physical examination and the arrangement of some laboratory investigations. Real or indeed perceived failure often results in a change of physician, or even system. Even now, this attitude can be reflected in the United Kingdom in the frequent changing of general practitioners, very often without any apprently good reason. It is not unusual to hear an Asian patient say, 'We are with you, doctor, for so many years. We have not changed.'—as if changing to another doctor is the usual practice.

It can be beneficial at the first encounter with new patients to briefly check out their understanding of the NHS. If appropriate, it can be useful to stress the benefits of continuity of care and the value of accumulated knowledge, and to dispel any misunderstandings about private patients' receiving 'better treatment'.

Appointment systems with one slot for each patient are now a standard part of British general practice. It is important that doctors and especially their receptionists realize that attitudes to time-keeping differ between cultures, and that patients unfamiliar with the organization of British general practice may assume that several family members' problems can be dealt with during a single appointment. Tact, sensitivity, negotiation, and appropriate education can avoid conflict in situations which can initially provoke irritation.

Attitudes to health professionals

The concept of the primary helath-care team may be unfamiliar to some Asians. In general, doctors are held in high regard, but the nurse's status may be lessened by the fact that she has to mix with male doctors and other health professionals, and to have physical contact with strange men. Gender preferences reflect prevailing cultural attitudes. Non-Asian women prefer to attend a female doctor for contraceptive advice (Preston-Whyte *et al.* 1983), and this preference is even stronger among Asian women, especially Muslims (Zaklama, 1984; McAvoy and Raza 1988). Wherever possible, Asian women should always be offered the opportunity to be examined by a female doctor. If this is not possible, a non-Asian male doctor, who is not part of the culture of the patient, may be more acceptable than a fellow Asian. Similarly, older Muslim men are often unaccustomed to dealing with women in positions of authority, and may sometimes be embarrassed by female health workers, especially nurses (Henley 1982). Again, in these circumstances, cultural awareness and understanding, tact, and sensitivity on the part of doctors and other health professionals are required in order to avoid conflict or misunderstandings.

Modes of communication

In any interaction with a patient the doctor should be aware of the significance of the verbal and non-verbal components of communication, as well as the paralinguistics. There is potential for confusion in each or all of these components in any consultation, but once again the opportunities for misunderstanding are greatly increased when the individuals are from different social and cultural backgrounds.

The most obvious barrier to verbal communication occurs when there is no common language between the doctor and the patient. Methods of dealing with this situation are described later in this chapter. Even when there is a common language, however, misunderstandings can still occur. In addition to diverse meanings for the same word, as with 'subway' in Britain and the USA, different accents can readily lead to stereotyping. Another source of difficulty can be the use of inappropriate language—for example, addressing an unmarried woman as 'Mrs', or calling a ward sister 'nurse'. Appropriateness of language can be of crucial importance where status is at stake, but is culturally determined (Owusu-Bempah 1988). An all-too-common example of this is when a patient answers 'yes' to all questions because he or she feels it would be impolite or hostile to disagree. This response can also result from a combination of failing to understand what is being said and wishing to please the doctor by agreeing with all he says.

Probably the main source of confusion, however, relates to paralinguistics. A sudden lowering of the voice, a hesitation, a clearing of the throat, or a cough can provide valuable clues to the meaning of information being given. Tone, pitch, rhythm, pauses, emphasis, stress, and pace often reveal much about the feelings and attitude of the speaker. These features, however, and the way in which people organize their conversations, are not universal to all languages. For example, many Asians converse in an indirect or circular pattern, contrasting markedly with the direct, linear orientation of English. Such an approach can be misinterpreted as indicating shyness, verbosity, or evasiveness.

Non-verbal communication consists mainly of facial expressions, gestures, movements, proximity, touch, gaze, and eye contact, dress, and general appearance. These are predominantly culture-bound, and so can have different meanings or connotations in different cultures. It has been suggested that in a normal two-person conversation the verbal component carries less than 35 per cent of the social meaning of a situation, and more than 65 per cent is carried by the non-verbal component (Birdwhistell 1970). Indeed non-verbal cues are often the best indicators of an individual's true attitudes or intentions, irrespective of what has been said. The potential for confusion and misunderstanding here is considerable. For example, in Western culture eye-contact during conversation is considered polite and a sign of attentiveness, but is perceived as rude and indicating annoyance in Eastern culture; amongst Muslim women especially, sitting with somewhat bowed head and downcast eyes is a sign of great modesty. Gestures, too, are culture-based. Eye-winking, which in Western culture is often used to put someone at ease, can cause grave offence to many Asians, especially if directed at a women by a man. To Asians the 'thumbs up' sign symbolizes defiance, not success or good luck. Pointing the index finger during conversation, often used for emphasis or discipline in Western culture, is regarded as bad manners by many Asians. Finally, the ring formed by curving the thumb and index finger is an innocent gesture in the West, but for Asians this symbolizes the anus, and is therefore offensive.

Social conventions

Day-to-day behaviour associated with good manners and politeness is also cul-ture-based, and often is largely unconscious. Among indigenous members of the British population 'Hello' often means nothing more than a mere acknow-ledgement. By contrast greetings in the Asian community are a way of showing one's courtesy, respect, and affection. Words of greeting are almost always synchronized with appropriate body language, and vary between different religious groups. Joined palms raised to the bowed head, accompanied by the word 'Namaste'—'my humble greetings to you'—is the greeting of Hindus, and is almost universal in the Indian subcontinent. The reply is 'Namaste', as is the parting greeting. The simple addition of 'ji' after the word 'Namaste' makes it more respectful, courteous, and intimate.

Muslims greet each other with 'As-salamu Alaykum'—'peace be upon you'. The reply is 'Walaykum As-salam'—'peace be upon you as well'. This is accom-panied by handshaking. To show respect, the addressed person takes the right hand of the other in both his hands; this only applies to males. The parting greeting is again 'Salam', and shaking hands accompanied by the phrase 'Khoda hafiz'—'be in God's security'. The common Sikh greeting is 'Sat-Sri-Akal' which literally means 'Truth in the God', and is used both as a welcoming and a parting greeting. Many Sikhs use 'Namaste' to greet non-Sikhs.

Asians speaking English may rarely use the words 'please' and 'thank you' because these are only used in their mother tongue on very formal occasions. An unsuspecting Briton can misconstrue this as rudeness, reinforcing negative stereotypes. Failure to observe social conventions can cause offence, and ser-iously interfere with establishing rapport in a consultation.

Fluency and literacy

It is estimated that over 200 000 adults resident in Britain can speak English only slightly or not at all, the majority of these being Asian (Smith 1977). The proportion of Asians able to speak and understand English varies with gender, age, and ethnic background.

A survey of Britain's blacks by the Policy Studies Institute (PSI) (Brown 1984) discovered that within the adult Asian population 60 per cent of Bangladeshis and 48 per cent of Pakistanis spoke little or no English, compared with only 28 per cent of Indians and 18 per cent of 'African Asians'. The survey also found that within this population households facing the most serious class disad-vantage (such as chronic housing conditions and unemployment) were least likely to be fluent in English. Although this link is not necessarily causal, it suggests that a lack of English can often be an indicator of other disadvantages that give rise to poor health. Another national study (Smith 1977) showed that 77 per cent of Pakistani women and 60 per cent of Indian women spoke English only slightly or not at all. Age seems to be more closely related to fluency in English than length of domicile in Britain. The PSI survey discovered that about a quarter of adult Asians aged under thirty-five speak little or no English, compared to over half of those aged over fifty-five. For all age-groups men are on the whole more fluent than women. In time lack of English should become less of a problem, but certain factors make it difficult for individuals to learn to speak English (Mares *et al*. 1985):

- Lack of contact with English speakers.
- Lack of educational opportunity in the past.
- Lack of confidence.
- Age.
- Non-availability of English-speaking relatives and friends.

The majority of people whose first language is not English can read and write in their mother tongue, but only a minority can read and write in English. The Linguistic Minorities Project (LMP) surveyed eleven minority-language communities in Bradford, Coventry, and London (Stubbs 1985), and found that in all the communities literacy in English was lower than in the mother tongue. However, only 47 per cent of Pakistani Punjabi speakers in Bradford were literate in their mother tongue. A similar study of literacy among Asians attending clinics or community groups in Oldham revealed that 90 per cent of Bengali men and 52 per cent of Bengali women could read their mother tongue, while the figures for reading English were 41 per cent and none respectively. Among Pakistanis 85 per cent of men and 77 per cent of women could read their own language, but only 25 per cent of men and 4 per cent of women could read English (Learmonth 1980).

These studies underline the importance of considering local ethnic minority needs in the planning and delivery of health services, particularly with regard to preparing health education materials (see Chapter 10).

Overcoming the language barrier

You know, in this country if you don't know English they make you feel you are nothing, and that attitude makes you feel so small and insignificant. No matter how much you know in your home and with your family, outside you are zero—you are utterly insignificant. (Mrs Bisla, a Sikh who can speak Punjabi, Urdu, and Hindi, and write in Devanagri and Gurmukhi, but cannot speak or understand English (Ahmed and Watt 1986).)

Mares *et al*. (1985) have suggested five practical ways in which doctors can improve communication with people who speak little or no English, or who speak English as a second language:

(a) Reducing stress.
(b) Simplifying your English.

(c) Checking back properly.
(d) Using a qualified interpreter.
(e) Learning the client's language.

(a) Reducing stress

The stress of an illness or having to attend a doctor's surgery can interfere with a patient's ability to communicate. This is compounded for those who speak English as a second language. Mares *et al*. (1985) have suggested a number of ways of reducing such stress:

- Allow more time than you would for an English-speaking patient.
- Give plenty of non-verbal reassurance.
- Try to communicate some information about what's going to happen next, even at a very simple level.
- Get the patient's name right.
- Try also to pronounce the patient's name correctly.
- Keep fuller case notes (this avoids subjecting the patient to repeated unnecessary or complicated questioning).
- Try to ensure that the patient always sees the same staff as far as possible.
- Try and find out whether the patient has any specific fears or worries.
- Write down any important points clearly and simply on a piece of paper for the patient to take away.

(b) Simplifying your English

To avoid patronizing or offending patients it is important to adapt the following advice to the individual's needs (Mares *et al*. 1985):

- Speak clearly but do not raise your voice.
- Speak slowly throughout (but not too slowly).
- Repeat when you have not been understood.
- Use the words the patient is likely to know.
- Be careful of idioms.
- Simplify the form of each sentence.
- Don't speak pidgin English.
- Give instructions in a clear, logical sequence.
- Simplify the total structure of what you want to say in your mind before you begin.
- Stick to one topic at a time.
- Be careful when you use examples.
- Use pictures or clear mime to help get the meaning across.
- Judge how much people are likely to remember.
- Be aware of your language (both verbal and non-verbal) all the time.

Closed questions are best for obtaining facts or information.

(c) Checking back properly

This should be done regularly throughout the consultation, using the following simple techniques (Mares *et al*. 1985):

- Try not to ask 'Do not understand?' or 'Is that all right?' You are almost bound to get 'yes' for an answer.
- Try also to avoid questions to which a correct answer is 'yes'.
- Ask the patient to explain back to you what he is going to do.

In addition don't take nods and other gestures or expressions at face value.

(d) Using a qualified interpreter

This would appear to be an obvious way of overcoming the language barrier, but there still can be drawbacks (Fuller and Toon 1988):

- The interpreter may leave out a vital piece of information by accident. It may be difficult for the interpreter to see the importance of a particular phrase or piece of information used by a patient.
- The interpreter may not understand (or interpret) a word or concept.
- The interpreter may put in his or her own advice.
- The interpreter may interpret what she or he thinks the doctor wants to hear.
- The interpreter may become angry or impatient with the patient and criticize him or her.
- The interpreter may refuse to interpret something the professional says because it goes against his or her own beliefs.

In addition the patient may be reluctant to discuss sensitive subjects in the presence of a third party, or may be concerned about dangers to confidentiality. All these potential problems are more likely if untrained interpreters are used. A detailed study of four bilingual hospital out-patient interviews involving relatives as interpreters revealed that up to 52 per cent of questions were mistranslated or not translated at all (Ebden *et al*. 1988). In the 143 questions and answers there were more than 80 words or phrases which were mistranslated, misunderstood, or not translated by at least one interpreter. Not surprisingly technical terms were often mistranslated, with 'breathlessness' used for 'asthma' and 'being mad' for 'epileptic fit'. Two words caused particular problems: 'trouble' in Indian English means pain, and hence the question 'What is the trouble?' was mistranslated. 'Cough', in English, was confused with the Gujarati word 'kuf' meaning phlegm.

Unfortunately trained interpreters are not widely available, especially in a general-practice setting. Some social services departments maintain lists of interpreters. However, a survey of District Health Authorities in England and Wales with Asian populations greater than 500 revealed that only 14 per cent employed interpreters (Donaldson and Odell 1984). In the majority of settings heavy reliance was placed on informal solutions, such as the use of lay and volunteer interpreters, usually members of the family, and the language skills of staff. Using members of the family can introduce problems of distortion due to their close emotional involvement, particularly in the case of children. Indeed, Rack (1982) has stated that 'Under no circumstances should children be asked to interpret medical details for their parents. It appears to us to be unethical, unprofessional, uncivilized, and totally unacceptable.'

Mares *et al.* (1985) have described the characteristics of the interpreter who can best serve your needs:

- Is fluent in both English and the patient's language.
- Has some training in interpreting.
- Has some medical knowledge, and knowledge of how the health services work.
- Accompanies you every time you visit the patient.
- Is acceptable to you, and trusted by the patient.
- Is sensitive to both your needs and those of the patient.
- Takes a neutral role.
- Puts the patient at ease.
- Has a good memory and pays careful attention to detail.
- Can translate fine shades of meaning.
- Tells you when she or he has difficulty in translating what you have said, and explains why.
- Is aware of cultural expectations or attitudes—yours and your patient's—and can explain things to both of you when needed.
- Can tell you a good deal about the patient from his or her own observations after the interview.

The health professional and interpreter should work as a team, but this takes time, mutual trust, and co-operation (Henley 1979). Shackman (1984) has devised a useful checklist for interviewers using an interpreter:

Practical things to do:
- Check that the interpreter and client speak the same language or dialect.
- Allow time for a pre-interview discussion with the interpreter, in order to talk about the content of the interview and the way in which you will work together.
- Encourage the interpreter to interrupt and intervene during the interview when necessary.
- Use straightforward language.
- Actively listen to the interpreter and the client.
- Allow enough time for the interview.
- At the end of the interview check whether the client has understood everything and wants to know or ask anything else.
- Have a post-interview discussion with the interpreter.

Things to remember:

- The pressures on the interpreter.
- The responsibility for the interview is yours.
- Your power—as perceived by the interpreter and the client.
- To be patient and show compassion in a demanding situation.
- To be aware of your own racial attitudes.
- To be aware of your own shortcomings—for example, being monolingual.
- To show respect for the interpreter and his or her skills.

Points to check if things seem to be going wrong:

- Does the interpreter speak English and the client's language fluently?
- Is the interpreter acceptable to the client (same sex, similar age)?
- Is your client prevented from telling you things because of his or her relationship with the interpreter?
- Are you creating as good a relationship as possible with your client?
- Is the interpreter translating exactly what you and your client are saying, or is she or he putting forward her or his own views and opinions?
- Does the interpreter understand the purpose of the interview and what her or his role is within it?
- Have you given the interpreter time to get to know your client and explain what is going on?
- Does the interpreter feel free to interrupt you when necessary, to point out problems or to ask for clarification?
- Are you using simple jargon-free English?
- Is the interpreter ashamed of or embarrassed by your client?
- Are you asking too much of the interpreter?
- Are you allowing the interpreter enough time?
- Are you maintaining as good a relationship with the interpreter as you can?

Patient advocates These are trained members of ethnic minorities who both interpret the patient's needs and beliefs and provide an insight into the current beliefs of that community (Fuller 1987). They also interpret the needs of the medical community to the patient, and are available for advice on health education and training of staff. The idea originated in the United States; but advocacy schemes now exist in the United Kingdom, for example, the Hackney Multi-Ethnic Women's Project. A report of this project (Cornwell and Gordon 1984) describes the distinction between advocates and interpreters:

> The argument for advocacy is based on the proposition that the relationship between patient and staff in medical settings is not equal, and that the inequality

in the relationship works to the patient's detriment. There is a need for advocates amongst all types of patient, but . . . the need is particularly acute for female patients and patients who do not speak English.

To the people involved in the Project the distinction between interpreting and advocacy is crucial. Both aim to improve communication between patients and staff, but other than that the two types of service have very little in common. Interpreting services tend to be set up where hospital staff find it difficult to communicate effectively with patients who do not speak English. The interpreter's role is to find out from the patient the answers to the staff's questions, and to relay to the patient the staff's wishes/directives.

Advocacy, however, is based on the idea that it is always difficult for patients to negotiate what happens to them in hospital on their own terms. The advocate's role (the exact reverse of the interpreter's role) is to find out from the staff the answers to the patient's questions and relay to the staff the patient's wishes.

The Asian Mother and Baby Campaign (DHSS 1985) employed 96 link workers in Birmingham, Blackburn, Bolton, Bradford, Brent, Dewsbury, Huddersfield, Leicester, Newham, South Bedfordshire, Walsall, Wandsworth, and Wolverhampton health authorities. The aim was to make antenatal services for Asian women more accessible and more acceptable by overcoming cultural and linguistic barriers. The link worker's function goes beyond that of an interpreter, and involves an element of advocacy—answering questions, explaining procedures and 'the systems', and raising issues with health professionals on the mother's behalf. Some District Health Authorities have now employed link workers on a permanent basis. Further information is available from the address given at the end of Chapter 10.

Most organizations find it extremely difficult to accept new roles, and this type of initiative is bound to encounter concern and unease from other health workers about encroachment into professional territory; it is also likely to expose undercurrents of racism (Mares 1986). The experience of existing schemes has shown that certain key elements are essential to help minimize the difficulties of introducing a new kind of worker into a well-established hierarchy, and to ensure the success of the project (Mares 1986):

- Community involvement.
- Independent management structure.
- Active support from, and immediate access to, senior managers.
- Recognizing the need to challenge racism.
- Emphasis on advocacy.
- Personal qualities of the workers.
- Training and support for the workers.
- Promoting and explaining the scheme to other health workers.
- Secure funding.

(e) Learning the client's language

This is the most difficult of all the options, and is not practical for general practitioners with small numbers of Asian patients, or with several diverse language-groups in their practices. It can be helpful, however, to learn a few basic phrases and key words in the commonest language(s) of your Asian patients, and this will often be perceived as a gesture of goodwill. Several Education Authorities now provide short courses for professionals working with linguistic minorities.

Other measures

Some health authorities, although they are still in the minority, provide training for staff on transcultural issues. Most Education Authorities run English as a Second Language (ESL) classes, but it may be difficult for Asian women, especially Muslims, to attend these. English for Pregnancy classes are held in several parts of the country. The common experience is that tuition has to start in the home; later, when the confidence of the women and their families has been gained, small community-based classes do succeed (Karseras and Hopkins 1987). Finally, recruitment of ethnic minority staff by Health Authorities and general practitioners can also make a contribution to improving the accessibility and acceptability of services. The use of written materials, videotapes, and the mass media to improve communication and health education are dealt with in Chapter 10.

Conclusion

Communication skills are the most basic of all clinical skills, and an essential part of a doctor's clinical expertise. Improving such skills will increase patients' compliance with advice and treatment, and also their satisfaction. The cross-cultural consultation poses challenges, but these can be met with tact, sensitivity, and some practical efforts on the part of the doctor. The potential for misunder-standing, which exists in any consultation, is enhanced when different cultures and languages are involved. However, critical awareness of the significance and culture-based nature of verbal and non-verbal aspects of communication, including paralinguistics, can go a long way towards avoiding such confusion. Where there is also a language barrier communication can be improved by reduc-ing stress, simplifying English, and checking back properly.

Moreover, using a qualified interpreter can be helpful, but requires skills on the part of the doctor. Recently interest has grown in developing advocacy schemes for particular individuals or groups of patients. This acknowledges the fact that by treating everyone equally a service may fail to cater for unequal needs, a point emphasized in a report by the Wandsworth Council for Community Relations (1978):

If cultural background, language problems, feelings of alienation or particular health problems create special needs or even isolate the Asian population from the health service, thereby placing them at risk, it is imperative that services be adapted to take account of these factors. This may necessitate the creation of separate facilities for part of the Asian community or special provisions directed largely if not exclusively at Asians. Providing the same service to all in the face of differing needs is not an equitable service.

Indeed, section 35 of the Race Relations Act 1976 makes allowance for the provision of such services or facilities to meet the special needs of ethnic minority groups in regard to their education, training, welfare, or need for ancillary benefits.

Perhaps the final word should rest with former Minister of Health, Mr Tony Newton (DHSS 1988):

> What is needed is a willingness to adapt. It is not necessarily a case of providing extra or special services but where appropriate of considering different ways of providing existing services. It is not a case of giving more favourable treatment—of positive discrimination—but of taking positive action to ensure that treatment is not *less* favourable. It is a question of redressing the balance.

References

Ahmed, G. and Watt, S. (1986). Understanding Asian women in pregnancy and confinement. *Midwives Chronicle and Nursing Notes*, **99**, 98–101.

Birdwhistell, R. L. (1970). *Kinetics and context.* University of Pennsylvia Press, Philadelphia.

Bochner, S. (1982). The social psychology of cross-cultural relations. In *Cultures in contact: studies in cross-cultural interaction*, (ed. S. Bochner) pp. 5–44. Pergamon Press, Oxford.

Brown, C. (1984). *Black and white Britain: the third PSI survey.* Heinemann Educational, London.

Cornwell, J. and Gordon, P. (eds) (1984). *An experiment in advocacy, the Hackney multiethnic women's project.* King's Fund Centre, London.

DHSS (Department of Health and Social Security) (1988). *Ethnic minority health. A report of a management seminar.* DHSS, London.

DHSS (Department of Health and Social Security) (1985). *Maternal and child health: the Asian mother and baby campaign*, CMO **(85)2**. DHSS, London.

Donaldson, L. J. and Odell, A. (1984). Planning and providing services for the Asian population: a survey of District Health Authorities. *Journal of the Royal Society of Health*, **104**, 199–202.

Ebden, P., Bhatt, A., Carey, O. J. and Harrison, B. (1988). The bilingual consulation. *Lancet*, **i**, 347.

Fuller, J. (1987). Contraceptive services for ethnic minorities. *British Medical Journal*, **295**, 1365.

Fuller, J. H. S. and Toon, P. D. *Medical practice in a multicultural society.* Heinemann Medical, Oxford.

Hampton, J. R., Harrison, M. J. E. and Mitchell, J. R. A. (1975). Relative contributions of history-taking, physical examination and laboratory investigation to diagnosis and management of medical out-patients. *British Medical Journal*, **2**, 486–9.

Henley, A. (1979). *Asian patients in hospital and at home*. King's Fund, London.

Henley, A. (1982). *Caring for Muslims and their families: religious aspects of care*. DHSS/King's Fund, London.

Hussain, M. F. and Gomersall, J. D. (1978). Affective disorders in Asian immigrants. *Psychiatrica Clinica*, **11**, 87–9.

Karseras, P. and Hopkins, E. (1987). *British Asians' health in the community*. Wiley, Chichester.

Learmonth, A. (1980). Asians' literacy in their mother tongue and English. *Nursing Times*, February 28, 27–28.

Ley, P. (1983). Patients' understanding and recall in clinical communication failure. In *Doctor-Patient Communication*, (ed. D. Pendleton and J. Hasler), pp. 89–107. Academic Press, London.

McAvoy, B. R. and Raza, R. (1988). Asian women: (ii) contraceptive services and cervical cytology. *Health Trends*, **20**, 14–17.

Mares, P. (1986). Improving communication. *Health and Race*, **4**, 1–5.

Mares, P., Henley, A., and Baxter, C. (1985). *Health care in multiracial Britain*. Health Education Council/National Extension College, Cambridge.

Owusu-Bempah, J. (1988). Cross-cultural communication problems: a racist ploy. *Racial Justice*, **8**, 3–12.

Preston-Whyte, M. E., Fraser, R. C., and Beckett, J. L. (1983). Effects of a principal's gender on consultation patterns. *Journal of the Royal College of General Practitioners*, **33**, 654–8.

Rack, P. (1982). *Race, culture and mental disorder*. Tavistock, London.

Sandler, G. (1979). Costs of unnecessary tests. *British Medical Journal*, **2**, 21–4.

Shackman, J. (1984). *The right to be understood*. National Extension College, Cambridge.

Smith, D. J. (1977). *The facts of racial disadvantage*. Penguin, Harmondsworth.

Stubbs, M. (ed.) (1985). *The other languages of England: Linguistic minorities project*. Routledge and Kegan Paul, London.

Wandsworth Council for Community Relations (1978). *Asians and the Health Service*. Wandsworth Council for Community Relations, London.

Zaklama, M. S. (1984). The Asian community in Leicester and the family planning services. *Biology and Society*, **1**, 63–9.

Zborowski, M. (1952). Cultural components in response to pain. *Journal of Social Issues*, **8**, 16–30.

Zola, I. K. (1966). Culture and symptoms—an analysis of patients' presenting complaints. *American Sociological Review*, **31**, 615–30.

6 Asians in Britain: the population and its characteristics

Liam Donaldson and Luise Parsons

Introduction

The first steps in the process of assessing the health needs of a population involve assembling information to describe: its size and growth; its structure (in terms of factors such as age, sex, social class, housing, and geographical distribution); and the pattern of mortality and morbidity within it.

Even these simple first elements of assessment are made difficult when addressing the Asian population in Britain, because of the absence of comprehensive and valid data on ethnicity within the information systems which are conventionally used to describe the general population in this way.

Epidemiological studies of the health of Asians are still relatively small in number, bearing in mind the length of time the communities have now been established in Britain and given the valuable opportunity which presented itself to study the disease experience of a population at various stages of adaptation to living in another culture.

This chapter seeks to draw attention to the sources and limitations of data on this population and, notwithstanding difficulties of interpretation, to provide a profile of the Asian population in Britain.

Population

Estimating the size of the ethnic minority populations

The two most widely-used sources of data about the Asian population are the decennial census and the Labour Force Survey. The national Census of Population, undertaken every ten years on behalf of the Government, is the most comprehensive source of statistics routinely collected on the total population of Britain. These statistics not only form the basis of many planning and policy decisions both at national and local level, but also describe the characteristics of our society and the changes which are taking place within it.

The decennial census of population

In every census since 1841, data have been collected on the place of birth of each resident. A question on nationality was introduced into the census in 1851, and remained in use for more than a century until its discontinuation after the

1961 census, when it was not well answered—nor particularly relevant, as many immigrants had British passports. For over a century, therefore, it has been possible to enumerate those born outside the United Kingdom. However, it had not been possible to count children of migrants until 1971, when a question was also included on parents' place of birth. Hitherto, given the relatively small number of immigrants to Britain, this did not cause particular problems; but it became important when there was large-scale immigration, beginning in the late 1950s, mainly from the Caribbean countries, East Africa, and the Indian subcontinent.

The inclusion of a question on parents' place of birth was helpful; but there were still difficulties even with this, because the place of birth of a person's parents is not a completely reliable guide to their ethnic origin. The Office of Population Censuses and Surveys (OPCS) has carried out some detailed analyses of the 1981 census, including cross-tabulations of ethnic origin (from the Labour Force Survey) and country of birth of the head of household. These showed that 90 per cent of people of New Commonwealth and Pakistan (NCWP) origin live in households where the head was born in the New Commonwealth or Pakistan, and, at the same time, 15 per cent of people in households with the head born in the NCWP are not of NCWP ethnic origin (OPCS 1982). In addition, about 35 per cent of the 1971 population of NCWP ethnic origin were born in the United Kingdom, and it was not long before some of these were old enough to have children of their own. For the 1984 Labour Force Survey further showed that 15 per cent of all non-white children aged 0–14 years had UK-born mothers.

In preparation for the 1981 census, the Office of Population Censuses and Surveys investigated the possibility of asking direct questions on a person's racial and ethnic origin. After careful field tests it was considered untimely to pursue the ethnic question in a survey where response is compulsory. In announcing this decision in Parliament, the Secretary of State for Social Services said that the Government would look to voluntary surveys such as the Labour Force Survey to provide statistics on the size and composition of ethnic minorities in future.

Labour Force Survey (LFS)

The first Labour Force Survey (LFS) was conducted in Britain in 1973. It was commissioned to comply with the European Economic Community policy of monitoring patterns of employment. It also supplies a considerable amount of information about the Labour Force in Britain, including data on ethnic composition.

The LFS is a continuous survey conducted throughout the year of a sample of approximately 1 in 350 of the households in Great Britain. It has the disadvantage of not providing complete coverage of the population, and the estimate of population by ethnic group is subject to a relatively high sampling error.

This is because many ethnic groups are largely concentrated in certain geographic areas and within households (the LFS is a survey of households). Nevertheless, it does ask direct questions about ethnic group as well as country of birth, and is carried out on a regular basis. Since 1983 this basis has been annual.

Conceptually, information from the LFS, in which people say what ethnic group they consider themselves to belong to, is quite different from information about the country of birth, which is all that was available in the 1970s; so some discontinuity between new and old estimates is unavoidable. (OPCS 1986a).

The LFS question on ethnic origin first used in 1979 was found to be defective, and a modified form of question has subsequently been introduced.

The question asks 'to which of the groups listed (on a card) do you consider you belong?' The categories listed are: White, West Indian or Guyanese, Indian, Pakistani, Bangladeshi, Chinese, African, Arab, Mixed Origin, and Others.

The LFS thus provides an estimate of the size of the Asian population nationally or in the larger conurbations. The LFS does not provide estimates of ethnic minority population size at health authority level.

Population size and structure

The estimated average size of the ethnic minority population of Great Britain during the period between 1984 and 1986 was around 2.4 million, or 4.5 per cent of the total population. Of these 1.3 million, or 2.4 per cent, were from the Indian subcontinent (India, Pakistan, Bangladesh). Details are shown in Table 6.1.

Table 6.1 *Estimated size of the population by ethnic group in Great Britain, average for the period 1984–86*

Ethnic group	Population (thousands)
White	51 107
Indian	760
Pakistani	397
Bangladeshi	103

Source: Shaw 1988a

Trends indicate that the ethnic minority population has doubled in size since 1971, and the increase since 1981 suggests that it is currently growing by between eighty and ninety thousand people a year (Fig. 6.1).

The largest single minority group is the population of Indian origin. Together, Asian (Indian, Pakistani, or Bangladeshi) groups are 51 per cent of the total ethnic minority population (Fig. 6.2).

The LFS also enables comparisons to be made between ethnic origin and

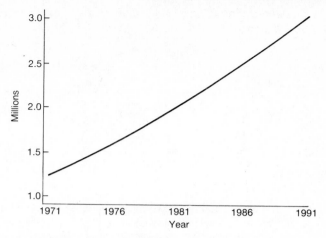

Fig. 6.1 Estimated and projected population of NCWP origin. Great Britain, 1971–1991.
Source: Adapted from LFS and OPCS 1986*b*.

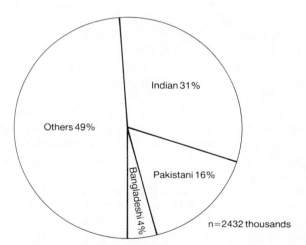

Fig. 6.2 Composition of ethnic minority population of Great Britain (1984–86 average).
Source: LFS 1984–86 from Shaw 1988*a*.

country of birth. Table 6.2 shows that approximately one-third of the Asian
population was born in the UK. This emphasizes the dangers of relying on
country of birth to estimate Britain's Asian population.

The distribution of the main Asian population in Britain is shown in Fig.
6.3, which shows that here Asian communities are far from homogeneous: for
example, the West Midlands Asian community has a majority of Indian people,

Table 6.2   *Country of birth of people belonging to different ethnic groups (per-centages), Great Britain 1984 – 86 average*

Ethnic group	Country of birth			All countries
	UK	NCWP	Rest of the world	
White	96	1	3	100
Indian	37	61	3	100
Pakistani	43	56	1	100
Bangladeshi	34	66	0	100

Source: Shaw 1988*a*

and the Bradford Asians are mainly Pakistani, while those living in Inner London districts such as Tower Hamlets show a relatively high proportion of Bangla-deshis.

The age-structure of the Asian population in 1985 is shown in Fig. 6.4, and illustrates that it is much younger than the indigenous white population. For example, nearly half the Pakistani and Bangladeshi population was under the age of sixteen, and 70 per cent were under thirty. In contrast, the elderly popula-tion was small. Only about 3 per cent had reached retirement age. The differing age-structures are largely a reflection of the pattern of immigration.

The LFS also analyses persons born overseas by country of birth and year of entry into the UK (Fig. 6.5), and indicates the different periods of settlement of the various overseas-born populations. Only 10 per cent of those persons born in the NCWP who stated their year of entry entered the UK before 1955, and most of these were white persons born in the Mediterranean Commonwealth or in India. The majority of people born in India and Pakistan entered the UK in the late 1960s and early 1970s. People born in Bangladesh were more recent entrants to the UK, and more than one-third first entered the UK during the 1980s, largely as children.

The problems of trying to plan without accurate data on the demography and distribution of different ethnic groups, together with growing acceptance of the importance of recording the size of the ethnic population, have emphasized the need for an ethnic question in the 1991 census. This issue is currently being investigated (HMSO 1988).

Birth and perinatal deaths

Limitations of data on birth registration

Most data on the fertility of the population are derived from birth registration, which also records the birthplace of the mother of the child. This provides information on the number of babies produced by Asian women, but only by

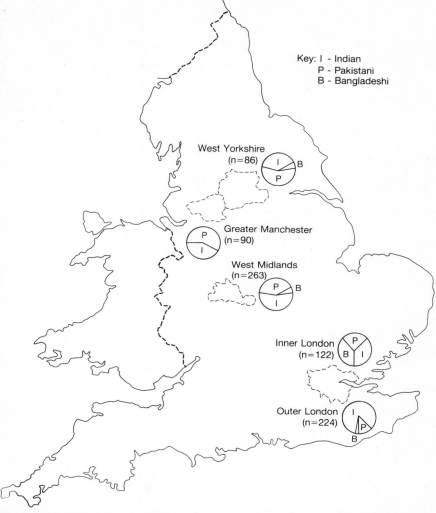

Fig. 6.3 Distribution of certain Asian communities in urban conurbations in England, 1985. Percentages within each category; total Asian populations (n) for each conurbation are in thousands. *Source:* Extracted from OPCS 1986c.

those born overseas. Also the number of births to women born in the Indian subcontinent will include some to women who were not of Asian origin. Since birth registration does not record ethnicity directly, the true fertility pattern of the ethnic minority population is not known with certainty, because of the growing proportion of mothers who have themselves been born in Britain.

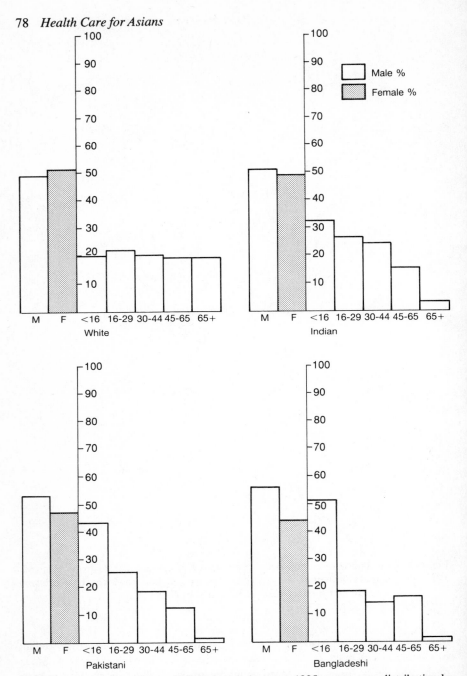

Fig. 6.4 Population of Great Britain by ethnic group 1985: percentage distribution by age-group, and proportion of males and females in each case. *Source:* Extracted from OPCS 1986*c*.

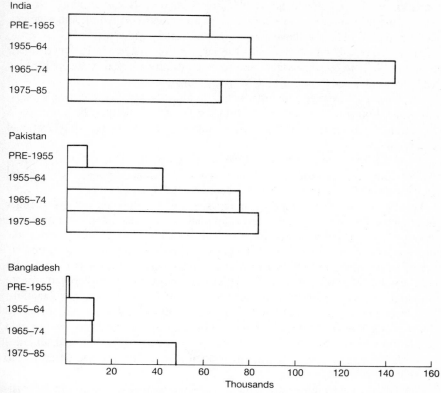

Fig. 6.5 Persons born outside the UK by year of entry and country of birth, Great Britain 1985. *Source:* Extracted from OPCS 1986c.

Trends in fertility

There were 28 991 births to mothers born in India, Pakistan, and Bangladesh in 1985, which represented 4.4 per cent of the total number of births. It has been estimated that the number of births to UK-born Indian, Pakistani, or Bangladeshi women might have amounted to approximately 3000 per year in Great Britain during the period 1984 to 1986 (Shaw 1988b). This number will grow as greater numbers of Asian women in their late teens reach peak childbearing ages.

The General Fertility Rate (GFR) for Asian women in 1985 was 110 per 1000 women aged 15–44 years. This was considerably above the comparable figure of 60 for mothers born in the United Kingdom.

However, there is also variation in fertility within the Asian population: the GFR for women born in India was 100 per 1000, whilst mothers born in Pakistan and Bangladesh had a GFR of 210 (OPCS 1986d). This again illustrates the need to avoid generalizations about Asians based on the assumption that they are a homogeneous group. In addition, these estimates of GFR omit Asian women born in the UK, who may have a very different pattern of fertility.

Fertility rates of ethnic minority women who have lived in Britain all their lives are likely to be somewhere between the rates for women in the appropriate NCWP country and those for all UK-born women.

While religion may be a factor which will influence fertility in certain groups, for other groups the country of birth of the parents is likely to be a much less important determinant of fertility than factors such as social class or educational qualifications.

The GFR for Asian women in 1985 was not dissimilar to the peak GFR of 93 per 1000 women aged 15–44 years seen in the whole population of England and Wales in 1964, during a period of economic prosperity.

Fertility rates can fluctuate quite rapidly, and usually this reflects changes in society. For instance, low levels of natural increase of population were recorded during parts of the First and Second World Wars, and during the economic depression of the 1930s. High levels were recorded in the 'baby booms' which followed the Second World War and in the period of economic prosperity during the mid 1960s. The lowest levels of natural increase of population of the century, however, were recorded in the mid-1970s. A number of explanations have been put forward to account for the changes in fertility which have occurred since World War II. Three common interpretations of the trends are: widespread availability of modern contraceptive methods; levels of income and attitudes towards future prosperity; and more women of childbearing age going out to work.

The factors determining the fertility rate in Asians have not been comprehensively studied. However, it is known that the fertility of recent immigrants tends to be relatively high, but as immigrant communities have been in Britain longer, their fertility has tended to move closer to that of the indigenous population. It has been suggested that the initial higher rates reflect the pattern of fertility in the country of origin, and the fact that families are often reunited after a period of separation. For instance, the Caribbean-born population is relatively long-established in Britain, and their fertility pattern is now similar to that of UK-born women. However, Asian groups are much more recent arrivals, particularly women from Pakistan and Bangladesh, and their fertility levels remain much higher than those of the indigenous population.

Perinatal mortality

Since 1975, infant death records have been linked to their corresponding birth records, in order to obtain information on the social and biological aspects of a baby's family. Only a limited amount of information (some of which is confidential) relating to the parents of the deceased infant is obtainable from death registration; but a considerable amount of information is given at birth registration, including age of parents, number of legitimate children, occupation of parent (usually father), country of birth of parents, institution of birth, and whether the baby was a singleton or not.

Since 1980, this linkage has been over 90 per cent complete, and OPCS now publish tables of mortality statistics by social and biological factors. These have revealed the marked differences in Perinatal Mortality Rate (PNMR) by mother's country of birth, as shown for 1985 in Table 6.3. The PNMR of mothers born in the New Commonwealth and Pakistan is 50 per cent higher than that of those born in the UK, the greatest excess mortality (75 per cent) being seen in the babies born to mothers born in Pakistan. This worrying finding has been consistently observed since perinatal mortality statistics have been analysed by country of birth of mother.

Table 6.3 *Perinatal deaths—numbers and rates per 1000 total births: by country of birth of mother; 1985*

Place of birth of mother	Number	Rate
All	6463	9.8
United Kingdom	5493	9.5
Irish Republic	81	12.7
Australia, Canada, New Zealand	24	10.1
New Commonwealth and Pakistan	675	12.7
New Commonwealth		
Bangladesh	55	12.9
India	113	10.1
East Africa	77	10.8
Rest of Africa	49	13.5
Caribbean Commonwealth	72	14.7
Mediterranean Commonwealth	19	6.8
Remainder of New Commonwealth	43	7.9
Pakistan	247	17.9
Remainder of Europe	77	9.0
Not stated	22	144.7
Other	91	8.1

Source: OPCS 1985

Many of the extra deaths are accounted for by stillbirths and congenital malformations. Increased genetic defects associated with a high proportion of consanguineous marriages amongst Muslims have been suggested as a mechanism for the high rate of stillbirths and neonatal deaths, and this is a subject discussed by Young in Chapter 12 of this book.

Perhaps the single most important determinant of PNMR is birthweight. Low birthweight infants, weighing less than 2500 grams at birth, make up 6 per cent of total deliveries in the UK, but nevertheless account for 60 per cent of perinatal deaths. Approximately 11 per cent of babies born to Asian mothers are below 2500 grams in weight (OPCS 1988).

Concern about ethnic differences in birthweight and outcome grew with the immigrant population in the late 1960s and early 1970s. However, at that time, routine statistics were not available by mothers' country of birth. *Ad hoc* studies in centres such as Leicester, Birmingham, Hillingdon, and Bradford found that babies of Asian mothers were approximately 300 grams lighter than their Caucasian counterparts at term. The question was, did it matter?

OPCS record-linkage provided the opportunity to answer this question. Birthweight-specific mortality tables are now published routinely, and include analyses by mother's country of birth. The rates are based on small numbers in some of the cells, so interpretation must be cautious (Table 6.4).

The main observation is that Indian and Bengali babies tend to do slightly better at the lower birthweights (less than 2500 grams), and worse at the higher birthweights (more than 3000 grams), while Pakistani babies do consistently worse at all birthweights compared to babies born to mothers born in the UK. The 300 gram difference in mean birthweight alone does not seem to be significant once the birthweight-specific mortality rates are known.

Detailed local studies in areas with large Asian populations, such as the Leicestershire perinatal mortality study described by MacVicar in Chapter 11 of this book, have allowed the further elucidation and exploration of risk factors for perinatal death in the Asian community.

Patterns of disease

Studies of disease in Asians

There are records of Asians living in Britain for over five hundred years, yet the first collection of papers on medical aspects of immigration did not appear until 1966. Since then, there have been a number of different approaches to describing the pattern of disease in Asians.

Until the Second World War, the majority of Asians in Britain were sailors

Table 6.4 *Perinatal mortality rates by birthweight and mother's country of birth, 1986. England and Wales*

Mother's country of birth	Birthweight (grams)									
	All weights	Under 2500	Under 1500	1500–1999	2000–2499	2500–2999	3000–3499	3500–3999	4000– and over	Not stated
Numbers										
All	6388	4141	2487	799	855	798	748	367	162	122
United Kingdom	5469	3590	2174	681	735	668	642	321	140	180
India	113	74	45	13	16	22	11	3	2	1
Bangladesh	46	24	11	7	6	4	8	7	1	2
Pakistan	231	145	88	21	36	36	32	12	3	3
Rates										
All	9.5	86.4	345.5	85.0	27.3	6.6	3.0	2.0	2.7	187.1
United Kingdom	9.4	88.3	351.2	84.3	27.9	6.6	2.9	1.9	2.6	219.5
India	10.5	59.2	340.9	64.4	17.4	6.7	2.6	1.8	6.3	111.1
Bangladesh	9.7	47.1	289.5	92.1	15.2	2.6	4.4	9.7	6.4	117.6
Pakistan	16.9	105.4	417.1	91.7	38.5	10.4	5.9	4.5	4.2	333.3

Source: OPCS 1988

or residents of seaport towns such as Cardiff, Liverpool, and South Shields. This may account for the emphasis in early studies on exotic diseases, the import-ation of illness, and the prevention of the spread of infectious disease to the host population. Such 'port medicine' continued to dominate ideas about Asian health care through the peak of immigration in 1962 and the parallel expansion of the National Health Service, which did little else to adapt to different ethnic groups.

Another medical focus of interest in relation to the Asian community has been called 'eugenic'. Biology, genetics, and heredity clearly do have a place in medicine for a multi-ethnic community. Certain haemoglobinopathies, such as sickle-cell disease and thalassaemia, have been extensively studied, and are of great concern to the communities at risk and to their medical practitioners. This is a theme taken up by Young in Chapter 12 of this book.

During the late 1960s and 1970s, concern was expressed about nutritional deficiency diseases, particularly rickets. This led to demands for health education against 'faulty' cultural and dietetic practices, which developed into a campaign described by one sociologist as verging on 'moral panic'.

Published research work dealing with the health of Asians has tended to reflect these different areas of clinical concern through which the medical profession in Britain has perceived the main health problems of the Asian community. Thus, the majority of research reports have dealt with: the incidence of tuberculosis, its prevention and control; problems of pregnancy and infancy; nutritional-deficiency disorders, particularly rickets; and mental illness. Studies of chronic disease such as heart disease, stroke, and diabetes have begun to emerge, and some of these are covered by Sturman and Beevers in Chapter 9 of this book.

Presently, there is an interest in appropriate health-care provision, but with an emphasis on the effects of differential provision and need. The relationship between use of general practitioners and social class is well documented, and this factor needs to be taken into account, along with income and need, in studies which find higher usage of the services by ethnic minorities. When these are taken into account, Asian patients seem to be rather more like white working-class patients in their use of the NHS, except in their use of emergency night calls and hospital out-patient services (lower) and child health and vaccination clinics (probably higher). More studies are required that seek to examine patterns of accessibility, treatment, outcome, and acceptability of the service to patients of different ethnic origins.

Much research work in this field still falls into the category of descriptive epidemiology, from which the research workers concerned have drawn inferences about aetiology to a greater or lesser extent. When causal inferences are drawn, they are usually attributed to ethnicity directly. There is a marked paucity of formal epidemiological studies of the disease-experience of the Asian community, in which ethnic origin can be distinguished from other variables, such as social class, when exploring disease associations.

Deaths

Death registration also provides data on country of birth. In 1985, 8033 (1.3 per cent) of the 590 734 deaths which occurred in England and Wales were recorded amongst people who had been born in the NCWP. This again reflects the young age-structure of the Asian population.

A first stage in examining the disease-experience from an epidemiological viewpoint is to examine the distribution of causes of death, and make comparisons.

In 1984, the first major Immigrant Mortality Study in England and Wales was published (Marmot *et al.* 1984). The mortality rates for most immigrant groups were lower than those of their countries of birth, possibly indicating that healthier than average individuals 'selected' themselves for immigration.

In addition, a detailed analysis for the years 1975–7 confirmed the findings of the Immigrant Mortality Study, and provided further insight into mortality differences. Observed mortality was higher than expected for Asians, owing to infective and parasitic diseases, diseases of the endocrine system (particularly diabetes mellitus), diseases of the circulatory system (particularly coronary heart disease and stroke in men), and some diseases of the digestive system. Fewer than expected deaths were due to cancer (notably lung cancer) and chronic bronchitis (Balarajan *et al.* 1984).

Bhopal (1988) has argued that too great an emphasis has been placed upon comparing differences between the Asian and the non-Asian population in terms of mortality experience, pointing out that the similarities are much greater than the differences. Table 6.5 shows the common causes of death for the two populations, and indicates that causes of death are broadly similar.

Morbidity

Routinely available morbidity data within the health service, which collect information on morbidity or illness, are relatively limited, as there is no systematic recording of data by ethnic group.

Reports based on health-service information systems which have examined the pattern of morbidity in Asians have usually assigned ethnic group to records as a special exercise.

A comparison of morbidity amongst Asians and non-Asians based on hospital discharge data showed apparent differences in disease pattern (Fig. 6.6). Conclusions from such data should be cautiously drawn, because of the previously referred-to difficulty of comparing data, and because of potential selection of hospital admissions. However, if this is the explanation for any of the differences found in the study shown in Fig. 6.6, then there would have to have been a greater likelihood of being admitted to hospital for one ethnic group compared to the others.

A similar exercise conducted on cancer registration data showed an apparently

Table 6.5   *Ten commonest causes of death in* Asian *and* non-Asian *men*

Indian subcontinent *Asian* men in England and Wales 1970–72 (20 and over)		All men in England and Wales 1971	
Cause of death	Number of deaths	Cause of death	Number of deaths
Ischaemic heart disease	1533	Ischaemic heart disease	77 521
Cerebrovascular accident	438	Cerebrovascular accident	29 005
Bronchitis, emphysema, and asthma	123	Carcinoma of the lung	23 891
Carcinoma of the lung and bronchus and trachea	218	Bronchitis and emphysema	19 242
Pneumonia	214	Pneumonia	16 477
Motor-vehicle accidents	134	Carcinoma of the stomach	6733
Arterial disease	101	Motor-vehicle accidents	4489
Hypertensive heart disease	85	All other (non-motor-vehicle) accidents	4915
Leukaemia and other neoplasms of lymphatic and haema-topoietic system	74	Hypertensive heart disease	3795
Suicide	69	Diabetes	2906

Source: Bhopal 1988

increased incidence of cancer compared to that expected at certain sites (tongue, oral cavity, pharynx, oesophagus) for Asians compared to non-Asians (Fig. 6.7). For most sites, though, there were fewer Asian cases than would be expected. The statistical methodology in this study was complex, once again because of the absence of valid data on the age- and sex-distribution of the Asian population, and the resulting difficulty in constructing denominators for rates.

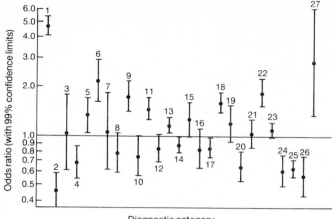

Fig. 6.6 Pattern of hospital morbidity for Asians compared to non-Asians in Leicester-shire. Diagnostic categories where the plot and the confidence limits lie above or below the horizontal line denote a significant excess (or deficit) of Asian cases in that category. Ratio of odds (with 99% confidence limits) of Asians being discharged from hospital in a particular diagnostic category compared with non-Asians. 1 Infective and parasitic diseases (ICD No 000–136), 2 all malignant neoplasms (140–199), 3 neoplasms of lymphatic and haematopoietic tissues (200–209), 4 benign neoplasms and neoplasms of unspecified nature (210–239), 5 endocrine, nutritional and metabolic diseases (240–279), 6 diseases of blood and blood forming organs (280–289), 7 mental disorders (290–315), 8 diseases of nervous system (320–358), 9 diseases of the eye (360–379), 10 diseases of the ear and mastoid process (380–389); 11 rheumatic fever, hypertensive disease, and heart disease (390–429), 12 diseases of peripheral circulatory system (430–458), 13 diseases of respiratory system (460–519), 14 diseases of digestive system (520–577), 15 diseases of urinary system (580–599), 16 male genital disorders (600–607), 17 diseases of breast and female genital system (610–629), 18 conditions of pregnancy, childbirth, and puerperium (630–678, Y60–Y61), 19 diseases of skin and subcutaneous tissue (680–709), 20 diseases of musculoskeletal system and connective tissue (710–738), 21 congenital anomalies (740–759), 22 certain causes of perinatal morbidity (760–779), 23 symptoms and ill-defined conditions (780–796), 24 fractures, dislocations, and sprains (800–848), 25 other injuries and reactions (850–999), 26 people undergoing preventive procedures (Y40–43, Y45, Y50, Y52, Y62–79), and 27 unclassified.
Source: Donaldson and Taylor 1983.

Conclusion

Asian communities now make up a significant minority of the population in Britain, particularly in certain conurbations. The age-structure reflects a high birth-rate, and the wave of immigration that occurred in the 1960s and early 1970s. The disproportionately large number of young people in the Asian population, particularly women in their child-bearing years, means that these communities will continue to grow for some time despite restrictions on immigration.

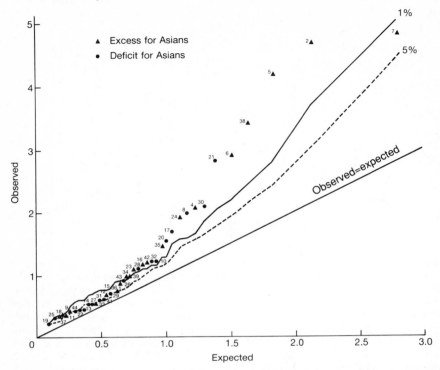

Fig. 6.7 Comparisons of cancer incidence at different sites: Asians compared to non-Asians in Leicestershire. Plots show sites where there was an excess of Asian cases or a deficit of Asian cases (where plots fall above the 1% or 5% lines this denotes statistical significance at these levels). Contributions of each cancer site to the overall chi-squared test, with simulation envelopes for 1% and 5% levels of significance log units.

Site of cancer: 1 Lip, 2 tongue, 3 salivary glands, 4 gum, floor of mouth, other mouth, 5 oro-, naso-, hypopharynx, 6 other oral cavity, 7 oesophagus, 8 stomach, 9 small intestine, 10 colon, rectum, 11 liver, bile ducts, gallbladder, extrahepatic bile ducts, 12 pancreas, 13 peritoneum, 14 other and ill-defined (digestive organs, and peritoneum), 15 nasal cavities, etc, 16 larynx, 17 trachea, bronchus, lung, 18 pleura, thymus, heart, 19 bone and cartilage, connective tissue, 20 malignant melanoma, 21 other skin, 22 breast, 23 uterus unspecified, 24 cervix, 25 placenta, 26 body of uterus, 27 ovary and tubes, 28 other female genital, 29 prostate, 30 testis, 31 penis and other male genital, 32 bladder, kidney, ureter, 33 eye, 34 brain, other nervous system, 35 thyroid, 36 other endocrine, 37 other ill defined sites, 38 lymph nodes, other and unspecified, 39 secondary of respiratory and digestive system and other site, unspecified site, 40 lymphosarcoma and reticulosarcoma, 41 Hodgkin's disease, 42 other lymphoid, 43 multiple myeloma, and 44 leukaemia.

Source: Donaldson and Clayton 1984.

The youthful nature of the population, a legacy of disease from under-developed countries, and poor socio-economic status in Britain all contribute to a pattern of disease that has some important differences from that of the host community. This pattern of disease may change as the Asian population ages and adapts to the lifestyle of the host community. It is important to understand these factors if we are to improve the delivery of health care and plan appropriate services for an often deprived section of society.

References

Balarajan, R., Bulusu, L., Adelstein, A. M., and Shukla, V. (1984). Patterns of mortality among migrants to England and Wales from the Indian subcontinent. *British Medical Journal*, **289**, 1185–7.

Bhopal, R. S. (1988). Health care for Asians: conflict in need, demand and provision. In *Equity: a prerequisite for health*, proceedings of the 1987 Summer Scientific Conference, pp. 52–5. Faculty of Community Medicine and WHO, London.

Donaldson, L. J. and Clayton, D. G. (1984). Occurrence of cancer in Asians and non-Asians. *Journal of Epidemiology and Community Health*, **38**, 203–7.

Donaldson, L. J. and Taylor, J. B. (1983). Patterns of Asian and non-Asian morbidity in hospitals. *British Medical Journal*, **286**, 949–51.

HMSO (1988). 1991 Census of Population. White paper presented to Parliament by the Secretary of State for Social Services and the Secretary of State of Scotland by Command of Her Majesty, July 1988. **430**, HMSO London.

Marmot, M. G., Adelstein, A. M., and Bulusu, L. (1984). *Immigrant mortality in England and Wales 1970–78*, OPCS Studies on Medical and Population Subjects, **No. 47**. HMSO, London.

OPCS (Office of Population Censuses and Surveys) (1982). Sources of statistics on ethnic minorities. (Editorial) *Population Trends*, **28**, 1–8. HMSO, London.

OPCS (1985). *Mortality statistics: biological and social factors*, Series DH3 **No. 18**. HMSO, London.

OPCS (1986*a*). Estimating the size of ethnic minority populations in the 1980s. Population Statistics Division, OPCS. *Population Trends*, **44**, 22–27.

OPCS (1986*b*). Ethnic minority populations in Great Britain. *Population Trends*, **46**, 18–21.

OPCS (1986*c*). Labour Force Survey 1985: ethnic group and country of birth. *OPCS Monitor*, LFS 86/2 and PP1 86/3. HMSO, London.

OPCS (1986*d*). FMI. No. 12. Birth statistics, 1985. HMSO, London.

OPCS (1988). Infant and perinatal mortality 1986: Birthweight. *OPCS Monitor*, DH3 88/1. HMSO, London.

Shaw, C. (1988*a*). Latest estimates of ethnic minority populations. *Population Trends*, **51**, 5–8. HMSO, London.

Shaw, C. (1988*b*) Components of growth in the ethnic minority population. *Population Trends*, **52**, 27–31. HMSO, London.

Clinical aspects

Clinical reports

7 Alternative/complementary medicine

Bashir Qureshi

Introduction

The aim of this chapter is to inform the service general practitioner and other health professionals about: why an Asian patient may have great faith in alternative medicine; whom he is likely to consult; what effect an alternative therapy may have on some drugs—interaction, counteraction, or potentiation caused by alternative therapies; and what a doctor can do when caring for such a patient.

An overview of alternative medical therapies is presented, describing their principles and practices, along with the patient's perceptions, and approaches to them which might be adopted by the NHS doctor. The underlying goal is recognition of the need for greater mutual understanding and tolerance of differing beliefs and perspectives. If this can be achieved then western and traditional approaches to health and disease can be truly complementary, and the western doctor and his Asian patient can have a harmonious relationship.

Historical perspective

The art of healing was continually practised by the founders of all six major religions of the world: Hinduism (The Vedas—2000 BC), Judaism (Moses—586 BC), Buddhism (Buddha—563 to 483 BC), Christianity (Jesus—AD 0 to AD 33), Islam (Muhammad—AD 570 to 632), and Sikhism (Nanak—AD 1469 to 1539). Religion has played a healing role throughout human history.

Religion deals in subjectivity and intuition, whereas science is concerned with objectivity and reason. It should be remembered that they complement each other in the real lives of the vast majority of our patients.

Medical history testifies that the first surgeon in the world was Sasruta, 500 BC, a Hindu from India (Wijesinha 1985); and the first physician was Imhotep, 2800 BC, an Egyptian (Anon. 1978). Modern medicine—allopathy—was founded by Hippocrates (460–377 BC), a Greek physician, and it was strengthened by Galen (AD 130–200), a Graeco-Roman physician. Medicine has thus been advanced from the beginning by both the East and the West.

'Homoeopathy' was introduced by the German doctor, Samuel Hahnemann (1755–1843). Indian Hindu medicine ('*Ayurveda*') dates back to 2000 BC, and Muslim medicine ('*Hikmat*') originated in India, under the Mogul ruler Baber (1483–1530). *Ayurveda* is still more popular among Hindus, whereas *Hikmat* is used more often by Muslims. Allopathy and homoeopathy are equally used by both.

Asian practitioners—*hakims* and *vaids*—number close on 300 in Britain; they mainly serve Asian patients, but some Europeans also attend their clinics (Bourne 1985).

It is true that Asians as well as Europeans have developed their own orthodox systems of medicine, and are proud of their history. Nevertheless, both sections of the British community—ethnic majority and minority—do not hesitate to use alternative medicine, while enjoying the benefits of allopathic medicine. This fact should be clearly understood by the service GP: that Asian patients will often consult alternative practitioners, by preference homoeopath, *hakim*, or *vaid* in the UK; and it is not uncommon for them to obtain their remedies simply by postal consultations.

Why choose alternative medicine?

When faced with a doctor from a western culture, the average Asian patient who is not sufficiently westernized experiences a cultural barrier in both verbal and non-verbal communication. For example, an Asian woman is unused to being touched by a male doctor; nor is an Asian man accustomed to being examined by a female doctor. Such basic cultural inhibitions pose a real dilemma, and are in part the reason why some Asian patients will turn to a familiar alternative medicine practitioner. In the hands of a British doctor who tries to understand their culture and religions, they will however feel confident: Asian people like to have faith in British medicine, and given a sympathetic and understanding approach will be only too pleased to consult a western doctor.

Another reason why patients may turn to a traditional healer has to do with the differences in the lay and medical concepts of illness which are embodied in the western approach to medicine. A doctor trained in the 'bio-medical' model, even if this is broadened to encompass the physical, psychological, and social aspects of illness, may not be capable of taking account of culture, religion, and ethnicity in an appropriate way when assessing and meeting his patients' needs.

In emergencies, especially surgical, Asian patients will tolerate an unsatisfactory relationship with their doctor; but in the treatment of chronic physical and emotional problems, lack of immediate relief or care may lead to the use of alternative health-care providers. Lack of communication and understanding between patient and doctor may make this more likely.

Asian patients are particularly likely to consult alternative health workers when suffering from:

(a) anxiety states and depression;
(b) pain;

(c) allergies, for example, food allergies;
(d) chronic conditions, such as arthritis, multiple sclerosis, anaemia, asthma, hay fever, and eczema;
(e) psychosexual problems, such as impotence; and
(f) terminal illness.

Alternative therapies

Asian patients in the United Kingdom are likely to have access to and consider any of the twenty alternative therapies which are commonly available to their communities: aromatherapy, astrotherapy, Ayurvedic medicine, dream guidance, faith-healing, food therapy or health foods, folklore remedies, herbal medicine, *Hikmat*, homoeopathy, magic, music therapy, osteopathy and massage therapy, over-the-counter medicine and tonics, palmistry, religious rituals, spa therapy, transcendental meditation, urinotherapy, and yoga.

Religion governs the lives of orthodox Asians. Muslims are likely to consult a *hakim* and Hindus as well as Sikhs may go to a *vaid*, but Buddhists (and some Hindus) may prefer transcendental meditation or yoga. Nevertheless, almost all Asians have confidence in homoeopathy. These five alternative therapies are more commonly used at present than the other fifteen.

Acupuncture, acupressure, the Alexander technique, applied kinesiology, art therapy, autogenic training, Bach flower remedies, biofeedback, biomagnetism, chiropractice, hypnotherapy, Kirlian photography, metamorphic technique, reflexology, and zone therapy, although increasingly popular alternative therapies among the indigenous population, are not yet widely used by ethnic Asians.

Aromatherapy

Theory

Incense, aromatic herbs, perfumes, and oils have been frequently used by Asians since ancient times. Incense such as joss-sticks (*agarbati*) is burnt by Hindus. Saffron (an aromatic herb) is burnt for its smoke by Muslims. The scented smoke is meant to mask any unpleasant smell, and is believed to have antiseptic properties. A similar approach was adapted during the Industrial Revolution in nineteenth-century Britain, particularly at times of epidemics such as cholera. Popular perfumes are 'rose' and 'jasmine' extracts. The scented water is used as an air freshener. *Sarsoon* (or mustard) oil—which has a strong smell—is used as a cleansing agent prior to having a bath, as a protective suntan oil, as a hair cream, and in the treatment of dry skin and mild eczema.

Saand oil—an extract from the testes of a bull—is applied locally by some middle-aged men for the treatment of impotence. Its smell and massage, along with self-reassurance, is said to restore the erection.

Practice

Scented smoke is used in almost all Asian religious rituals, and scented water is often sprayed, during a sermon, on the audience, who may have to sit for many hours. Some Asians may use these at home to welcome a British doctor making a home visit. Sesame oil is used locally as a panacea for skin ailments, but its strong smell may be off-putting for Europeans, and can cause problems in waiting rooms.

In the Indian subcontinent, *saand* oil is traditionally sold by Pathan travelling salesmen, who put up their stalls on a footpath in a busy street to attract the attention of passers-by. These substances can be purchased over the counter from many Asian corner shops, and, in order to provide the best quality, they are often imported. Talking about sex is taboo in Asian culture; and therefore a customer may be directed to go elsewhere to obtain *saand* oil.

Asian perceptions

An Asian patient who asks his GP for some oil to rub on a bruise, rash, or painful joint, is likely not to receive prescribed medication on the grounds that such an approach will be thought by the practitioner to have no therapeutic basis. Similarly, an Asian man, anxious about his failure to achieve an erection, or about premature ejaculation, may ask for an injection or a local treatment with some oil; but the approach taken by his doctor may be based on reassurance or counselling.

These differing expectations, together with the resulting heightened anxiety on the patient's part, may lead him to turn to alternative medicine and consult an Asian aromatherapist.

Doctor's approach

A GP will do well to realize that he or she is dealing with a patient from a different culture with different beliefs, behaviour, and expectations.

An NHS doctor should arrange for some social education and counselling, perhaps involving other members of the primary-care team, to enable patients and the doctor to communicate on the same wavelength. Negotiation is often necessary. For example, olive oil could be suggested instead of sesame oil, on the understanding that if it is not successful in improving a patch of mild eczema, the patient returns for further advice.

Astrotherapy

Theory

Astrology is based on the belief that a person's character, destiny, and fate in everyday life is influenced by the position of the stars and planets, not only at the time of birth but also during life. Professional astrologers devise birth charts showing the precise position of the planets in the zodiac at the time of birth, so as to understand a person and foretell his or her future.

Practice

As with the Chinese and the Druids, some south Asians, especially Hindus, have great faith in astrology. Hindus use this knowledge in giving a name to a newborn baby and in choosing a date for a marriage. During an illness, especially with psychological problems, many Hindu and Sikh patients consult an astrotherapist, who often practises near a temple. Muslims do not believe in the stars, but may attribute the cure of any illness to the will of Allah. An astrotherapist builds up his clients' self-confidence by telling the good fortune first, thereby raising hopes as well as motivation. Later he imparts less desirable features, and prepares the client to face these possibilities by working through his problems. This 'anticipatory learning' is compatible with the concepts of Carl Jung and, to some extent, Sigmund Freud. Such a counselling technique is based on a sound scientific principle.

Asian perceptions

An Asian may religiously believe in God's will in healing, and that a doctor is a medium through whom God exercises his healing powers. An astrotherapist reinforces this ancient fatalistic conviction, and provides such a client with a listening ear, a caring attitude, and sympathetic counselling. Often, a Hindu patient will not tell his GP about this consultation, in order to avoid any awkward confrontation.

Doctor's approach

A British doctor should understand the religious and psycho-therapeutic value of his or her patient's belief in astrotherapy. Through respecting the patient's faith and through persistent counselling, a doctor can achieve good rapport, and expect compliance with his own therapy from his Asian patient. The gap may not be so wide as was first thought at the beginning of the cross-cultural consultation. The belief of Muslims in the will of Allah can be used by the doctor with therapeutic benefit: for example, in helping terminally ill patients and their relatives to come to terms with their condition.

Ayurvedic medicine

Theory

This ancient Hindu system of medicine is derived from the Vedas, the holy books written in Sanskrit dating back to 2000 BC. *'Ayur'* means life, and *'Veda'* stands for science. It is a philosophy of prolonging life, and the science of preventing and treating disease.

Three energies known as *doshas—Vata, Pitta*, and *Kapha*—are believed to have originated from five elements: *Vata* from space and air; *Pitta* from fire; and *Kapha* from water and earth. Any imbalance of these energies in the body can precipitate illness. *Kapha*-dominated people are prone to diseases of the musculo-skeletal system. *Pitta*-dominated people tend to get gastro-intestinal disorders. Those who are *Vata*-dominated can get respiratory and neurological conditions. *Ayurveda* is very akin to the humoral theory of the ancient Greeks.

Practice

A *vaid* (practitioner) often prescribes for local use: nasal oils, blood-letting, oil massage, manipulation; and for systemic: medicinal herbs, heavy metals (for example gold leaf), and special diets. Ayurvedic theory accepts the very powerful role of the mind in the cause and cure of a disease, and the *vaid* uses the power of suggestion. The Ayurvedic pharmacopoeia contains 3000 plants, of which 500 are used either simply or in concoctions and syrup compounds. The Indian and Sri Lankan Governments sponsor Ayurvedic medical schools (running five-year courses), and the World Health Organisation recognized *Ayurveda* in 1980. Although there are as many as 160 000 Ayurvedic practitioners in India, in Britain there are only a few qualified *vaids*. *Ayurveda* cannot be used to treat emergencies, and no longer includes surgery. It is said to deal with all ailments; but it is in chronic diseases—rheumatic and orthopaedic conditions, jaundice, gut disorders, and terminal illness—that it is claimed to be more successful.

Asian perceptions

Hindu patients have great faith in this system, and it is naive to think that they will abandon it because they now live in the UK. Contrary to common belief, any duress in fact strengthens a religious conviction. An Asian is invariably accustomed to expect fast cures from Western medicine, but will also happily accept the unhurried approach of Eastern therapies. Indeed, such a patient may use both systems of medicine, and sometimes even both concurrently.

Doctor's approach

A GP may encounter three problems: firstly, an Asian patient may not comply with the prescribed medical treatment, because an Ayurvedic practitioner, like other alternative practitioners, usually advises the avoidance of synthetic drugs. He rather involves the patient and his or her family in the preparation of a remedy. However, some patients may use both therapies, and may experience side-effects due to interaction, counteraction, or potentiation. Secondly, Ayurvedic remedies may appear bizarre to Western eyes. For instance, the treatment for asthma is: ghee in increasing doses with a strict vegetarian diet; sudation in a sauna bath on the seventh day; emetics on the ninth day, until the patient has vomited seven times; and a special diet for several weeks (Glynn and Heyman 1985).

Finally, there may be some cases of acute, sub-acute, and chronic poisoning or allergic dermatitis from the medicinal herbs and heavy-metal compounds used in Ayurvedic remedies. These can be diagnosed by taking a detailed and frank history, followed by a thorough examination.

Dream guidance

Theory

Freud (1865–1939) developed the method of interpretation of dreams and free association which is still a basic technique of psychoanalysis. In the East, the interpretation of dreams in foretelling the future and the prognosis of disease is a centuries-old custom.

Practice

As psychiatry has always been considered taboo in Asian culture this work was taken over by faith-healers or religious teachers. It is not uncommon for an Asian to consult an ancient book for dream interpretation, or see an expert at his customary place of worship, especially if he or she has had a nightmare. The expert will invariably reassure the patient: for example, by saying that the death of a loved one in a dream in fact means an extension of life, its opposite.

Asian perceptions

A Muslim may consult an Imam in a mosque, a Hindu may seek the advice of a Pandit in a temple, and a Sikh may turn to his Guru in a *gurdwara*.

Doctor's approach

It is reasonable for a GP to explain that foretelling the future or prognosis from dreams does not feature in modern medical thinking. Such a frank explanation will be accepted by the Asian patient, who may still consult a traditional healer for interpretation or reassurance concerning dreams. The Western doctor should be tolerant of this aspect of this patient's need.

Faith-healing (spiritual medicine)

Theory

Faith-healing means healing by prayer, religious faith, and suggestion, without using medical skills. For example, there is a Christian belief, based on James, Chapter 5, verse 15, that sickness is a spiritual disorder, and may be cured without medical appliances or advice if the prayer is accompanied in the sufferer by true faith using the power of the mind:

> And the prayer of faith shall save the sick man: and the Lord shall raise him up.

There are three doctrines: firstly that of 'reincarnation', held in Hinduism, Buddhism, Sikhism, and Jainism—Indian-originated religions: that after death the soul continues to live on in another body, of a human or an animal, on earth, and this cycle can only be broken when a person has reached spiritual perfection or Nirvana, so that failure of any treatment indicates the effect of sins in an earlier life. Secondly, the 'resurrection' doctrine, adhered to by Jews, Christians, and Muslims: that the souls of all men and women will rise from the dead on the Day of Judgement, and that some souls, after being made perfect, will be reunited with their bodies on the way to Heaven; whereas others with dreadful sins, after this reunion, will be sent to hell. Muslims believe that any cure is only granted by the will of Allah, and that suffering during an illness could go some way to perfecting the soul, and that a martyr earns eternal life and is guaranteed the bliss of Heaven with God. Finally, there is the 'spiritual' theory accepted by clairvoyants: that a body has three components—the physical, the lower etheric, and the soul (higher etheric)—and that a disease is caused by disharmony between these three components; and that a clairvoyant can see the lower etheric component as an aura or halo a few inches from the physical body. The colours of the aura indicate the physical, mental, and psychic health of a person.

Practice

Asians in the UK belong mainly to the Hindu, Muslim, Sikh, Buddhist, and Catholic religions. Faith-healing differs from religion-therapy in that the former is practised by faith-healers, but the latter by religious priests. A faith-healer actually performs major rituals such as exorcisms; whereas a religion-therapist carries out only ceremonial rituals, such as baptisms or giving charms (see later); but both play important roles in the prevention and treatment of disease, especially chronic and psychiatric problems, encountered among Asian patients. Exorcisms are commonly performed in psychiatric conditions to chase out the devil. They can sometimes be quite alarming, as the faith-healer may severely beat the patient in order to drive the evil influence out of the body.

Asian perceptions

Asians consult a faith-healer as a last resort. The treatment is based on ritual, varying from suggestion to a kind of psychotherapy, and from desensitization to flooding. An Asian may consult a faith-healer for three conditions—evil eye (phobia), *latah* (hysteria), and the possession syndrome (obsession). Very rarely, stimulatory drugs can be used by these healers, who are called *fakirs* or *saeen babas*.

Although faith-healing is based on religious doctrines, priests do not support faith-healers, and are more in favour of medical or other drug-orientated therapies.

Doctor's approach

Some cases of schizophrenia or personality disorders can be missed or remain untreated. A GP whose patient (or his family) will not permit treatment should keep such a patient under surveillance, and monitor the progress of the faith-healing. Where medical intervention is considered necessary, a doctor should approach the appropriate religious priest—a Pandit, Guru, Imam, or Holy Father—who can override the patient's choice of using a faith-healer by persuading his or her family to use medical or even psychiatric treatment. Asians often live in close-knit families, and, contrary to the English custom, the interest of the family takes precedence over the choice of the individual. This authority can be used by a caring family doctor in pursuing the correct management of an illness.

Food-therapy (health foods)

Theory

Health foods are thought to have health-giving qualities—for example, natural unprocessed foods that are grown and prepared without artificial fertilizers or chemical additives. In addition to their nutritional value they are useful in the treatment of constipation, which is a common problem for those eating a mainly British diet. They are not so popular among Asians, who usually eat Indian food, with spices and a high fibre content. Nevertheless, Asians are very fond of using food, or the avoidance of certain foods, during a particular illness as a therapy. This is a cultural tradition.

Practice

An Asian food-therapist will recommend a wide range of remedies based upon alterations to the diet of his patient. For example, honey licked from a finger during acute tonsillitis is considered to have a local action of forming a protective coating on the tonsils (just as a dressing protects a wound). Yoghurt is perceived as a soothing agent, relieving irritation of surfaces, especially the mucous membranes; and for this demulcent action it is taken on an empty stomach for the treatment of gastro-enteritis, and can be eaten with every meal to prevent curry gastritis. Garlic is used freely, as it contains essential oils with antibacterial, antifungal, and antithrombotic effects; these effects are now thought to be due to diallyl disulphide and methyl allyl trisulphide (Beely 1986). Sesame seeds (*sesamum indicum*), known as 'mustard', are taken orally for the treatment of whooping cough. Some foods are avoided: for example, milk during a cough and red or green chillies in gut disorders are forbidden.

Asian perceptions

Despite strong external influences, Asian culture has not changed much over centuries, and inevitably old habits will die hard. An Asian may not trust a doctor who does not make recommendations about food as part of his management of a clinical problem; but he will not let the doctor know, so as to avoid hurting his feelings. Nevertheless, such a patient may not comply with the therapy prescribed.

Doctor's approach

If a doctor has some knowledge of food-therapy, he or she should use it. If that advice is not possible, it is tactful to allow an Asian patient to take a specific food or to avoid certain foods, as taught by his parents or friends. Specific diets are still used in treating various diseases in allopathic medicine, and it is not unreasonable to accept the role of food as a mitigating or aggravating factor in an illness.

Folklore remedies

Theory

A folklore remedy is like a poem. A poet writes a poem but never explains what he means, only to find that different people read different meanings into it. Nevertheless, poetry is handed down through generations, and such too is the life-history of a folk remedy. Every region and village in the world has local remedies—available locally, easy to use, and, of course, effective—and the Asian subcontinent is no exception. The list of Asian folklore medicines is endless, and their use is empirical. Some are very useful, some are placebos, and some are downright dangerous. People may use them with blind faith.

Practice

Some families have a tradition of cooking a dish made from mouldy chapatis known as '*tukras*' ('mean pieces')—and we now know that penicillin is extracted from moulds. The application of an onion poultice to an inflamed or sore area of skin or a boil is an old Indian remedy. No one knows why, but piercing the tragus and inserting an ear thread can alleviate some symptoms of asthma in certain children. Deadly nightshade, meadowsweet, and foxlgove were all used in Asia as well as in Europe, and now we use their extracts as atropine, salicin, and digitalis respectively.

Doctor's approach

A doctor should ask if a folklore remedy has been used, so as to exclude possible side-effects which may complicate the clinical picture. A careful history will help to establish the most probable underlying cause, which may be iatrogenic. However, encouraging or directly dabbling in such approaches are best avoided by the Western doctor, who should adopt a neutral approach to this form of alternative medicine.

Herbal Medicine (green pharmacy)

Theory

> Excellent herbs had our fathers of old,
> Excellent herbs to heal their pain,
> Alexander and Marigolds,
> Eyebright, Orris and Elecampagne,
> Basil, Rocket, Valerian, Rue,
> Vervain, Dittany, Call-me-to-you,
> Cowslip, Melilot, Rose of the Sun.
> Rudyard Kipling

Kipling (1865–1936) was born in Bombay, India. His jingoistic imperialism had a counterbalancing sensitivity and admiration of Indian life, and he appreciated Indian herbs. Herbal medicine is as old as man himself. Asians have been using herbs in their food and as medicines since ancient times. Herbs are considered natural and therefore harmless; but nothing is further from the truth, and in fact some can be dangerous (Madge 1987). Nevertheless, their beneficial effects outweigh the risks.

Practice

In the UK, a herbal practitioner is usually a European Protestant, a *hakim* is an Asian Muslim, and a *vaid* is an Asian Hindu. Broadly speaking, each of these practitioners attract patients from their respective ethno-religious groups. The British Herbal Medical Association publishes the British Herbal Pharmacopoeia. The National Institute of Medical Herbalists, founded in 1841, has about 100 members. The recently-formed College of phytotherapy runs a four-year course in herbalism. The Medicines Act 1968 and the Retail Sale and Supply of Herbal Remedies Order 1977 S.I. No. 2130 (HMSO) control the green pharmacy. Some 341 herbal medicines are included in the General Sales List, and are available without prescription. About 550 herbal remedies are in general use in the United Kingdom, and these include 75 potent plants.

Some examples are: *Aerva lanata* (from Sri Lanka) used for cystitis; Indian bazaar snake root (*Rauwolfia serpentina*—reserpine) used for hypertension; liquorice used as an expectorant and an anti-rheumatic; peppermint for indigestion; blackcurrant for colds and as a source of Vitamin C; rhubarb as a laxative; and *Gossypium* used for male contraception.

Asian perceptions

Attracted by the Asian faith in herbs, many herbal practitioners have opened up their Green Pharmacy shops in inner-city areas. As Asian who cannot find a *hakim* or *vaid* should easily be able to find a herbalist.

Doctor's approach

Many herbs are beneficial, but may have side-effects, and a herbal remedy can potentiate, or interact or counteract with a manufactured therapy. It is important that the doctor is aware of these potential problems, which add a further dimension to the question of vigilance in minimizing the effect of 'drug' interactions.

Hikmat (Tibe-Unani)

Theory

'*Hikmat*' means 'wisdom', and its synonym '*Tibe-Unani*' means 'Greek medicine'. Although *Hikmat* had Greek origins, probably from when Alexander the Great (356–323 BC) invaded Northern India, and it was influenced by Persian and Egyptian medicine, its practitioners, known as *hakims*, established themselves in India during Muslim rule under the Mogul Empire (1526–1857). *Hakims* are licensed to practise by the Pakistani Government. The leading institution, *Hamdard Dawakhana*—Karachi and Delhi—publishes the Hamdard Pharmacopoeia, which list over 3000 preparations. In India and Pakistan, some wards in large hospitals are provided for patients to be treated by traditional medicine.

The central concept is a humoral theory derived from the Greek idea that all matter was formed from fire (hot and dry), air (hot and wet), earth (cold and dry), and water (cold and wet). The *hakim's* four humours—*Safra, Khun, Soda,* and *Balgham*—correspond to the medieval physician's concepts of yellow bile (fire), blood (air), black bile (earth), and phlegm (water). The dominance of a particular humour is thought to cause a disease. A *hakim* looks at a patient's appearance and listens to the symptoms, and makes a very detailed examination of the pulse while taking the history from the whole family.

Practice

The *Hikmat* pharmacopoeia contains herbal medicines, and heavy metals, such as gold, silver, tin, copper, barium, lead, traces of arsenic, mercury, zinc, antimony, and iron. The tonics are called *kushtays*. These are all potent medicines, and have beneficial effects in the recommended doses. However, as with a GP's drugs, they may have side-effects, and it is essential that they are used under the supervision of a qualified *hakim*.

In addition to herbal or mineral therapy, a *hakim* often suggests a diet, and asks the patient to avoid certain foods as part of the treatment. He uses his skills in counselling, psychotherapy, and social support, and provides continued personal care. Not only Asians but also some Europeans consult *hakims* for chronic conditions such as eczema, asthma, arthritis, and for anxiety, depression, stress, and psychosocial and psychosexual problems. A *hakim* provides not only aphrodisiacs for men but also a contraceptive pill for women. One pill made from the seeds of the shrub *Abrus precatorius*, which grows in Asia and Africa, is taken on the seventh day of the cycle, and it is claimed to give contraceptive protection for a whole month (Eagle 1980).

It is now being realized that a patient may think that if a little is good, more must be better, and may exceed the recommended doses of *kushtays* made from heavy metals. Moreover, an Asian in Europe may not have easy access to a *hakim*. A tonic in large doses can become a poison; and to avoid this possibility, the use of heavy metals is being replaced by eggshells, seashells, musk plant, oyster shells, and pearls. For those who cannot afford the high price of these exotic tonics, there is *gulkand*—a sugary preparation of rose petals ground in a mortar with a pestle.

Asian perceptions

Asking an Asian point-blank to give up consulting a *hakim* (or a *vaid*) is unlikely to be successful. In the UK, it is not uncommon for an Asian to use dual treatment—from a GP as well as a *hakim*—and tell neither practitioner, so as to avoid alienating them.

Doctor's approach

Three things should be borne in mind: firstly, an Asian patient might traditionally consult a *hakim*, and this does not necessarily mean a lack of trust in the GP; secondly, the adverse side-effects of Eastern medicine may have been exaggerated by Western commentators; finally, it is essential to be vigilant about the dual treatment causing any iatrogenic problems or any toxicity as a result of excessive use of a *hakim's* remedy. Mutual understanding and compromise between the doctor and an Asian patient is fundamental to the process.

Homoeopathy

Theory

Homoeopathy is a means of restoring health by exciting similar symptoms to those of the disease, and thus stimulating the body's healing response, preventing the recurrence of illness, and regaining the body's balance and harmony through natural remedies, which are thought to work somewhat like inoculation and counter-irritant therapies. The principle is 'like treats like' and 'a smaller dose has higher potency'.

The concept was conceived by Hippocrates (460–377 BC), who stated that there were two methods of treating disease; one, the treatment by opposites, when a medicament was used to oppose or counteract the symptoms; the other, by stimulating healing in the body by giving a substance which will mimic the symptoms and signs of the disease. Allopathy attacks the disease, or the seed, whereas homoeopathy strengthens the body, or the soil. Paracelsus (1493–1541) tried to revive the idea of treatment by similars, but it was Dr Samuel Hahnemann (1755–1843) who founded homoeopathy (Gibson and Gibson 1987).

It is interesting to note that allopathy, homoeopathy, and *Hikmat* (*Tibe Unani*) all originated in Greece. As with religions, each system claims to be the only right one!

Practice

Out of 2000 homoeopathic remedies, about 500 are in common use. These are available on the National Health Service, and all patients have the right to such treatment. In Britain, over 300 doctors practise and 400 pharmacists dispense homoeopathic remedies, and there are six homoeopathic hospitals, with 8000 in-patients and 60 000 out-patients annually.

The Faculty of Homoeopathy, recognized by the 1950 Act of Parliament, provides extensive education at the London School of Homoeopathy for doctors, and grants postgraduate diplomas (Madge 1987). Graduates from homoeopathic colleges in Asia who are not qualified doctors are not accepted by the Faculty, but can practise, as all other alternative practitioners can practise, in the UK under the common law right to ply their trade, as they do in Asian countries.

Some popular remedies include: Arnica 6 orally for all cases of injury, bruises, haemorrhage, shock, and sprain; Rhus Tox 6 for muscular stiffness; *Urtica Urens* 6 for nettle-stings, plant stings, and sunburn; Arsenicum Album 6 for food-poisoning.

Asian perceptions

Asians may prefer 'natural' remedies, and believe these to have no side-effects. They may go still further, and accept even a placebo, as long as it has no side-effects. Homoeopathic remedies are thought to be free of untoward reactions, even if their effectiveness is questionable. The concept that the side-effects of a drug can be treated has not yet caught on with less westernized Asians. They prefer risk-free treatments, and homoeopathic medicine seems to fit the bill. It is probably a reasonable generalization that many Asians consult a homoeopathic practitioner as their second choice, even more so than a *hakim* or a *vaid*. Parents may take a schoolchild with eczema or asthma to a local homoepath, who invariably advises them to stop the GP's medication during homoeopathic treatment.

Doctor's approach

Homoeopathy is a subject likely to raise antipathy on the part of someone with a modern western medical school training. It is, however, so firmly rooted in Asian culture and beliefs that it cannot be ignored. It is best for the GP who is sceptical, or even hostile, to try to adopt a neutral stance and avoid the situation where the patient is made to feel guilty about his choice. If possible the patient should be welcomed back if he decides to return to the GP at a later date.

Magic

Theory

Magic has two forms: firstly, the demonstration of a phenomenon, presumably with the powers of supernatural beings; secondly, bringing a curse on someone by using occult forces in nature or people. Magic is beyond the understanding of modern science.

Practice

A magic practitioner employs rituals to persuade supernatural forces such as gods, demons, spirits, or occult forces to produce beneficial or harmful effects—physical, mental, or spiritual—especially upon the enemy of his client.

Asian perceptions

An Asian woman may come to see her GP with the complaint that her in-laws have arranged to have a curse or magic put upon her and that she is ill.

Doctor's approach

A doctor should exclude mental illness—for example, schizophrenia—and then contact the appropriate religious priest, who will be happy to help.

Osteopathy and massage therapy

Theory

Osteopathy is a system of manual adjustment of the disordered skeletal framework which sustains a disease. It was founded by an American doctor, Andrew Taylor Still, in 1874, and is a Western therapy. Massage is a Western but also an Eastern therapy, practised since ancient times.

Practice

An osteopath deals with back troubles, injuries, aches, arthropathies, neuralgia, torticollis, cervical spondylosis, postural defects, tension headaches, and digestive problems, including constipation (Thomson 1986). There are no known massage therapists in the United Kingdom.

Asian perceptions

Asians are not familiar with osteopathy and are apprehensive of bone manipulation, but will be attracted by soft-tissue manipulation, as it is similar to massage—a popular Asian custom. A son is obliged culturally to massage the head, arms, legs, and back of both parents, especially when they fall ill. The feeling of touch, reassurance, relaxation, and increased blood-supply in a tense muscle is thought to be of therapeutic value in such an extended family. Massage is commonly used in the treatment of muscle weakness and strokes.

Doctor's approach

If an Asian patient asks the GP whether he or she can have the affected musculo-skeletal part massaged by a younger relative, provided there are no contraindications, it will gain him respect to grant this request for additional therapy. The prescription of ointments and rubs (where indicated) is often particularly welcomed by Asians.

Over-the-counter medicine

In India, Pakistan, Bangladesh, and Sri Lanka, almost all medicines are sold over the counter, and a doctor's prescription is used as an advice slip. Therefore self-medication with medicines purchased from a chemist is part of a long-standing tradition of self-care among Asians.

Practice

There are three categories: prescription-only medicine, unrestricted-sale preparations, and pharmacist-permitted medications.

Asian perception

Some Asians will buy over-the-counter medicines even for serious conditions by simply asking for a preparation without even talking to the pharmacist.

Doctor's approach

The GP's approach will be much the same as with any other patient: to ask the patient at the outset about the nature and extent of any self-medication.

Palmistry

Palmistry is an ancient art, and the lines or signs in one's hands are supposed to indicate one's health, character, and future. Carl Jung is said to have had the handprints of his patients interpreted, in order to gain extra insight into their strengths and weaknesses (Sheridan 1970).

Practice

Hindus, Buddhists, and some Sikhs have great faith in palmistry; but Muslims, Jews, and Christians take it very lightly.

Asian perceptions

An Asian worried about his health, future, finances, friends, and relatives may consult a palmist, known as a '*jotishi*', who may also be an astrologer.

Doctor's approach

An Asian patient may be worried about the prediction of the death of a close relative by a palmist; a similar anxiety, fear, or obsession may lead to illness. A doctor should take this seriously and provide reassurance and, if the problem is recurrent, suggest psychotherapy.

Religious rituals

Theory

Religious rituals are—in scientific terms—psychotherapy (individual and group), behaviour therapy, and drug therapy, where mineral, vegetable, or animal foods are served. All prophets were the healers of their times. The aim has been to promote physical and mental health, prevent a disease, treat a disorder, provide spiritual guidance, prepare someone near death to accept it, and provide bereavement counselling. Every religion includes a degree of the 'sanctity of life' doctrine that all killing is wrong, no matter what the circumstances are, because the giving or taking or life is believed to be the right of God, who is the creator of the universe. This doctrine can be used by a British doctor having difficulty in treating a devoutly religious person (Qureshi 1984).

Practice

Pakistanis and Bangladeshis are usually Muslims, Sri Lankans are either Buddhists (Sinhalis) or Hindus (Tamils), and Indians are Hindus, Muslims, or Sikhs. Anglo-Christians, contrary to popular belief, do not have a mixed-race background; they are usually Catholics. They all speak different languages and have different dietary customs, and therefore can present diagnostic and management problems to the British doctor (Qureshi 1986).

For example: some patients will wear holy threads and charms so as to prevent accidents and disease—the removal of these before an operation or during an examination can be very upsetting for the patient; a Sikh may wear a *kirpan* (ritual dagger), and this could be very alarming for the Western doctor; a patient may take longer to undress if he or she wears a religious costume; a baby may not be given a name for up to six weeks after birth, pending astrological or religious decisions; Asians celebrate death anniversaries rather than birthdays, and may not know their dates of birth.

The therapeutic value of religious rituals is enormous. For example: prayers provide psychotherapy and self-audit; fasting requires self-discipline; confessions clear guilt-feelings; and a priest is always on hand for the followers of his religion, giving social and spiritual support.

Asian perceptions

Asians are generally religious people, and some tend to adhere to their religions more when in the UK than when they were living in their countries of origin. Some devout parents have conflicts with their westernized children, especially the girls. They religiously contact their respective priests for birth, marriage, and death ceremonies. Other religious customs include baptism, head-shaving, and male circumcision.

Doctor's approach

Knowledge of a patient's religious beliefs can be helpful, and enable the GP to be more sensitive to that individual's expectations and needs.

Spa therapy

Theory

Spa water is supposed to have soothing, cleansing, massaging, and overall healing properties. The temperature and mineral contents of a spa, and its attractiveness to vistors, given proper maintenance to keep it open, could be of benefit to patients suffering from rheumatism and other disorders. The patients' faith in a spa, particularly if it is attached to a holy shrine and is in the presence of a caring healer, increases its therapeutic value.

Practice

There are many springs used for spa therapy in Japan, the Indian subcontinent, Austria, France, and Germany. All but one—Leamington—of the British spas are closed. British rheumatologists disapprove of spa therapy; but many patients with rheumatic conditions wish to have these spas reopened (Thomson 1982).

Asian perceptions

In India, many spas are attached to holy shrines. Some spa waters contain sulphur, and some have medicinal contents in the underlying mud. Many leprosy patients are said to have been healed from these waters. Many Asians still believe in a pilgrimage to a spa, and have family reunions during the journey—all this attention, reassurance, and faith is likely to contribute to healing.

Doctor's advice

An Asian woman may seek her GP's approval to travel to a spa. Unless there is a specific contraindication, perhaps it is wise to allow such treatment to take place. However, such patients should be reminded to continue their medical treatment.

Transcendental mediation

Theory

This is a technique of creating a relaxed but wakeful condition during which anti-anxiety metabolic changes occur that are said to improve resistance to stress, learning ability, creativity, and efficiency. In a person's life, disagreeable events are stresses, and the resultant palpitations, hypertension, anorexia, or duodenal ulcer are strains (Freedman 1987). Some people cannot cope with their everyday stress and become distressed, and it is for these people that transcendental meditation (TM) is indicated. In Asian culture, where psychiatry is taboo, it takes the place of psychotherapy in treating mental illness, psychosomatic problems such as insomnia or tension headache, and stress-induced diseases such as hypertension, heart disease, migraine, peptic ulcer, and asthma. Although it is attributed to a Hindu philosopher, Shankara (500 BC), transcendental meditators do not need to have any religious beliefs.

Practice

TM is practised in sessions of twenty minutes' duration twice a day. A meditator sits in a relaxed mood, breathing normally and focusing attention on a mantra, which is a short phrase or a word such as '*ome*' (god) or 'one', and is repeated constantly, so as to clear the mind of unnecessary thoughts. It was popularized in the West by the Maharishi Mahesh, an Indian religious teacher, who came to the public attention through his influence on the Beatles for a time in the 1960s.

The psychological effects of TM have been shown to include: low respiration rate, less oxygen consumption, decrease in blood lactate, changes in galvanic skin response, effect on brain waves demonstrated by EEG (leading to a feeling of energy-flows), reduced heart rate, and decreased blood-pressure in hypertensives. It is very effective in reducing anxiety and treating insomnia. Its critics say its effects are not significantly different from other relaxing practices such as listening to music (Crook 1983).

Asian perceptions

TM attracts Hindus and Sikhs, as well as some individuals from white ethnic groups. Devout Muslims, Buddhists, Jews, and Christians are less inclined to practise it because they have their own religious meditation systems.

Doctor's approach

Some Asian patients who are reluctant to accept psychotherapy—in the surgery or in a psychiatric clinic—and for whom drugs are to be avoided, can be offered sympathy and counselling. But if this is insufficient to let them develop their own way of coping with the problems and pressures of their lives, they could be encouraged to attend a transcendental meditation centre that is not too commercialized.

Urinotherapy

Theory

One of the most seemingly bizarre forms of alternative therapy adopted by Asian patients is urinotherapy, an ancient Indian therapy. Urine contains 96 per cent, water, salts, and hormones that are considered of therapeutic value by the urinotherapists. A glass of a person's own urine taken each day is claimed to have prophylactic properties, particularly against infections, and local application is supposed to have a healing effect.

Practice

Urine is used orally to treat: cancer, diabetes, gallstones, genital herpes, heart disease, leprosy, multiple sclerosis, myopia, orchitis, pyorrhoea, renal stones and ulcers. Its local application is claimed to heal bee stings, scorpion stings, snake bites, and wounds. It is said to keep the skin smooth, and is used in beauty treatment. In the UK, some therapists give urine by injection so as to overcome aesthetic objections (Walton 1983).

Asian perceptions

Urinotherapy made the news headlines in the 1980s when it was revealed that the then Prime Minister of India, Mr Murarji Desai, not only drank his own urine but also applied it to his own skin daily, believing it to prevent disease.

Doctor's approach

A GP will very rarely come across a patient who is adopting this form of therapy. Urinotherapy is not, however, exclusive to India—it is a well-known English folklore treatment for rheumatism and gout.

Yoga

Theory

Yoga has two meanings: in Mahayana and Vajrayana Buddhism, it simply means 'meditation'; in Hinduism, it is one of the six orthodox schools of Hindu Philosophy based on eight parts of a whole—personal morality, social ethics, physical position or posture, breath control, command over the senses, concentration, meditation, and samadhi (inner happiness and freedom of the soul). In the west it is known as Hatha Yoga, and deals with physical positions and exercise which expand the limits of endurance of the body and mind. This philosophy was introduced by an Indian preacher, Patanjali (who lived in 150 BC), aiming to achieve a mystical union with a personal deity through hypnosis and by rising above the sense through the adoption of postures, meditation, and induced relaxation. A Hindu guru, Ianga, introduced yoga to Britain in 1918, and it is estimated that a quarter of a million people practice yoga in the United Kingdom.

Practice

Pauline Dowling (1982) a yoga teacher, claimed that 'yoga is not alternative, fringe, or even holistic medicine. In fact it is not medicine at all, any more than life is an illness. It certainly should not be thought of as treatment for all stress-related conditions such as spastic colon. For the essence of yoga is becoming master of yourself and accepting complete responsibility for yourself. Yoga is true liberation, stability, and relaxation.' However, its meditation and relaxation component is said to help in reducing hypertension, especially in pregnancy, and in natural birth and asthma. Its postural exercises—standing, sitting, bending, twisting, and balancing—are meant to extend stamina, strength, balance, and flexibility, leading to physical, psychological, and emotional stability.

Asian perceptions

As expected, being an active Hindu philosophy, it is practised predominantly by Hindus, by some Sikhs, and by many white ethnic group followers.

Doctors' approach

Some teachers accept yoga as a form of meditation, but others point out that meditation is only a small part of this Hindu philosophy: a doctor should bear this in mind when referring a patient for yoga. An appropriate and duly qualified teacher should be sought. When treating hypertensives and asthmatics who are practising yoga (or other meditation), an allowance should be made in drug therapy. This dual treatment necessitates more careful surveillance.

Conclusion

Healers have practised their skills since the beginning of time. The Indian subcontinent in particular has been a rich source of wisdom and inspiration to the healing arts. Knowledge and awareness of the large variety of alternative therapies available to Asian patients is essential for the general practitioner, and should enable him to develop a less ethnocentric approach, which recognizes the complementary nature of many such therapies.

References

Anon. (1978). Imhotep, the first known physician. *Hospital Update*, **4**, 235–7.

Beely, L. (1986). Do the antithrombotic, antibiotic and other medicinal properties disappear when garlic is boiled or fried? *British Medical Journal*, **293**, 1090.

Bourne, S. (1985). Asian medicine: traditional remedies or health risks? *The Listener*, **28 November**, 8–10.

Crook, J. (1983). Meditation. *Update*, **30**, 48–54.

Dowling, P. (1982). Before you prescribe, read on . . . *World Medicine*, **17**, 37–40.

Eagle, R. (1980). Your friendly neighbourhood Hakim. *World Medicine*, **15**, 19–22.

Freedman, B. (1987). *Just a word, doctor*. Oxford University Press, Oxford.

Gibson, S. and Gibson, R. (1987). *Homoeopathy for everyone*, pp. 84–97. Penguin, Harmondsworth.

Glynn, J. and Heyman, T. (1985). Factors that influence patients in Sri Lanka in their choice between Ayurvedic and Western medicine. *British Medical Journal*, **291**, 470–2.

Madge, M. (1987). *Alternative or complementary medicine*. (Booklet obtainable from: Marshalle Publications, Chelfam House, Saltburn Road, St Budeaux, Plymouth. Tel: 0752 361832.)

Qureshi, B. (1984). Muslim patients and the British general practitioner. *The Medical Annual*, **1984**, 259–71.

Qureshi, B. (1986). Management of ethnic Asian patients in general practice. *The Medical Annual*, **1986**, 155–65.

Sheridan, J. (1970). It's all in the hands. *Woman*, **January 17**, a supplement, 1–15.

Thomson, J. (1986). Osteopathic practitioners ready to help the GP. *London Medicine*, **1**, 16–17.

Thomson, W. (1982). The over-all value of spas and spa treatment. *Journal of Royal Society of Health*, **102**, 185–9.

Walton, P. (1983). 'Water of Life' pours health by the glassful. *Doctor*, **12** (March 17), 27.

Wijesinha, S. (1985). Sasruta: surgeon of ancient India and pioneer of plastic surgery. *Surgery*, (Oxford), **1**, 380.

Recommended Books

1. Gibson, S. and R, Gibson, R. (1987). *Homoeopathy for everyone*. Penguin, Harmondsworth.
2. Madge, M. (1987). *Alternative or complementary medicine*. Marshalle Publications, Plymouth.

3. Munro, R., Trevelyan, J., and West, R. (1987). *Mind—body therapies: a select bibliography of books in English*. Mansell Publications, London.
4. Qureshi, B. (1989). *Transcultural medicine: dealing with patients from different cultures*. Kluwer Academic Publishers, Lancaster.
5. Rolt, F. (1985). *Pills, policies and profits*. (Bangladesh). War on Want, London.
6. Khan, S. (1987). *Islamic medicine*. Routledge and Kegan Paul, London.
7. Brown, E. G. (1921). *Arabian medicine*. Cambridge University Press, Cambridge. (Reprinted 1983, Hyperion, Connecticut.)
8. Elder, E. and Samuel, O. (1987). '*While I'm here, doctor*'. Tavistock Publications, London.

Useful Addresses

The Faculty of Homoeopathy, 2 Powys Place, Great Ormond Street, London WC1N 3HT. Telephone: 01-837-9469.
Osteopathic Education Foundations, 16 Buckingham Gate, London SW1.
The National Insitute of Medical Herbalists, 41 Hatherley Road, Winchester, Hampshire. Telephone: 0962 68776.
Transcendental Meditation, Central London Centre, 26 Craven Street, London WC2.
Association of Ayurvedic Practitioners, 7 Ravenscroft Avenue, London NW11 0SA.
Hakim Hamdard Dawakhana, Karachi, Pakistan.
Tibbi Foundation, 446 East Park Road, Leicester.

8 Diet and Nutrition

Bashir Qureshi

Introduction

Aside from the British people who served in the Far East during the Second World War, the majority of the British population will have become familiar with Asian cuisine largely through the growth in popularity of the Asian restaurant, and latterly through the wider dissemination of Asian recipes in cookery books and television programmes. These Asian culinary experiences provide only a limited insight into the great diversity of diet enjoyed by people living in the United Kingdom whose origins or traditions are within the Indian subcontinent.

Diet and health are often related. A doctor should therefore be aware of the diet his patients usually follow. This varies between individuals, depending on their religion and regional background (Table 8.1).

Table 8.1 *Regional differences in staple diet among Asians*

	Origin	Food
I	Pakistan	
	(a) Punjabis	Meat curry and chapati
	(b) Pathans	Tandoori meat and nan
II	India	
	(a) Punjabis	Meat curry and chapati
	(b) Gujaratis	Vegetarian or vegan
	(c) Bengalis	Fish and rice
	(d) South Indians	Fish and rice
III	Bangladeshis	Fish and rice
IV	Sri Lankans	Fish and rice
V	Kenyan or Ugandan Asians	
	(a) Punjabis	Meat and wheat
	(a) Gujaratis	Vegetarian or vegan

Source: Qureshi 1986

Table 8.2 shows some staple foods, which are chosen for many reasons, including availability, acceptability, price, storage facilities, and personal and community preferences. Occasionally problems can arise which may concern the general practitioner, and these will be described in the sections on specific diseases linked to dietary factors and on medical emergencies.

Table 8.2   *Staple foods*

• Nan

A soft triangular or round bread, resembling pizza, usually an inch thick, made from white flour leavened with bicarbonate of soda and yeast, and bound with yoghurt. Cooked in an oven without fat, on charcoal, it is the staple food of Pathans.

• Chapati

A thin unleavened bread made from whole wheat flour. It is cooked in an Indian pan called a *tawa* without fat. It is the staple food of Punjabis, but popular all over the Indian subcontinent. Its modified form cooked in fat is called *paratha*.

• Bhatura

A leavened bread made from white flour with bicarbonate of soda and a little sugar; after making a dough with yoghurt, it is deep-fried. It is a favourite breakfast bread of Punjabis and other Asians.

• Plain pilau

Patna or Basmati rice fried in butter. It is seasoned with butter and salt, and simmered with fried onion. Almonds or cashew nuts may be added before serving. It is the staple food of Gujaratis (Hindus), Bangladeshis (Muslims), South Indians (Hindus and Anglo-Christians), and Sri Lankans (among whom are the Tamils who are again Hindus, some Anglo-Christians, and the majority Sinhalis, who are largely Buddhists).

Source: CRE 1977

An Asian patient with religious reservations regarding food is likely to come from one of three religions: Islam, Hinduism, or Sikhism. Almost all Muslims are 'meat and wheat' eaters, (although Bangladeshis prefer rice); whereas Hindus, Buddhists, and Sikhs can be vegetarians, vegans, or selective omnivores.

Islam

The Quran determines dietary restrictions, the principal one being the total prohibition of pork and pork products.

General dietary observations

Islam recommends that a lawful animal such as cow, goat, or sheep should be slaughtered in a ritual humane way with a quick cutting of the throat while invoking the name of Allah and draining all the blood away before cooking;

this method is called '*halal*', meaning 'allowed'. Any meat not obtained in this way is '*haram*', meaning 'forbidden'.

The fear of consuming non-*halal* meat is often very great: some Muslim mothers will decline English meat and tinned dishes; schoolchildren may leave a meal untouched if there is *haram* meat on the plate; workers may bring their own food in order to avoid canteen facilities; and patients may well refuse hospital food. Politeness may prevent the Muslim person explaining this behaviour, and therefore a great deal of understanding and compromise is required from British health professionals.

Fish must be alive when taken out of the river or sea, but does not have to be slaughtered by a ritual, because it has no neck, and so cannot be drained of blood, as with other animals. However, only fish that have fins and scales are recommended.

A Muslim is expected to fast from dawn to dusk at certain times, particularly during the holy month of Ramadan, but to continue to be at work. This self-discipline has spiritual and physical advantages. However, side-effects such as hypoglycaemia, lack of concentration, and lethargy can bring such a person into contact with medical services, and it is important to recognize that the fast is a possible underlying cause for these clinical presentations.

Food is generally considered as a gift from God, and should all be consumed. A clean plate after eating may be misunderstood as greediness by those who are not aware of this.

Festive foods

Mithai—festive sweets; honey—a tonic; vermicelli pudding—a pasta for sustained release of energy; all can be used at occasions such as the feast of *Eed*.

Forbidden foods

A number of foods are specifically forbidden in the Islamic religion, often for reasons which are soundly rooted in traditions of good hygiene and the avoidance of illness.
Examples are:

- Pork and pork products—the pig is avoided because of its uncleanliness;
- blood—because of the belief that to consume it is absorbing the spirit of another being;
- alcohol—because of its intoxicating effects, causing immoral acts and accidents; and
- eels and the shark family, through fear of infection, and also because of their not having scales (Hunt 1975).

Knowledge of these forbidden dietary products can also have important applications in the therapeutic field. Pork insulin is perhaps the most obvious example;

but there are also over sixty preparations listed in the Monthly Index of Medical Specialities (MIMS) which contain alcohol. All are strongly taboo. It must be remembered that some patients will avoid taking medicines because of a fear that they may contain the forbidden, and that this can be an important cause of non-compliance. It is better to give a specific assurance to a patient about the content of a medication than to leave this to chance. If it is not possible to avoid a preparation, and its administration is life-saving, a doctor should seek the help of a local Imam (priest), who can persuade the patient to accept it by using the umbrella of the 'sanctity of life' doctrine—that Allah says life must be saved, that suicide is taboo in Islam, and that the priest as well as the physician share in the decision, so as to avoid painful feelings of guilt on the part of the patient.

Hinduism

Hindus believe in *ahimsa*—the sanctity of life doctrine that killing is always wrong. They also believe in reincarnation, and that the cow is sacred as a source of milk and ghee, which can also provide the manure, used in rural parts of India as fuel.

General dietary observations

Strict Hindus are either vegans, who not only exclude flesh, fish, and fowl from their diet, but also milk and dairy products (cream, butter, cheese), as well as eggs; or vegetarians, who, while they will not eat flesh, fish, or fowl, are permitted cow's milk and its products in their diet. A quite common variation for less orthodox Hindus is to be 'ovo-lacto-vegetarians', a group who will eat eggs (especially if infertile) and milk, or 'pesco-vegetarians', in whose diet white fish only is allowed. Westernized Hindus who do eat meat such as lamb or mutton will still abstain from beef.

Vegetarians receive their protein from various pulses. A vegetarian diet can be a balanced diet if it includes some vitamin B_{12} preparation, and is wide in its variety. Similarly, essential nutrients can be obtained in a vegan diet from cereals, pulses, nuts, fruits, vegetables, vegan margarine, soya protein foods, nutmeats, yeast extracts, and plant-milks (DHSS 1980). Fasting is considered spiritually and physically beneficial. It often involves restrictions on certain foods, rather than total abstention, in Hindu religion.

Festive foods

Particular foods are also associated with Hindu festivals. Examples are: *laddoo* (sweet balls), made of pulse flour, sugar, and ghee; *jalaibi* (sweet rings), containing white flour, sugar, and ghee; and *gajer halwa* (a carrot sweet). Ghee (clarified butter) is generally used to sanctify food.

Forbidden foods

For vegetarians, all meat, and, for vegans, even milk products, are taboo. However, some who are otherwise omnivores will consider the following food taboo: beef (the cow is considered as sacred as the mother); pork (for its uncleanliness); oily fish (a rich source of vitamin D, but considered dirty); and eggs (as a potential source of life).

Jainism, the non-theistic Hindu sect that originated 5000 years ago in Gujarat, is founded on a belief in the total sanctity of life. This has a bearing on diet; although Jains are generally lacto-vegetarians (the cow is sacred, but its milk is acceptable), they will not eat root vegetables such as potatoes, carrots, and radishes. This seems to be because the act of pulling them from the soil puts at risk the lives of insects and worms. A Jain may even sweep the floor before walking on it so as to spare the life of insects: living creatures such as these are also sacrosanct. Anaemias, particularly of the iron and vitamin B_{12} deficiency type, are not uncommon among Jains and other Hindu vegetarians, especially vegans. Many vegetarians will not accept egg- or chick-based vaccines, such as those for measles, mumps, influenza, and yellow fever.

Two particular dietary issues may concern Hindu patients. Firstly, beef insulin is taboo, and if a patient is allergic to other forms of insulin this can cause very great difficulty and distress. The wide availability of human insulins has reduced this problem. Secondly, any baby milk which says 'animal oil' on its label may, in fact, contain beef fat, which is strongly taboo, and would pollute the baby's religion. In the latter case, a different milk that does not contain 'animal oil' should be substituted. Details of the composition of some commonly used baby milks are shown in Table 13.1, p. 213. A doctor should not hesitate to seek the assistance of the Pandit from the local Hindu Temple or another professional if necessary; and it is better to do this rather than attempt to hide the truth. The later discovery by an Asian person that he has unknowingly taken a forbidden substance, even in the form of a medication, can have a serious psychological impact, and may jeopardize the doctor–patient relationship.

Sikhism

Sikhism developed as an offshoot of Hinduism in the sixteenth century. In general, Sikhs observe fewer dietary prohibitions than Hindus, although some devout Sikhs fast on certain days.

General dietary observations

Sikhs are taught to use a ritual method of killing an animal such as a lamb, goat, or sheep, called '*jhatka*' which entails killing by one blow to the head. This is similar to the British practice of killing by stunning, and is very different from the Muslim (*halal*) and Jewish (*kosher*) methods. Orthodox Sikhs will not eat *halal* or *kosher* meat because of the different method of slaughter. Some Sikhs are vegetarians, but others are omnivores.

Festive foods

A communal meal is served at the *gurdwara*, and the festival dish is '*karah parshad*', made of semolina cooked in water, butter, and sugar.

Forbidden foods

As with Hindus, the fact that the cow is regarded as sacred means that Sikhs will not eat beef. Some will not eat pork or drink alcohol, for the same reasons as Muslims.

Lacto-vegetarianism occurs amongst Sikhs; and this group does not eat eggs, which are a potential source of life. Smoking is forbidden to Sikhs; and, in taking a history, the doctor should remember this, because to ask a Sikh man, or particularly a woman, whether they smoke can cause offence.

Other cultural aspects of diet

Two particular dietary concepts are adhered to by many Asian patients: the classification of foods as 'hot' and 'cold', and food avoidance (*perhaiz*). This classification is not related to a food's temperature, or even how spicy it is, but more to its effect on the human body. The idea that groups of foods have different properties is a concept derived from ancient Hindu medicine.

'Hot' foods are considered good for treating the common cold, but harmful in pregnancy (causing miscarriage) and in feverish illnesses. 'Cold' foods have the reverse properties, and these are also avoided during lactation.

Examples of 'hot' foods are: meat, eggs, fish, lentils, onions, dates, aubergines, chillies, ginger, carrots, honey, brown sugar, tea, coffee, nuts, potatoes, radishes, garlic, and mangoes; and of 'cold': orange juice, milk, buttermilk, yoghurt, fruits (such as the lemon), white sugar, rice, vegetables (such as spinach), and carbonated drinks.

There is some scientific basis for such a classification, in that the effect of food in the gut results in changes in splanchnic blood-flow, gastric emptying, and gastric secretion. Splanchnic blood-flow is increased by high-protein meals, whereas it is transiently decreased by high-glucose liquid meals. The rate of blood-flow will affect the absorption of nutrients and drugs (Dickerson and Booth 1985).

The concept of food avoidance of *perhaiz* is based on centuries of experience of Muslim medicine. There is a strong belief that food can result in allergy or infection, and thus be a cause of disease. It is widely accepted that almost every food can cause allergy.

These concepts are unfamiliar to those trained in Western medicine; but the Asian patient may expect his doctor to take this into account when advising or treating, as would be the case in traditional Asian medicine. An Asian patient will invariably ask the doctor 'What food should I avoid?' If this question is dismissed or not responded to, the patient may lose faith in the competence of the doctor to help him, and turn to alternative medicine.

A number of habits and customs which are part of Asian culture may be unfamiliar to the indigenous population, and may give rise to negative reactions or misunderstandings. These are matters which the well-informed doctor can be aware of and can discuss with an Asian patient, though it is important not to seek to weaken cultural identity merely as a convenience.

The strong smell and stains of curried food can cause cross-cultural problems. Simple advice concerning hygiene, when sensitively given in the appropriate situation, is often enough to solve most problems. It should be remembered that hygiene has a high value amongst most Asians. Turmeric stains should not be confused with henna stains, which are ritual.

Spices are used as a rich source of iron, and herbs have carminative as well as flavouring properties. However, they can be irritant to the buccal and also to the gastric mucosa. The Asian habit of rolling a piece of *chapati* or *nan* round a piece of spiced meat, as if making a small sandwich or roll, is meant to protect the buccal mucosa. The custom of using yoghurt in cooking and taking it with meals may also protect the gastric mucosa and the gut.

After using one's hands for eating, it is customary to wash them, and also to rinse the mouth thoroughly. It is said that this latter habit is one reason for strong, healthy teeth. Some Asians are not accustomed to eating with a knife and fork, but are happy to use a spoon. Schoolchildren and patients in hospital may refuse to eat meat or peas if they are not allowed to use their hands or a spoon.

Some Asian patients do not trust hospital food, in case they are given pork, lard, beef, or non-*halal* meat, even inadvertently; and it is customary for relatives to bring in some Asian food. On the one hand, a home-cooked Asian meal should be checked by a dietitian or an experienced ward sister to eliminate any potential food–drug interaction or disease exacerbation, such as may occur for instance with a peptic ulcer; but on the other hand every effort should be made to provide acceptable ethnic dishes on the hospital menu.

A DHSS (1980) publication 'Catering for minority groups' recommends many menus suitable for Muslim, Hindu, Sikh, Jewish, vegetarian, and vegan patients. For example, a menu for one day for a vegetarian patient on a normal diet is shown in Table 8.3. Many English or Scottish patients like to eat ethnic dishes if given the choice. Food that is appealing and acceptable helps morale and saves wastage.

Table 8.3   *Typical daily hospital menu for a vegetarian patient*

Breakfast:	Fruit juice or cereal with milk.
	Poached egg on toast.
	Wholemeal bread, butter, and marmalade.
Mid-day:	Cream of vegetable soup.
(or evening)	Cottage cheese, sultana, and nut salad.
	Apple pie and custard
	(or vegetable curry, *chapati*, and *halawa*).
Evening:	Spaghetti Bolognese (soya protein).
(or midday)	Green salad.
	Apricot fool or yoghurt
	(or lentils, rice, and ice cream).

Source: DHSS 1980

Specific diseases linked to dietary factors

There are ethno-cultural aspects of three groups of diseases, prevalent among Asian patients, which can be prevented and managed by a British general practitioner and the wider primary-care team: bone diseases, anaemias and other deficiencies, and gift food-poisoning. The reader may find it helpful when considering this section of the chapter to consult the list of further reading shown at the end.

(a) Bone diseases

Rickets (fetal, infantile, and childhood) and osteomalacia (in adolescents, pregnant women, and the elderly) are far more common in Asians than in any other ethnic group in Britain. In children, bony deformities, and in women, a contracted pelvis—necessitating a Caesarean section in childbirth—are areas of great health-care concern; and these are preventable diseases. Prevention (and treatment) depends on understanding the causes specific to this particular ethnic group.

These are diseases of calcium and phosphorus metabolism resulting in softening of the bone due to a defiency of vitamin D or of calcium, or of both. No single factor appears to be responsible for the susceptibility of Asian women and children to vitamin D defiency. However, the following might be involved:

    (i) increased requirements;

   (ii) a dietary defiency of vitamin D;

  (iii) the high phytate content of *chapati*, impairing calcium absorption (see below);

  (iv) lack of exposure to sunlight, to allow endogenous production of vitamin D;

(v) cultural/religious factors, for example, vegans avoiding milk and Hindus eschewing oily fish; and

(vi) genetic predisposition.

It is advisable that Asian children should receive daily vitamin D supplements of 400 i.u., especially during the first five years of life or more. Routine supplements of 1000 i.u. have been recommended for pregnant Asian women (Williams and Qureshi 1988). Asian adolescents should also be given such supplements. Vitamin drops and tablets and cod-liver oil are recommended. Vitamin-D-containing foods should be promoted.

Chapati is eaten as the main bread source by almost all Asians, especially those from the Punjab (see Table 8.1). *Chapati* flour, often imported from India, contains phytic acid, which combines with dietary calcium to form calcium phytate, which cannot be absorbed. This factor, combined with a lack of vitamin D and calcium supplements, is the most likely cause of these bone diseases. Moreover, phytic acid also binds iron and zinc in a similar way, leading to a deficiency of these minerals.

Interestingly, there is a way of dealing with phytic acid—as so often happens, a remedy to a cultural problem is found within the culture itself! Fisher (1983), a home consultant, has described how *chapati* (wholemeal) flour should be used according to Indian recipes, which advise that it should be mixed with warm water and allowed to stand for two to three hours, before kneading, rolling, and shaping. In this way the texture and nutritive value of the diet is improved, because when warm dough is allowed to stand, a naturally-occurring enzyme developes in the dough—phytase—which destroys the phytic acid and liberates the calcium, iron, and zinc. It should be noted that the same effect is obtained when doughs are mixed with yeast, as in bread.

(b) Anaemias and other deficiencies

(i) Iron Iron deficiency is by far the commonest cause of anaemia throughout the world, and among Asians is possibly due to their religious and cultural restriction on foods such as meat and eggs. In Britain, iron-defciency anaemia is very common among Asian children, because many infants are introduced to cow's milk earlier than is advisable, either for convenience or through lack of trust in western tinned milk and foods—Hindus are concerned about beef fat, Muslims are forbidden foods with pork or lard content, and vegetarians keep well away from both. However, there is also an Asian custom of prolonged breast-feeding, for up to two years. Milk is a poor source of iron. However, Mahatma Gandhi, who was a lacto-vegetarian, is said to have lived solely on goat's milk in later years; but he supplemented this with bananas, believed to be a rich source of iron. The role of *chapati* in diminishing absorption of iron has already been described.

Iron supplements and iron-containing food—lentils, pulses, meat and eggs for omnivores, dried fruits, bread, cocoa, peas, spinach, cabbage, and Brussels sprouts (Beal 1976)—should be given. However, there is an exception to this rule, and that is thalassaemia. Not only Middle Easterners but also Asians suffer from this condition, in which dietary iron is contraindicated.

(ii) Folic acid It is an Asian custom to cook food—vegetables or meat—slowly over a long period, to improve the taste and kill any parasites. This method results in the total destruction of vitamin C, folic acid, and vitamin B_{12}. Fortunately, every Indian meal is customarily served with green salad and fresh fruit. A health professional should ensure that Asian patients are eating enough leafy green vegteables, milks, nuts, yeast, and pulses; and—for omnivores—white fish and liver should be advised.

(iii) Vitamin B_{12} This vitamin is said to be found in animal foods alone. Nevertheless, research in India has led to the isolation of vitamin B_{12} from certain green leaves. This perhaps explains why evidence of vitamin B_{12} deficiency is rare in most vegetarians. (Williams and Qureshi 1988).

It is advisable that an omnivore should eat enough meat, liver, and oily fish. A vegetarian should eat yoghurt and cheese, and drink at least two pints of milk daily, so as to avoid this type of anaemia.

Finally, protein deprivation, vitamin C deficiency, and hookworm infestation (in those returning from holiday in Asia) should be watched out for.

(c) Gift food-poisoning

Every year many Hindus visit the holy river Ganges in India, and many Muslims go on pilgrimage, to Mecca, where there is a holy spring called 'Zam Zam'. It is customary to bring back holy water as a present to be distributed among relatives and friends in Britain. Moreover, ordinary holidaymakers visiting Asian countries often bring back food presents, such as *halawa*.

Such products may be contaminated at source; or if the weather is hot and refrigerating facilities during travel are inadequate, organisms (such as *Salmonella typhimurium*) may multiply. This should always be considered as a possible cause of apparently unexplained food-poisoning in an Asian patient.

Medical emergencies precipitated by dietary factors

There are three important emergency clinical presentations which can occur among patients who eat Asian food as a staple diet: prolonged hypoglycaemia, hypertensive reactions, and postbulbar duodenal ulcer.

(a) Prolonged hypoglycaemia in diabetic patients

This can occur in a diabetic on oral hypoglycaemics who eats a large amount of '*karela* curry', which is a tasty Indian dish. It is customary to use varying amounts of garlic and onion in Indian cuisine.

Karela (*Momordica charantia*), garlic (*Allium sativum*), and onion (*Allium capa*) are all hypoglycaemic agents. Recent research (Leatherdale 1981) has warned doctors supervising Asian diabetics in particular to be aware of the hypoglycaemic properties of *karela*. As serum insulin concentrations are not increased, *karela* may directly influence hepatic or peripheral glucose disposal.

Karela, in small amounts, may cause lethargy and lack of concentration; and, if included in a diabetic diet, it may well improve glucose tolerance. However, in large amounts it can potentiate the action of chlorpropamide or tolbutamide, and cause prolonged hypoglycaemia, leading to faintness or coma. A similar but less severe hypoglycaemic action can occur with garlic and onion.

(b) Hypertensive reactions in patients on monoamine oxidase inhibitors (MAOIs)

The interaction of MAOI antidepressants with sympathomimetic tyramine-containing foods (for example, cheese, game, liver, chocolate, certain wines, broad beans, pickled herrings, Bovril, Marmite, Oxo, yeast, and yoghurt, as well as stale food) is well known. Unfamiliarity with Asian cuisine on the part of the doctor and/or failure to properly explain the potential danger to an Asian patient can lead to this complication. It is not widely appreciated that many Asian dishes are cooked and served with yoghurt as a matter of course; and that *nan* bread, a common accompaniment to many Asian meals, contains relatively large amounts of yeast. It is important that special attention is paid to dietary screening, and providing appropriate advice to the small number of Asian patients who will be on MAOIs.

(c) Postbulbar duodenal ulcer

The eminent British radiologist Oscar Craig, in an unpublished tutorial 'Barium meal X-rays of the gut', delivered at the Royal College of Surgeons (1978) first pointed out the apparent clinical association between postbulbar duodenal ulcer and habitual rice-eating populations such as South Indians. It should be borne in mind that rice is the staple diet of Bangladeshis, Sri Lankans, Afro-Caribbeans, and Chinese, and that this lesion can occur commonly amongst them.

A posterior duodenal ulcer carries a risk of secondary haemorrhage by the erosion of a large vessel, and an early referral to hospital can be life-saving.

Conclusion

The roots of education are bitter but the fruit is sweet (Aristotle).

It is essential for a health professional to undertand his or her patient's lifestyle, dietary habits, and genetic characteristics. Some dietary habits can cause health problems. A doctor should take a dietary history as part of the clinical interview, and look out for any signs of nutritional deficiency or excess. It is good practice to observe the six variables: age, sex, social class, ethnic origin, religion, and region. All directly influence a patient's health, nutritional status, cause and course of disease, expectations from a doctor, and compliance with treatment.

In this chapter, regional diets, ethnic characteristics, religious beliefs, and aspects of culture among Asian patients have all been highlighted. Some acute and chronic diseases are described from a cultural angle, as these may present to a general practitioner in a clinical consultation with an Asian patient. It is hoped that this chapter will assist the general practitioner in caring for all his patients—ethnic majority and minority; and particularly those from the Asian subcontinent.

References

Beal, G. (1976). *Asian diet and health.* Ealing Community Education Team, Southall (Middlesex).

CRE (Commission for Racial Equality) (1977). *A guide to Asian diets.* CRE, London.

DHSS (Department of Health and Social Security) (1980). Catering for minority groups. In *Health Service Catering*, **6**, DHSS, London.

Dickerson, J. and Booth, E. (1985). *Clinical nutrition for nurses, dietitians and other health care professionals.* Faber, London.

Fisher, P. (1983). *Samosa.* Forbes Publications, London.

Hunt, S. (1975). *Asians in Britain.* Van den Berghs and Jurgens, Burgess Hill, Sussex.

Leatherdale, B. (1981). Improvements in glucose tolerance due to Momordica charantia (Karela). *British Medical Journal*, **282**, 1823–4.

Qureshi, B. (1986). Management of ethnic Asian patients in general practice. *The Medical Annual*, **1986**, 155–65.

Williams, C. and Qureshi, B. (1988). Nutritional aspects of different dietary practices. In *Nutrition in clinical management of disease*, (ed. J. Dickerson and H. Lee), pp. 422–39. Edward Arnold, London.

Recommended reading

Baird, J. D. and Truswell, A. S. (1987). Nutritional factors in disease. In *Davidson's principles and practice of medicine*, (ed. J. Macleod, C. Edwards, and I. Bouchier), pp. 49–83. Churchill Livingstone, Edinburgh.

Black, J. (1985). *The new paediatrics.* BMJ Publications, London.

Dunnigan, M., Glekin, B., Henderson, J., McIntosh, W., Summer, D. and Sutherland,

G. (1985). Prevention of rickets in Asian children: assessment of Glasgow campaign. *British Medical Journal*, **291**, 239–42.

Helman, C. (1984). *Culture, health and illness*. Wright, Bristol.

Henley, A. (1979). *Asian patients in hospital and at home*. King's Fund, London.

Lobo, E. de H. (1978). *Children of immigrants to Britain: their health and social problems*. Hodder and Stoughton, London.

Qureshi, B. (1989). *Transcultural medicine: dealing with patients from other cultures*. Kluwer Academic Publishers, Lancaster.

Smith, R. and Jones, W. P. T. (1987). Nutrition. In *Oxford textbook of medicine*, 2nd ed., (eds. D. J. Weatherall, J. G. G. Ledingham, and D. A. Warrell, Sections 8.1–8.61. Oxford University Press, Oxford.

Useful addresses

The Vegan Society, 47 Highlands Road, Leatherhead, Surrey.
The Vegetarian Society (UK), 53 Marloes Road, Kensington, London W8.

9 General medical problems

Stephen Sturman and D. G. Beevers

Introduction

The differences in disease patterns between blacks, whites, and Asians in Britain are striking; but it must be stated clearly that these differences are cultural or environmental rather than racial. There are no diseases which are genetically related to any particular racial group; even sickle-cell disease is seen in non-black people. It follows that any ethnic patterns in disease are predominantly of environmental origin. Factors like housing conditions, employment or its lack, urban overcrowding, dietary habits, alcohol and smoking, and lack of awareness or availability of medical care are all alterable, and are the main causes of both ethnic and social-class differences in disease.

Much attention has been paid to the use of traditional medical practices by Asian migrants to Britain. These problems have largely been overstated. While there is some use of native *hakims* (untrained, often self-appointed healers) most Asian people simply wish to avail themselves of good primary and secondary medical care. They frequently attend Asian doctors because of their greater understanding of cultural factors in health-care use, and also because of the bonds of common language. Further details on alternative medicine are contained in Chapter 7.

Despite the many similarities in the health patterns of whites and Asians, there are also some important differences in the incidence of certain diseases, for reasons that frequently remain obscure. Most of the common cancers seen in whites are rare in first-generation Asian migrants in Britain. By contrast coronary heart disease, often regard as a 'western' epidemic, is unduly common in Asians, and hypertension and hyperlipidaemia are equally common in both groups. While type II (non-insulin-dependent) diabetes mellitus is unduly common in Asians, there is a striking deficit in true type I (insulin-dependent) diabetes.

The purpose of this chapter is to review some of the commoner medical conditions seen in clinical practice, where an awareness of the role of ethnic factors can improve clinical diagnoses and effective medical treatment.

It must be remembered that most data which are available routinely about illness are based on hospital in-patients' data and death certifications, and that for many diseases this represents an incomplete and atypical part of the extent of that particular disease in the population. Moreover, such health-service information systems do not routinely record ethnic origin as a variable.

Great caution must therefore be exercised in drawing firm conclusions about how common particular diseases are in the Asian community. However, given these limitations, the systematic examination of data based on clinical experience can provide a valuable insight into the disease-experience of this ethnic minority community. Further details on demography and epidemiology are covered in Chapter 6.

Coronary heart disease

Studies of mortality statistics for England and Wales (Marmot *et al.* 1984) as well as surveys from both London and Birmingham have all confirmed an excess of coronary heart disease in migrants from the Indian subcontinent (Cruickshank *et al.* 1980). This excess, representing between thirteen and twenty per cent, is seen in both sexes and in all ages (Fig. 9.1). While different ethnic groups

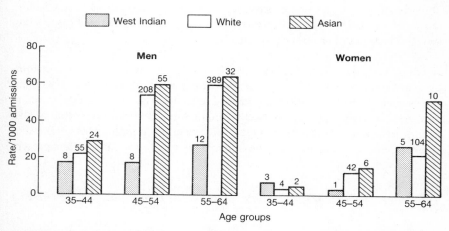

Fig. 9.1 Admissions to Dudley Road Hospital for myocardial infarcts 1975–1979 by place of birth. *Source:* Cruickshank *et al.* 1980.

may respond to chest pain in different ways, and this tendency may explain why more Asians are admitted to hospital for chest pain, it does not explain the excess death rate. A recent study of Asians in five different London boroughs (McKeigue and Marmot 1988) has confirmed a mortality from coronary heart disease fifty per cent higher than the national average. The communities were very diverse in terms of religions, countries of origin, economic status, smoking, and dietary habits, but it has been suggested that the one factor they may have in common is disturbed insulin metabolism (McKeigue *et al.* 1988). Chest pain in Asians should, therefore, be taken seriously.

Coronary angiographic studies also reveal a tendency for Asians to have more extensive coronary artery damage than whites. It is interesting to note that in

Asians with proven coronary disease, as many as 35 per cent had normal ECGs. (Lowry *et al.* 1984). This indicates that the diagnosis must depend on good history-taking, and, as suggested earlier, language problems may be a limiting factor.

The implications of this excess incidence of coronary heart disease are that there is a need for a ready availability of facilities for coronary angiography and coronary artery by-pass grafting in inner-city areas where Asians have tended to congregate. This is frequently a problem, particularly outside London, but doctors should consider lowering their threshold for referral to cardiac investigation centres when dealing with Asians with possible or definite coronary heart disease.

Coronary risk factors

The observed ethnic differences in coronary heart disease have led several observers to investigate ethnic differences in the three main coronary risk factors (cigarette-smoking, high blood-pressure, and hyperlipidaemia) as well as to study less well recognized or rarer causes of atheroma deposition.

Cigarette-smoking   Most studies have shown that cigarette-smoking is uncommon in Asian men in the UK, and practically unheard of in Asian women. (Jackson *et al.* 1981). This most potent and reversible risk factor does not explain why Asians have more heart attacks (Table 9.1). However as coronary risk factors have a multiplicative or synergistic effect on mortality rates, cigarette-smoking, on top of the other known or unknown risk factors, must when present be regarded as particularly dangerous.

Table 9.1   *The presence of cigarette smoking. The Birmingham Factory Project*

	Males			Females		
	Black	White	Asian	Black	White	Asian
Percentage of smokers	54	50	21	15	49	5

Source: Cruickshank *et al.* 1985

Hypertension   Population surveys have in general reported no important differences in the prevalence of hypertension in Asians and whites. High blood-pressure appears common in both groups (Cruickshank *et al.* 1985). There is, however a worrying tendency (Table 9.2) for Asians to be less likely to have had a blood-pressure check in general practice. Failure to diagnose hypertension, as well as other early symptomless disease, might explain why Asians in general do suffer as much or at times more vascular disease than whites. A different

Table 9.2 *The Birmingham Factory Screening Project. The frequency of blood-pressure measurement at work or in general practice. Men and women below age 65 years*

	Whites		Asians		Blacks	
	M	F	M	F	M	F
Total number of examinees	449	240	149	17	146	97
Number (%) ever had BP measured by general practitioner	205 (46%)	169 (70%)	43 (29%)	11 (65%)	76 (52%)	74 (76%)
Number (%) ever had BP measured at work	256 (57%)	128 (53%)	75 (50%)	9 (53%)	95 (65%)	63 (65%)
Number (%) never had BP measured before	94 (21%)	29 (12%)	61 (41%)	2 (12%)	26 (12%)	7 (7%)

Source: Cruickshank *et al.* 1985

picture emerges when analysing the ethnic origin of people admitted to hospital for hypertension, or referred to a blood-pressure clinic. Here Asians are seen more commonly than expected. This almost certainly reflects a tendency for doctors to refer known Asian hypertensives, either because their hypertension is very severe, or, more probably, because it is resistant to drug therapy. The commonest reason for failing to control blood-pressure is poor compliance, and this may frequently be related to poor understanding of the need for continuous therapy or of complex drug regimes, which may often be related to language barriers.

Practical points

1. Coronary heart disease is unduly common in Asians, and is associated with higher than average mortality.
2. Chest pain, even if atypical, should always be taken seriously.
3. Because of the high prevalence special care must be taken to control known cardiac risk factors.

Hyperlipidaemia   The high prevalence of coronary heart disease in Asians has lead to a search for ethnic differences in coronary risk factors. Cigarette-smoking is less common in Asians than in whites or blacks, so this clearly is not the explanation. Studies of plasma lipids are few. Asian-style food frequently has a high content of saturated fats, particularly clarified butter and other dairy products. However no consistent excess of the hyperlipidaemias has been reported in Asians. Recently it has been postulated that clarified dairy products, like ghee, and also Indian sweets, including *burfi*, *kulfi*, and *mawa*, contain a high proportion of cholesterol oxide, which may increase the deposition of atheroma in vessel walls (Raheja 1987). This problem is compounded if there is coexistent diabetes mellitus, and the coronary risk score is further elevated if the patient has also got a raised blood-pressure.

Diabetes

First-generation migrants from Asia and East Africa now living in London and Leicester have been found to have a particularly high prevalence of non-insulin-dependent diabetes mellitus (NIDDM) (Mather and Keen 1985; Samanta and Burden 1986). By sharp contrast true insulin-dependent diabetes (IDDM) is relatively uncommon. Those Asians who are receiving insulin therapy are not really insulin-dependent (Type I) cases, but rather are those in whom dietary caloric restriction or oral hypoglycaemic agents have been unsuccessful (Mather and Keen 1985).

It is possible that the low prevalence of insulin dependency is due to selective non-migration of young people who owing to type I diabetes were too ill to travel. The genetic inheritance of type I diabetes is such that this condition may remain rare in western countries.

Type II diabetes, however, remains a big problem. In many cases it is related to obesity, and compounded by a high prevalence of hyperlipidaemia. Treatment is rendered difficult in part because dietetic advice is difficult to administer, when taking into account Asian-style foods, many of which have a high content of carbohydrate (Odugbesan and Barnett 1985; Peterson *et al.* 1986). It is important that diabetic clinics in inner-city areas should employ dietitians of Asian origin who can give the appropriate advice. Furthermore here, as with so many conditions, language problems may mean that patients are insufficiently instructed in the management of their disease. Most diabetics when first diagnosed are not particularly ill, and their motivation to lose weight or take their tablets may be poor. Where dietary manoeuvres fail and oral therapy is unsuccessful insulin therapy may be necessary, and again compliance with insulin regimes may be hard to achieve. Special efforts and specially trained staff are necessary. There is no evidence of any true ethnic differences in diabetes between Asians and whites. The complications suffered are the same. By contrast there does seem to be a genuine excess of hyperosmolar non-ketotic diabetic coma in Afro-Caribbeans, many of whom present in middle age, and when treated remain non-insulin-dependent on a long-term basis.

Practical points

1. Non-insulin-dependent diabetes mellitus is common.
2. True insulin-dependency is rare.
3. Compliance with dietary restriction requires specially trained dietitians.
4. Treatment compliance may be poor.
5. Insulin regimes are hard to achieve, so special training and staff are necessary.

Renal disease

The diagnosis and treatment of renal disease in Asians is similar to that in non-Asians. However the clinician should remember that tuberculosis is common in Asians, and when present is frequently extra-pulmonary. A common presentation of renal tuberculosis is sterile pyuria. A mid-stream specimen of urine with more than 50 leucocytes but 'no growth' must be followed up with three early-morning urine collections for acid-fast bacilli. Advanced renal tuberculosis may present with fevers, urinary obstruction, loin pain, or a calcified partially cystic renal mass.

As hypertension is common, and diabetes is very common, in Asians, hypertensive nephrosclerosis and diabetic glomerulosclerosis are common, proceeding to chronic renal failure. Proteinuria and diabetic renal disease is commoner in Asian than white diabetics attending the diabetic clinic in Leicester (Samanta *et al.* 1986). The management of chronic renal failure, with dietary protein restriction and later haemodialysis or chronic ambulatory peritoneal dialysis proceeding to renal transplantation, requires highly motivated and well trained patients. Language, cultural, and dietary factors need careful attention, but should not be regarded as contraindications to dialysis.

Cancer

Neoplasia, in general, appears to be less common worldwide in Asians compared to whites (WHO 1982). In the few studies that are available this pattern seems to persist in Asians who have migrated to the UK (Potter *et al.* 1984; Donaldson and Clayton 1984). An Asian patient is therefore just under half as likely to be discharged from hospital with a diagnosis of malignancy as a white patient (Donaldson and Taylor 1983). To the academic oncologist changes in the incidence of cancer in migrant populations are a matter of great interest, because of the clues they give as to the causes of cancer. As yet there is little published information on changes in cancer incidence over the last twenty years in the Asian population specifically in the UK, and the pattern of disease at present reflects that of the populations of origin, although in many instances incidence is even lower, because of the 'healthy cohort effect' and the relative youth of migrants.

From published studies it appears that the incidence of lung cancer is about two-thirds that expected; the incidence of colorectal cancer one-half to one-eighth that expected, and the incidence of breast cancer is about one-half that expected (Fig. 9.2). However the number of actual cases involved in these studies are small. Stomach, testis, and skin malignancies are also significantly less common in Asians.

There are however some important exceptions to this general rule. Studies of standardized mortality ratios for Asians in the UK shows an unexpected excess of deaths from carcinoma of the cervix (Marmot *et al.* 1984). There appears to be a one-and-a-half times to fourfold excess of cases of carcinoma of the cervix among Asian women in the West of Scotland when compared with the general population (Matheson *et al.* 1985). The overall picture, however, is not clear, and is discussed in more detail in Chapter 10. Clearly, regular cervical smears are of the utmost importance in Asian women; but there is evidence of particularly poor uptake of the service in this group (McAvoy and Raza 1988). The administration of this service is likely to be difficult, and female medical or nursing staff will usually be preferred by the patient.

At least one British study has shown that there is a significant excess of tumours of the tongue, oral cavity, pharynx, and oesophagus in UK Asians (Donaldson and Clayton 1984). This is consistent with studies from India, Singapore, and South Africa, where a similar high incidence of these tumours has been noted

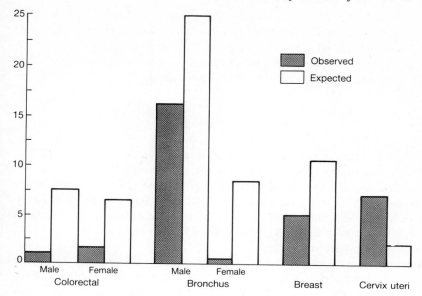

Fig. 9.2 Observed and expected cases of tumours in Asians 45–64 years living in the west of Scotland. *Source:* Adapted from Matheson *et al.* 1985.

in Asians living there. This excess has been related to chewing betel nut mixed with lime and tobacco; although the role of betel in carcinogenesis has been contested.

While breast cancer is less frequent in Asians than in whites, the mean age of presentation is said to be twelve years younger than the mean in whites, and the disease is more advanced; for instance in one study 66 per cent of Asian cases presented with stage III and IV disease (Potter *et al.* 1983). Again, perhaps, more intense screening is required, and better health education, so that Asian women are aware of the importance of seeking early medical advice regarding breast lumps.

Lung cancer too has been said to be present at an earlier age in Asians. Mean age at presentation has been said to be about twelve years younger than in whites, that is, 53.5 years in Asians versus 65.6 years in whites (Potter *et al.* 1984). The incidence of smoking is equally common in white and Asian lung-cancer patients, thus confirming its role in the aetiology of the disease.

Practical points

1. Cervical cancer may be commoner in Asian women.
2. Breast cancer may occur earlier and be more advanced in Asian women; regular breast-screening by self-palpation should be taught, and early self-

referral encouraged. Breast-cancer screening programmes in areas with large Asian populations should place particular emphasis on tailoring health-education material to encourage high levels of acceptance.

3. Treat oral lesions in Asians, and dysphagia, with a high index of suspicion, as they may represent early oro-pharyngeal cancer.

Respiratory disease

Discussion of respiratory disease in Asians is dominated by tuberculosis. The standardized mortality ratios for TB are threefold and ninefold greater for men and women respectively than for the white population (Marmot *et al.* 1984). Furthermore, TB in Asian people is more often also found in extrapulmonary sites, including the abdomen, the cervical lymph nodes, and the vertebral column (Honeybourne 1987). Since the topic is fully dealt with in Chapter 15 it will not be further discussed here.

The prevalence of asthma in the general population has not been accurately assessed. A recent survey of factory workers in Birmingham showed prevalence rates of 5.5 per cent for Caucasians and 3.2 per cent for Asians, but the differences were not statistically significant (Honeybourne 1987). Analyses of hospital admissions suggest that there is a disproportionate number of Asians admitted with asthma as the principal diagnosis (Jackson *et al.* 1981). It seems, however, that this excess is because Asian asthmatics are admitted more frequently to hospital, rather than because the prevalence of asthma in the Asian community is increased (Ayres 1986). Poor drug compliance, imperfect inhaler technique, and inaccurate assessment of symptoms because of language problems are cited as causes for this observation. There are no studies of objective criteria of the severity of asthma in Asians.

It is not uncommon for asthma to develop for the first time in Asians shortly after arriving in the UK. There is substantial evidence from Africa showing that asthma incidence rises to 'western' levels with the urbanization of rural communities, but the reasons for this are unclear. Positive skin tests to grass pollen and domestic animals are less frequent in Asians when compared with whites, but Asian children are more frequently positive for house-dust mite (Morrison-Smith and Cooper 1981). Asian patients with asthma are more likely to be allergic to moulds, especially *Aspergillus*, which tend to flourish in old and damp houses (Javaid and Ayres 1988). One could conjecture that poor-quality inner-city housing is to blame for these phenomena, but from a practical point of view it is important to recognize that the Asian asthmatic may present slightly later in life than the Caucasian (twenty-six years versus nineteen years respectively) (Partridge *et al.* 1979), and may be totally unfamiliar with the concept of asthma and the need for prophylactic treatment having migrated from an area with a low incidence. A thorough programme of patient education may well reduce the excess admission rate seen in Asians.

Sarcoidosis

Whilst it is well recognized that there are marked ethnic differences in the pattern, severity, and incidence of sarcoidosis, the picture is still not clear as regards the Asian community. From the limited work that has been done it appears that the incidence is somewhere between that of the British population (4 in 100 000) and the West Indian population (158 in 100 000) (McNicol and Luce 1985). Asians seem prone to more disseminated disease than whites, and consequently have a slightly poorer prognosis. This is roughly comparable with the pattern and prognosis seen in West Indians (Honeybourne 1987). It must be said, however, that these conclusions are drawn from small numbers of Asians from a particular subset of the Asian community. No good information on the natural history or incidence of sarcoid in India exists.

One important practical point is to remember that tubercle and sarcoidosis can co-exist in the same patient. This is a potent source of confusion in both diagnosis and treatment, but usually can be clarified by Kveim testing.

Prolonged steroid therapy in Asians for any condition, for example asthma or sarcoidosis, may result in reactivation of tuberculosis, with devastating consequences. While opinion on this is divided, many chest physicians suggest using prophylactic anti-TB therapy while the patient is on steroids.

Practical points

1. Poor compliance, especially with prophylactic treatment, may be the most important cause of inadequate asthma control.
2. Prolonged steroid therapy in Asians may re-activate TB; if it is needed, consider anti-tuberculous prophylaxis.

Haematology

In the late 1960s and early 1970s many cases of severe, megaloblastic anaemia were seen amongst Asians living in the UK. These have been extensively investigated (Britt *et al.* 1971; Chanarin *et al.* 1985); and interestingly the usual cause has been found to be nutritional vitamin B_{12} deficiency. Folate deficiency or combined folate/B_{12} deficiency account for a smaller number of cases. The Hindu vegetarian population seems particularly at risk of developing dietary B_{12} deficiency, since a vegetarian diet is said to contain between $0.3 \mu g$ and $1.5 \mu g$ of cobalamin (Stewart *et al.* 1970), while the daily requirement is $1-2 \mu g$. Whilst the number of reported cases of true Addisonian pernicious anaemia in Asians is small, a retrospective study has suggested that it occurs just as commonly as in the Caucasian population (Chanarin *et al.* 1985). An important practical point to note is that 10 per cent of cases of megaloblastic anaemia in this second study had a normal or low mean corpuscular volume (MCV), because of co-existing iron deficiency or haemoglobinopathy. Hence the diagnosis of B_{12} deficiency may require a strong index of suspicion.

The incidence of megaloblastic anaemia due to dietary deficiency seems to decline dramatically as western-type dietary habits are adopted, even if an essentially Asian 'menu' is retained. Iron-deficiency anaemia, however, remains very common, especially in females. Up to one-third of women may be anaemic, and three-quarters show features of iron deficiency (Britt *et al.* 1983). The high incidence of iron deficiency is thought to be due to dietary deficiency in most cases. In refractory cases it is important to consider primary gastro-intestinal pathology, or occasionally intestinal parasites, especially hookworm—although these are far less common now than when originally highlighted in the early 1960s as a problem among Asian immigrants.

In assessing the blood count of an Asian patient it is important, too, to bear in mind the effects of haemoglobinopathies. The most common, beta-thalassaemia trait presents as a mild anaemia (10.5–12.0 g/dl) with profound microcytosis (MCV circa 65 or less). Even though iron deficiency may be present, the abnormal parameters are not corrected with iron therapy. Haemoglobin electrophoresis shows an excess of haemoglobin A_2, with levels 3.5–7.0 per cent, and this is sufficient to confirm the diagnosis. If there is no excess of HbA_2, but the blood count remains abnormal, despite correction of iron deficiency, then alpha thalassaemia trait is the next most likely diagnosis.

In the Punjabi and Gujarati population haemoglobin D haemoglobinopathy is said to occur with a frequency of about 1 per cent (Griffiths *et al.* 1982), and presents as a mild haemolytic anaemia for which no treatment is required. Clearly the importance of recognizing all these minor abnormalities is in preventing unnecessary investigations of the mildly anaemic patient.

Glucose 6-phosphate dehydrogenase (G6PD) deficiency

Studies in India and among Indians living abroad have shown that G6PD deficiency does occur among Asians, although the frequency varies widely between individual communities. Bengalis have a frequency at the lower end of the range, at around 4 per cent, while the Parsees in Bombay have a frequency of 15 per cent (Chatterjea 1966). The agents likely to cause a haemolytic episode are shown in Table 9.3. In clinical practice in the UK, however, severe haemolysis is rarely seen, except when high doses of the drugs concerned are used. While G6PD deficiency is X-linked, and thus usually seen only in men, in areas of high prevalence a number of females will be homozygotes, and subject to the same hazards as men.

In practical terms, then, a high index of suspicion is needed to recognize G6PD deficiency in Asian men and women, in order to avoid both acute haemolytic crises and chronic haemolytic anaemia.

Table 9.3 *Agents which may cause haemolytic anaemia in G6PD deficiency*

1. Infections and other acute illnesses
2. Drugs:
    (a) antimalarials—for example, primaquine, pyrimethamine, quinine, and chloroquine;
    (b) analgesics: phenacetin, acetylsalycylic acid, and paracetamol;
    (c) anti-bacterials, such as sulphonamides, nitrofurones, penicillin, isoniazid, and streptomycin; and
    (d) miscellaneous: vitamin K, quinidine, and dapsone.
3. Fava beans

Practical points

1. Dietary B_{12} and folate deficiency are not uncommon, especially in 'new arrivals' from the Indian subcontinent.
2. Megaloblastic anaemia may not produce a macrocytosis in the peripheral blood-film in up to 10 per cent of cases.
3. In iron-deficiency anaemia refractory to treatment consider hookworm infestation.
4. Haemoglobinopathies may produce mild anaemia apparently refractory to iron treatment.

Alcohol-related disease

Those who work in areas where there are large Asian populations will be familiar with the patterns of alcohol usage within the community. Anecdotally it is thought that there is a very low level of alcohol usage amongst Muslim Pakistanis, but a high level of alcohol abuse amongst Hindu, and especially Sikh, men. Recently evidence has begun to accrue that this is not far from the truth. Although relatively imprecise indicators of the frequency of alcohol abuse, rates of admission to psychiatric hospitals for alcohol-related disorders have risen by 75 per cent among native-born patients, but by 121 per cent among Indian-born men between the years 1971 and 1981 (Cochrane and Bal 1989), and deaths from liver cirrhosis have been found to be twice as common in Hindu and Sikh men as in native-born men (Balarajan *et al.* 1984). There is also a slight excess of death from cirrhosis among Muslim men, but general-practice surveys in Liverpool and Manchester have confirmed that there is a very low level of alcohol usage in this group (Ghosh 1984). From a practical point of view it is probably worth questioning Hindu and Sikh men about their alcohol consumption routinely, so that advice can be offered before alcohol-related problems become serious. This is particularly important in the Asian man with coronary heart disease, whose drinking could be causing both hypertension and hyperlipi-daemia, thus compounding his risk factors. It must be remembered that hepatitis B is more frequent in Asians, and appropriate serology should be performed where liver function tests are abnormal.

Practical points

1. Heavy alcohol consumption is not uncommon among Sikhs and Hindus.
2. An alcohol history should be taken, and appropriate counselling started.
3. Hepatitis B is common in many Third World migrants.

Drug—metabolism—acetylation

It has been known for some years now that there are considerable inter-ethnic variations in the frequency (q) of the allele for slow acetylation of drugs and metabolites. Japanese and Polynesians are more frequently fast acetylators, with low q values of 0.3–0.45. From the limited data available, Asians and northern Europeans have a much higher frequency for slow acetylation, with q values of 0.70–0.88.

The best-known application of this knowledge is in treatment with isoniazid. In slow acetylators antagonism of pyridoxine (Vitamin B_6) is potentiated, and peripheral neuropathy may result. It is thus sound clinical practice to prescribe pyridoxine supplements with isoniazid in Asian patients (Karim *et al.* 1981).

General medical problems related to traditional Asian medicine

It is important to remember that Asian patients may consult a traditional practi-tioner, or *hakim*, in addition to their usual physician. It is important to ask about traditional remedies that may be being taken as well as conventional medi-cines. For example adult males may take metal-containing or metal-coated pills known as '*kushtay*' for treatment of sexual dysfunction (Aslam and Healey 1983). Whilst no adverse effect has yet been reported with this preparation, the potential for toxicity is clear, and will only be recognized if there is a high index of suspicion.

Better-documented is the occurrence of lead poisoning in mothers and children using *surma* as a cosmetic. This is crushed lead sulphide in the form of ore galena. An active public-health campaign has reduced the incidence of this prob-lem a great deal (Ali *et al.* 1978).

Another interesting observation has been on the interaction of *Karela* (*Momor-*

dica charantia, or bitter gourd) with oral hypoglycaemic agents. Karela has been shown to improve glucose tolerance in diabetics (Leatherdale *et al.* 1981), and has also been shown to interact with chlorpropamide. Doctors supervising Asian diabetic patients need to be aware of this interaction both for its beneficial and its potentially harmful effects.

Attention has recently been drawn to the use of mineral clay in the treatment of indigestion, and as a vitamin supplement amongst pregnant women in Asian communities (Lancet 1988). The clay, which is sold in food shops under the names of *sikor*, *mithi*, *patri*, *khurri*, and *khatta*, has been found to contain varying amounts of lead, and in many cases other poisonous substances, including arsenic.

Gastrointestinal disease

Peptic ulceration

Even within India there are wide variations in the incidence of peptic-ulcer disease and its complications. Duodenal ulcer is generally more common than gastric ulcer—with a mean ratio of 19:1, from 18 reported series (Tovey and Tunstall 1975). Duodenal ulcer is common in South India and parts of Kashmir and Assam, but rare in the Punjab and the rest of North India (Dogra 1941). In rural India duodenal ulcer is more likely to be complicated by pyloric stenosis than haemorrhage and perforation, while in the cities the reverse is true (Varma 1969).

Frequency of peptic ulceration increases with urbanization. Although reliable data on the size of the problem are not easily available, it seems to be rare in women, and the peak age of incidence is about ten years younger in Asians than in Europeans. It is not known how migration to the UK is affecting these patterns, but all the signs are that ulcer incidence in Asians will rise to western levels, with a western and urban disease pattern. A low incidence of gastric ulcer has been reported among one group of Asians in London (Glyn and Kane 1985), and studies of hospital in-patient analyses have not shown an excess of gastro-intestinal morbidity or mortality. Clearly further studies are required to see how the patterns change, and this might well give useful information on the aetiology and risk factors for peptic ulceration.

Inflammatory bowel disease

Inflammatory bowel disease is not uncommon amongst Asians. While parasitic causes of diarrhoea are common among those recently returned from the Indian subcontinent, a diagnosis of inflammatory bowel disease should never be excluded on ethnic grounds. The prevalence of ulcerative colitis (UC) amongst immigrants in Bradford is about 59 in 100 000, which is similar to that seen in native Britons (Mayberry 1985). In India information is less easily available, but UC is said to occur slightly more commonly in men of a younger age than in Europe, and with a lower incidence of systemic and local complications including carcinoma than in western Europeans (Sharma and Sarin 1985). It is not known whether this pattern persists amongst expatriate Indians.

Crohn's disease seems less common among Asians than among Europeans. It does occur, however, although the frequency is probably only one-third that in native Europeans (Keshavarzian *et al.* 1986). It is of prime importance however to exclude tuberculosis as a cause of ileitis in Asians before making a diagnosis of Crohn's disease (Burke and Zafar 1975). Crohn's disease is a rarity in India, with very few reported cases, so that the rise in incidence among expatriate Asians is of great interest. There do not appear to be any salient differences in the presentation and outcome of Crohn's disease in Asians as against Europeans.

Lactose malabsorption and intolerance

This is surprisingly more common among Asians than Europeans. Over 80 per centr of Indians and 50–80 per cent of Pakistanis are said to lose intestinal lactase in early adult life. The clinical effect of this deficiency is very variable; at worst it can cause abdominal distention, colicky abdominal pain, watery diarrhoea, and flatus. The lactose load required to induce symptoms is also very variable, varying between a quarter of a cup of cow's milk to over a cupful (Lancet 1979). In view of the relative frequency of this condition it should be considered in all Asians presenting with vague abdominal symptoms where no other diagnosis can be made. It can be confirmed by either a lactose tolerance test or a breath hydrogen test. Treatment consists of a milk-free diet, but not all dairy products need be avoided—yoghurts, cheese, and double cream contain little lactose, and can be freely used by most patients. Many tablets contain appreciable quantities of lactose as a base, and this too should be considered when a particular brand of a drug seems to cause excessive gastro-intestinal side-effects.

Practical points

1. Inflammatory bowel disease *does* occur in Asians.
2. Exclude parasites as a cause of diarrhoea, first—especially *Entamoeba histolytica* and *Giardia lamblia*.
3. Abdominal TB is common, and is more likely than Crohn's disease.
4. Lactose deficiency is common in Asians, and can cause many minor gastrointestinal symptoms.

Neurology

Certain neurological conditions are considered rare among Asians in the United Kingdom. Multiple sclerosis occurs less commonly in those who spent their childhood years in areas of low prevalence (such as the Indian subcontinent and tropical Africa). Consequently it is rarely if ever seen amongst first-generation immigrants, and the diagnosis should not be made unless all other pathologies have been excluded. In contrast it appears that MS occurs with equal frequency to that in the white population in UK-born children of immigrants. While this was first shown among children of West Indian immigrants in London (Elian and Dean 1987), a recent study has confirmed it also to be the case among UK-born Asians. MS should therefore be considered in the differential diagnosis in UK-born Asians, and not discounted on ethnic grounds.

Giant-cell arteritis and neurosarcoid are also both said to occur rarely in Asians in India. Whether this pattern will change with time spent in the UK remains to be seen.

Aortic arch syndrome, or Takayasu's disease, is common in India, and should be considered in the young Asian presenting with stroke (Wadia 1973). Subarachnoid haemorrhage is said to be less common in India than in the West, but is more frequently due to angiomatous malformation than Berry aneurysm.

Craniovertebral anomalies, including congenital atlanto-axial dislocation and basilar invagination are comparatively common (eight to ten each year in a major neurology centre in India) and may present with trivial symptoms of transient spinal cord dysfunction, although the majority have signs of ongoing cervical myelopathy. Clearly these are rare syndromes; but to miss them could be disastrous.

Epilepsy is thought to be slightly more common in the Indian subcontinent because of the effects of TB, encephalitides and birth trauma. One interesting variant has been reported, in which temporal lobe attacks are precipitated by pouring hot water over the head, the so-called 'hot water epilepsy'. 'Funny turns' in the shower or bath should perhaps not be dismissed, therefore!

Probably the most important neurological condition not to miss is tuberculous meningitis. While the presentation can be classical, with meningism, photophobia, fever, and headache, the course of the disease may be far more indolent, and could be easily overlooked in its early stages unless there is a high index of suspicion. One important variant is that of spinal meningitis, which may present chronically as a radiculomyelopathy, or may be acute and ascending, and mimic transverse myelitis or Guillain–Barre syndrome. Early diagnosis and treatment of TB meningitis is essential if disaster is to be avoided; and so early investigation if the diagnosis is suspected is the rule.

Practical points

1. Multiple sclerosis is exceedingly rare in first-generation immigrants.

2. TB meningitis is fatal if not treated early and aggressively—a high index of suspicion is needed to make the diagnosis.

Osteomalacia

Osteomalacia was first recognized as a major problem among Asians living in the UK in the 1960s, when a high incidence of clinical rickets was found amongst Pakistani children in the Glasgow area. Since that time it has become well recognized that osteomalacia is common among Asian adults. A frequency of 22–25 per cent of biochemical vitamin D deficiency has been found in various studies (Shaunak *et al.* 1985; Peach *et al.* 1983); but the incidence of clinical disease is considerably less. Classically the patient is a middle-aged female with symptoms of hip and thigh pains and generalized 'weakness'. There is usually little to find on examination. Unless the diagnosis is actually considered the patient may be thought to be malingering. The diagnosis is easily confirmed by measuring serum alkaline phosphatase, which is usually elevated. Serum calcium and phosphate are much less useful as indicators of osteomalacia (Melikian 1981). Certain points from the history can be most useful in raising one's suspicion of osteomalacia. In particular a story of change of gait, with hip/leg pain, is suggestive; and other associated risk factors are vegetarianism, Hindu background, and Kenyan or Ugandan origin (Peach *et al.* 1983). Adolescent girls remain particularly at risk, as do pregnant women; and annual prophylaxis with one dose of ergocalciferol in the autumn has been advocated (O'Hare *et al.* 1984). It is also of some importance to note that the husbands of Asian women may have a similar degree of osteomalacia to their wives, and this condition has been described as a 'familial disorder' (Shaunak *et al.* 1985). Clearly if one member of a family is identified as having the condition enquiries about symptoms in the rest of the family might be fruitful.

The aetiology of the condition is a little obscure, and probably involves a complex combination of several factors. It has been contested whether the 'Asian' diet is actually deficient in vitamin D, and also whether patients with osteomalacia are exposed to less sunlight than average. It has been suggested that interruption of the enterohepatic circulation of vitamin D through the binding of it by dietary fibre might be an alternative explanation (Heath 1983). Whatever the course, however, treatment with calciferol is usually successful.

Practical points

1. Osteomalacia should be considered in the Asian patient presenting with vague body pains or change of gait.
2. Consider prophylaxis/screening in adolescent or pregnant females.
3. Consider screening other family members if osteomalacia is found in an Asian woman.

Conclusion

In general, Asian migrants to western countries have more health problems than the host population. Some of this excess is due to a higher incidence of specific diseases such as tuberculosis, diabetes and coronary artery disease. However, the common diseases which afflict whites also have a major impact on Asians. Special efforts are needed to improve the quality of health care to all disadvantaged groups, whether they are at risk as a result of low social class, poverty, ethnic origin, lack of motivation, or poor utilization of services. An awareness of disease-patterns in Asians is necessary for all doctors. It is a neglected topic, and it is the duty of all health-care workers to strive to correct these inequalities in health. Furthermore, the opportunities for practically useful epidemiological and clinical research are enormous.

References

Ali, A. R., Smales, O. R. C. and Aslam, M. (1978). Surma and lead poisoning. *British Medical Journal*, **1**, 915–6.

Aslam, M. and Healey, M. (1983). Asiatic medicine. *Update*, **9**, 1043–8.

Ayres, J. G. (1986). Acute asthma in Asian patients: hospital admissions and duration of stay in a district with a high immigrant population. *British Journal of Diseases of the Chest*, **80**, 242–8.

Balarajan, R., Bulusu, L., Adelstein, A. M. and Shukla, V. (1984). Patterns of mortality amongst migrants to England and Wales from the Indian sub-continent. *British Medical Journal*, **289**, 1185–7.

Britt, R. P., Harper, C. M. and Spray, G. H. (1971). Megaloblastic anaemia among Indians in Britain. *Quarterly Journal of Medicine*, **40**, 499–520.

Britt, R. P., Keil, J. E., Hollis, Y., Weinrich, M. and Keil, B. W. (1983). Anaemia in Asians in London. *Postgraduate Medical Journal*, **59**, 645–7.

Burke, G. J. and Zafar, S. A. (1975). Problems in distinguishing tuberculosis of the bowel from Crohn's disease. *British Medical Journal*, **4**, 395–7.

Chanarin, I., Malrowska, V., O'Hea, A-M., Rinsler, M. G. and Price, A. B. (1985). Megaloblastic anaemia in a vegetarian Hindu community. *Lancet*, **ii**, 1168–72.

Chatterjea, J. B. (1966). Haemoglobinopathies, glucose 6 phosphate dehydrogenase deficiency and allied problems in the Indian sub-continent. *Bulletin of the World Health Organization*, **35**, 837–56.

Cochrane, R. and Bal, S. S. (1989). Mental hospital admission rates of immigrants to England: a comparison of 1971 and 1981. *Social Psychiatry and Psychiatric Epidemiology*, **24**, 2–11.

Cruickshank, J. K., Beevers, D. G., Osbourne, V. L., Harper, R. A., Corlett, J. C. R. and Selby, S. (1980). Heart attack, stroke, diabetes and hypertension in West Indians, Asians and whites in Birmingham, England. *British Medical Journal*, **281**, 1108.

Cruickshank J. K., Jackson, S. H. D., Beevers, D. G., Bannan, L. T., Beevers, M. and Stewart, V. L. (1985). Similarity of blood pressures of blacks, whites and Asians in England. *Journal of Hypertension*, **3**, 365–71.

Dogra, J. R. (1941). Studies on peptic ulcer in South India, part IV: Incidence of peptic ulcer in India with particular reference to South India. *Indian Journal of Medical Research*, **29**, 665–76.

Donaldson, L. J. and Clayton D. G. (1984). Occurrence of cancer in Asians and non-Asians. *Journal of Epidemiology and Community Health*, **38**, 203–7.

Donaldson, L. J. and Taylor, J. B. (1983). Patterns of Asian and non-Asian morbidity in hospitals. *British Medical Journal*, **286**, 949–51.

Elian, M. and Dean, G. (1987). Multiple sclerosis among the UK-born children of immigrants from the West Indies. *Journal of Neurology, Neurosurgery and Psychiatry*, **50**, 327–332.

Ghosh, S. K. (1984). Prevalence survey of drinking alcohol and alcohol dependence in the Asian population in the UK. In *Alcohol related problems* (ed. N. Krasner, J. S. Madden and R. S. Walker), pp. 179–90. Wiley, Chichester.

Glyn, A. J. and Kane, S. P. (1985). Benign gastric ulceration in a health district: incidence and presentation. *Postgraduate Medical Journal*, **61**, 695–700.

Griffiths, K. K., Raine, D. N. and Mann J. R. (1982). Neonatal screening for sickle haemoglobinopathy in Birmingham. *British Medical Journal*, **284**, 933–5.

Heath, D. A. (1983). Thoughts on the aetiology of vitamin D deficiency in Asians. *Postgraduate Medical Journal*, **59**, 649–51.

Honeybourne, D. (1987). Ethnic differences in respiratory diseases. *Postgraduate Medical Journal*, **63**, 939–42.

Jackson, S. H. D., Bannan, L. T. and Beevers, D. G. (1981). Ethnic differences in respiratory disease. *Postgraduate Medical Journal*, **57**, 777–8.

Javaid, A. and Ayres, J. G. (1988). Asthma in ethnic communities. *Update*, **37**, 295–300.

Karim, A. K. M. B., Elfellah, M. S. and Evans, D. A. P. (1981). Human acetylator polymorphism: estimate of allele frequency in Libya and details of global distribution. *Journal of Medical Genetics*, **18**, 325–30.

Keshavarizian, A., Gupta, S., Saverytmuttu, S. H., and Hodgson, H. J. F. (1986). Are there ethnic differences in inflammatory bowel disease? *Indian Journal of Gastroenterology*, **5**, 95–7.

Lancet (1979). Lactose malabsorption and lactose intolerance. *Lancet*, **ii**, 831–2.

Lancet (1988). Concern over use of mineral clay. *Lancet*, **ii**, 1266.

Leatherdale, B. A., Panesar, R. K., Singh, G., Atkins, T. W., Bailey, C. J. and Bignell, A. H. C. (1981). Improvement in glucose tolerance due to *momordica charantia* (*Karela*). *British Medical Journal*, **282**, 1823–4.

Lowry, P. J., Glover, D. R., Mace, P. J. E., and Littler W. A. (1984). Coronary artery disease in Asians in Birmingham. *British Heart Journal*, **52**, 610–13.

Marmot, M. G., Adelstein, C. M., and Bulusu, L. (1984). Lessons from the study of immigrant mortality. *Lancet*, **i**, 1455–7.

Mather, H. M. and Keen H. (1985). The Southall Diabetes Survey: prevalence of known diabetes in Asians and Europeans. *British Medical Journal*, **291**, 1081–4.

Matheson, L. M., Dunnigan, M. G., Hole, D. and Gillis, C. R. (1985). Incidence of colo-rectal, breast and lung cancer in a Scottish Asian population. *Health Bulletin*, **43**, 245–9.

Mayberry, J. F. (1985). Some aspects of the epidemiology of ulcerative colitus. *Gut*, **26**, 968–74.

McAvoy, B. R. and Raza, R. (1988). Asian women: (ii) Contraceptive services and cervical cytology. *Health Trends*, **20**, 14–17.

McKeigue, P. M. and Marmot, M. G. (1988). Mortality from coronary heart disease in Asian communities in London. *British Medical Journal*, **297**, 903.

McKeigue, P. M., Marmot, M. G., Syndercombe Court, Y. D., Cottier, D. E., Rahman, S. and Riemersma, R. A. (1988). Diabetes, hyperinsulinaemia, and coronary risk factors in Bangladeshis in east London. *British Heart Journal*, **60**, 390–6.

McNicol, W. W. and Luce, P. J. (1985). Sarcoidosis in a racially mixed community. *Journal of the Royal College of Physicians*, **19**, 179–83.

Melikian, V. (1981). Adult Asian osteomalacia. *Postgraduate Medical Journal*, **57**, 784–6.

Morrison-Smith, J. and Cooper S. M. (1981). Asthma and atopic disease in immigrants from Asia and the West Indies. *Postgraduate Medical Journal*, **57**, 774–6.

Odugbesan, O. and Barnett, A. H. (1985). Asian patients attending a diabetic clinic. *British Medical Journal*, **290**, 1051–2.

O'Hare, A. E., Uttley, U. S., Belton, N. R., Westwood, A., Levin, S. D. and Anderson, F. (1984). Persisting vitamin D deficiency in the Asian adolescent. *Archives of Diseases in Childhood*, **59**, 766–70.

Partridge, M. R., Gibson, C. J. and Pride, N. B. (1979). Asthma in Asian immigrants. *Clinical Allergy*, **9**, 489–94.

Peach, H., Compston, J. and Vedi, S. (1983). Value of the history in diagnosis of histological osteomalacia among Asians presenting to the NHS. *Lancet*, **ii**, 1347–9.

Peterson, D. B., Dattani, J. T., Baylis, J. M. and Jepson E. M. (1986). Dietary practices of Asian diabetics. *British Medical Journal*, **292**, 170–1.

Potter, J. F., Terry, P., Dawkins, D. M. and Beevers, D. G. (1983). Breast cancer in blacks, whites and Asians in Birmingham. *Postgraduate Medical Journal*, **59**, 661–3.

Potter, J. F., Dawkins, D. M., Pandha, H. S., and Beevers D. G. (1984). Cancer in blacks, whites and Asians in a British Hospital. *Journal of the Royal College of Physicians*, **18**, 231–5.

Raheja, B. S. (1987). Ghee, cholesterol and heart disease. *Lancet*, **ii**, 1144.

Samanta, A. and Burden, A. C. (1986). Prevalence of non-insulin dependent diabetes mellitus (NIDDM) in Asian Indians. *Clinical Science*, **70** (suppl. 13), 19.

Samanta, A., Burden, A. C., Feehally, J. and Walls, J. (1986). Diabetic renal disease: differences between Asian and white patients. *British Medical Journal*, **293**, 366–7.

Sharma, M. P. and Sarin, S. K. (1985). Ulcerative colitis in a North Indian Hospital: current trends. *Journal of the Royal College of Physicians*, **19**, 99–102.

Shaunak, S., Colston, K., Ang, L., Patel, S., and Maxwell, J. D. (1985). Vitamin D deficiency in adult British Hindu Asians: a family disorder. *British Medical Journal*, **291**, 1166–8.

Stewart, J. S., Roberts, P. D. and Hoffbrand, A. V. (1970). Response of dietary vitamin B_{12} deficiency to physiological oral doses of cyanocotalamin. *Lancet*, **ii**, 542–5.

Tovey, F. I. and Tunstall, M. (1975). Duodenal ulcer in black populations south of the Sahara. *Gut*, **16**, 564–76.

Varma, R. A. (1969) Peptic ulcer in developing countries. In *After vagotomy* (ed. J. A. Williams and A. G. Cox), pp. 382–395 Butterworth, London.

Wadia, N. H. (1973). An introduction to neurology in India. In *Tropical Neurology* (ed. J. D. Spillane), pp. 25–36. Oxford University Press, Oxford.

WHO (World Health Organization) (1982) *Cancer incidence in five continents*. Vol IV (ed. J. Waterhouse, C. Muir, K. Shammugarathan and J. Powell). WHO, Lyon.

10 Women's health

Brian McAvoy

Introduction

Roles and attitudes are culturally determined, as are health beliefs. All these factors have considerable influence on women's health, their medical problems, and their utilization of health services. In Asian culture women are traditionally chiefly responsible for the comfort of their families, the upbringing and moral education of the children and the atmosphere and conduct of the home. Among Hindus, Muslims, and Sikhs behaviour between the sexes in public is influenced by a strong code of etiquette. Traditional female virtues such as decorum and modesty remain important to most Asian women. It is also traditional for men and women not to mix socially, and to be generally segregated from puberty (Henley 1983). The attitudes and behaviours summarized above will obviously vary considerably among Britain's Asians, depending on factors such as length of domicile in this country, social and educational background, geographical origins, and religious beliefs. For example, the role, duties, and rights of women are clearly defined in the Quran, and traditional Muslims practise purdah or physical seclusion of women from all men except very close relatives. By contrast, Sikh women were among the first Asian women in Britain to take up employment outside their homes.

Utilization of some health services by Asian women is poor. Uptake of cervical cytology, for example, is low (McAvoy and Raza 1988); but immunization rates for children are higher in Asians than non-Asians (Bhopal and Samim 1988; Baker *et al*. 1984). This may relate to the known lower rates of literacy in English among women (Brown 1984); but may also reflect the patriarchal structure of the traditional Asian family. Giving priority to the care of the husband and children may result in relative neglect of a woman's health.

Contraception

Little information is available nationally on the contraceptive practices and needs of the Asian population. Most national surveys on contraceptive usage do not provide data on ethnic background (Bone 1973, 1978; Dunnell 1976; OPCS 1985). Ann Cartwright's (1976) national study of family size and family spacing revealed marked differences in the contraceptive practices of Asians and non-Asians. Of mothers born in India or Pakistan, 33 per cent were using no contraception, 26 per cent the pill, and 21 per cent the sheath. Corresponding figures for mothers born in England and Wales were 9 per cent, 44 per cent and 23 per cent respectively. A survey of the domiciliary family-planning service in the London borough of Haringey from 1968 to 1976 (Christopher 1987) showed that among married Asians the IUCD was more popular than the sheath, which was in turn more popular than the pill. In contrast, unmarried Asians preferred the pill to the coil. In both these surveys, however, Asians constituted less than 5 per cent of the total study populations.

A small survey of 100 Bedford mothers (Beard 1982), which included 46 Punjabis and Bengalis, showed that the pill was more popular than the IUCD with the Asians, although nearly one-third of them were using no contraception at all. In Glasgow Rashid (1983) studied contraceptive use among 60 Asian women attending a family planning clinic. The sheath was by far the most popular method (53.3 per cent), followed by the IUCD (18.3 per cent) and the pill (11.7 per cent). She also found that the women tended to be directed almost entirely by their husbands in their choice of method. A similar study of 112 Asian women attending the antenatal and postnatal departments of a Leicester maternity hospital (Zaklama 1984) found that 40 per cent of them showed little or no understanding of the words 'family planning'. Among the 60 who had used contraception, the most popular method was the sheath, followed by the pill.

Not surprisingly the results of these studies on highly selected populations have been conflicing. Only one representative community-based study (McAvoy and Raza 1988) has been carried out, but this was confined to a single city, Leicester. Over 22 per cent of the city's population are of Asian descent or origin, and in 1986 they accounted for 33 per cent of all births in the city (OPCS 1987). Just under 30 per cent of Leicester's Asians were born in the United Kingdom, with half the remainder originating from the Indian subcontinent and half from East Africa. Nearly two-thirds are Hindus, with roughly equal numbers of Muslims and Sikhs among the remainder. The main findings of this survey were:

- 83 per cent of women approved of contraception, and 70 per cent had used it at some time.
- The most popular methods were the IUCD (33 per cent), the sheath (31 per cent), and the pill (26 per cent) (Table 10.1).
- Hindus favoured the IUCD most and the sheath least (Table 10.2).
- Muslims and Sikhs preferred the sheath to the IUCD (Table 10.2).
- Religion did not appear to be a bar to acceptance of or use of contraception.
- Knowledge of contraception varied considerably, but 75 per cent were satisfied with their present method.
- 73 per cent stated they had been able to get family-planning information as easily as they had wished.
- If seeking contraceptive advice 83 per cent would prefer a female doctor, but only 22 per cent would prefer an Asian doctor.
- Alternative service provision, such as a domiciliary service and an all-Asian

clinic, received limited support; but 82 per cent favoured an all-female clinic.

- Over half suggested improvements in contraceptive services, including provision of interpreters, information at the workplace, and production of more leaflets.

Table 10.1 *Methods of contraception in married women*

Method	Asian women Leicester (1985–86)		All women Great Britain (1983)		Significance
	No.	%	No.	%	
IUCD	53	33	224	8	$P < 0.001$**
Sheath	49	31	543	20	$P < 0.01$**
Pill	42	26	767	29	Not significant**
Female sterilization	10	6	447	17	$P < 0.001$**
Withdrawal	3	2	192	7	$P < 0.01$***
Safe period	1	1	64	2	Not significant***
Cap	0	0	64	2	$P < 0.05$***
Spermicides	0	0	32	1	Not significant***
Vasectomy	0	0	447	17	$P < 0.001$***
Base = 100%	158		2653*		

*Percentages add to more than 100 because of rounding and because some women used more than one method.
**Chi-square test.
***Fisher's exact test. The p value quoted is twice the one-tailed value.
Source: McAvoy and Raza 1988

Table 10.2 *Methods of contraception in different religious groups (n = 158)*

Religion	Sheath %	Pill %	IUCD %	Female sterilization %	Withdrawal %	Safe period %
Hindu	23	27	41	6	2	1
Muslim	42	25	23	10	2	0
Sikh	44	31	25	0	0	0
All women	31	26	33	6	2	1

Source: McAvoy and Raza 1988

Decisions on contraception are shaped by a number of factors—individuals' experience and future plans, the influence of peer groups, economic factors, and media publicity. Religious and cultural factors also play their part. For example, many Asian women use only one hand (the left) to touch the genital area. Attempting to insert a cap or spermicidal pessaries under these conditions poses considerable practical problems, and may well explain the relative unpopularity of these methods. Moreover, such factors may have effects in indirect and unexpected ways—for example, by emphasizing the importance of sperm, or attaching taboos to menstruation (Fuller 1987).

All the studies highlight the necessity for tailoring contraceptive services to the needs of local populations and showing sensitivity and understanding in dealing with individuals. For example, in families where husbands or older women are central to decision-making it is important to involve them in discussions about family planning.

Improving such services for ethnic minorities will also improve services for the majority, by improving skills in eliciting patients' beliefs and fears and in communicating, thus leading to more responsive and flexible services (Fuller 1987).

Sterilization and abortion

In general, sterilization and abortion are both disapproved of, especially by Muslims. Abortion is explicitly forbidden by the Quran:

> You shall not kill your children for fear or want. We will provide for them and for you. To kill them is a great sin.
>
> Quran, Chapter 17

If a woman has had to undergo abortion on medical grounds she will require considerable support afterwards to overcome feelings of guilt and remorse. From the limited information available, when sterilization is performed it is usually on the female partner—probably a reflection of the patriarchal structure of many Asian families.

In many societies, the birth of a son is seen as a greater blessing than that of a daughter. This is particularly so in the Indian subcontinent. Inheritance of land occurs through the male line. Sons can help with work on the farm, are expected to provide care and support for parents in their old age, and, amongst Hindus, are required to perform the death rites for parents. With such high value being placed on male children it is perhaps not surprising that prenatal sex determination and abortion have been seen as a means of enhancing the chances of having a son. In one study of 1000 terminations of pregnancy in India 97 per cent of the fetuses were female. Consequently in 1987 the government of Maharashtra in Bombay introduced legislation to ban prenatal sex-determination tests (Pandya 1988). There has been evidence of consultant obstetricians in the United Kingdom being approached by Asian patients requesting gender abortions. The Department of Health policy on this is clear—abortion solely on the grounds of unwanted fetal sex (gynicide) is illegal under the 1967 Abortion Act (Hansard 1988). In exceptional circumstances, however, it may be decided that continuing with the pregnancy would involve risk of injury to the mental health of the woman greater than if the pregnancy were terminated, thus complying with Clause 2 of the Act.

Sexual dysfunction

No figures are available on the prevalence of sexual dysfunction in Asian couples in the United Kingdom, but small descriptive studies have been published from psychosexual clinics. Bhugra and Cordle (1986) described 32 Asians couples attending the sexual dysfunction clinic in Leicester, a city where the Asian population is largely composed of Gujarati-speaking Hindus. The commonest male problems presented were erectile dysfunction (87 per cent) and premature ejaculation (61 per cent), the commonest female problems lack of interest (78 per cent) and dyspareunia (67 per cent). Christopher (1986) worked with two different groups (57 couples or individuals) at two psychosexual clinics in London. One clinic dealt with a poorer section of the Asian community, mainly Bangladeshis. Here male problems predominated, mainly premature ejaculation and secondary impotence, and successful outcome was rare. The other clinic dealt with a more educated and sophisticated group (mainly from East Africa, Pakistan, and India). Female problems predominated in this clinic, mainly non-consummation and non-responsiveness, which responded well to an eclectic approach, resulting in a 65 per cent success rate. In all three clinics, however, the drop-out rate was high—44 per cent in Leicester and about one-third among the men in London. This may have been due to 'loss of face' in a predominantly patriarchal culture, and a reluctance to explore emotional problems, or may have been related to seeing a female doctor, which may not be as acceptable to Asian men as to Asian women (Christopher 1986).

Bhugra and Cordle found that many of their patients seemed to insist on an organic explanation for the dysfunction, adding to the frustration of the therapist—and patients. They also felt that Asian couples were poorly motivated, thereby reducing the likelihood of a successful outcome. In both London clinics family problems, usually with in-laws, resulting in marital problems, were common, and great anxiety was expressed about confidentiality, lest the family discover the problem.

Cultural expectations affect attitudes to sex, which in turn influence sexual behaviour and also sexual dysfunction. Awareness of issues such as the cultural importance of sperm as a 'vital fluid', and the semen-losing syndrome (*Dhat* or *Jiryan*) is essential for the practitioner's understanding of problems which Asian patient may bring to him. Further discussion on this is contained in Chapter 17.

Cervical cytology and cervical cancer

Uptake of cervical cytology among Asian women seems to be poor. One study (McAvoy and Raza 1988) has shown that only 35 per cent of 309 women eligible for cytology reported ever having had a smear, a figure subsequently verified by cross-checking with the cytology laboratory. This low uptake, approximately half that of the indigenous population, applied equally to all three main religious groups. In this study only half the women (a random sample aged between sixteen and fifty years) knew what a cervical smear was, and over three-quarters were unaware how often a woman should normally have a test. When asked why they had never had a cervical smear, over half the women gave reasons related to lack of knowledge or awareness, with only a few stating religious or cultural reasons (Table 10.3). In a follow-up study to compare the effect of different health-education interventions on the uptake of cervical cytology, viewing a short multilingual videotape at home was found to be very effective in persuading women to attend for cervical smears (McAvoy, 1989). Indeed, the home video has been suggested as a particularly appropriate method of circulating health-education information amongst Asians, since watching films is known to be a popular pastime in the Asian community (Donaldson 1986), one study having shown that 81 per cent of women either possesed their own video or had easy access to one (McAvoy and Raza 1988). Health education is discussed further below.

Table 10.3 *Reasons given for never having had a cervical smear (each woman may have given more than one reason)*

Reason	%
Didn't know what smear was	27
Didn't need one	22
Couldn't be bothered	16
Didn't know where to go	8
Frightened	8
Dislike of internal examinations	7
Husband disagreed	5
Others	7
Number of women = 198	100

Source: McAvoy and Raza 1988

Cervical cancer is by far the commonest malignancy in women in the Indian subcontinent, with a crude incidence rate in 1975 of 24 in every 100 000 women (Parkin *et al.* 1984). This is one-and-a-half times the current incidence rate in England and Wales. A study of the Asian population of Natal in South Africa

(77 per cent Hindu, 16 per cent Muslim), who have been resident there as a community for over a hundred years, demonstrated a greater incidence of cervical cancer in both groups compared with England and Wales (Schonland and Bradshaw 1968). Detailed, large-scale comparative studies have not been conducted in the United Kingdom. A study of immigrants in England and Wales, based on census data and death certification (Marmot *et al*. 1984*a*), found a standardized mortality ratio of 115 for cervical cancer in those from the Indian subcontinent. Their figures, however, contained a significant number of women of British descent, and these alone accounted for the excess deaths. When these are extracted, the proportional mortality ratio (PMR) for Indian immigrants is 69. (Marmot *et al*. 1984*b*.) A further study of causes of deaths in immigrants from the Indian subcontinent (Balarajan *et al*. 1984) showed that Muslims have a particularly low PMR (19) for cervical cancer.

A smaller study (Donaldson and Clayton 1984), comparing cancer registrations in Asians and non-Asians over seven years in Leicestershire (62 per cent Hindu, 18 per cent Muslim, and 17 per cent Sikh), estimated a standardized registration ratio (SRR) of 1.20 for cervical cancer. Interestingly, many of these Asians originated from East Africa, where their communities, like those in Natal, had been resident for over a hundred years. They were therefore not representative of the majority of the Asian population, who migrated directly from the Indian subcontinent in the 1960s and 1970s. Furthermore, in the west of Scotland cancer of the cervix has been estimated to be four times commoner in the Asian than in the indigenous population, with an incidence rate much closer to that found in Bombay (Matheson *et al*. 1985). The numbers in this study, however, were very small.

By contrast in Bradford (70 per cent Muslim, 15 per cent Hindu), Barker (personal communication) has demonstrated an SRR of 14 for *in situ* cancer of the cervix, and 42 for invasive cancer. The overall picture is therefore not clear, once again reflecting the heterogeneous nature of Britain's Asian community. The reported lower uptake of cervical cytology, however, could have serious consequences in future years for Britain's Asian women.

Breast cancer

Age-adjusted incidence and mortality rates for breast cancer are highest in Western Europe, the United States, Canada, Australia, and New Zealand, intermediate in Eastern and Southern Europe, and lowest in Asia, Latin America, and Africa (Waterhouse *et al*. 1976). The incidence in Japan and other Asian countries (but not India) increases to a perimenopausal plateau, but declines progressively thereafter, in contrast to the continuing increase among older women in Western countries. This suggests that environmental factors play a more important role in the aetiology of postmenopausal breast cancer, whereas genetic, endocrinological, and other endogenous factors strongly influence the premenopausal disease

(Petrakis *et al.* 1982). Daughters of European immigrants to the USA reach the incidence rates of daughters of American-born parents within one generation; whereas Japanese women appear to require more than one generation. We do not know whether this is the case with Asians coming to Britain. There are no ethnic national figures for breast cancer available in Britain, but local studies have confirmed a lower incidence among Asians.

In the west of Scotland breast cancer has been estimated to be about half as common in the Asian as in the indigenous population, with an incidence rate much closer to that found in Bombay (Matheson *et al.* 1985). As with cervical cancer, however, the numbers in this study were very small. Donaldson and Clayton (1984), studying cancer registrations in Asians and non-Asians over seven years in Leicestershire, estimated a standardized registration ratio of 0.65 for breast cancer.

Potter *et al.* (1983, 1984) used Hospital Activity Analysis over twelve years to conduct a retrospective study of cancers in blacks, whites, and Asians attending a Birmingham hospital. Of 883 women recorded as having breast cancer only 17 (1.9 per cent) were Asian, and 30 (3.4 per cent) black. The Asians, however, presented at an earlier age compared to whites, but had more advanced disease. This may simply be a reflection of the younger age-distribution of Asians in this population, but could also be related to their higher parity and lower rate of breast-feeding. A similar trend has been suggested by an exploration of breast-cancer registrations in Leicestershire (H. Botha—personal communication). The UK National Breast-Screening Programme is aimed at women aged between fifty and sixty-four; but among Asians this is not the age-group in which the disease in commonest. Consequently it has been suggested that it may be prudent to target a lower age-group amongst Asians (Potter *et al.* 1983).

Child rearing

This section will cover three areas:

(a) postnatal rites and customs;
(b) infant feeding; and
(c) family systems.

(a) Postnatal rites and customs

These may vary according to religion, and have been described by Henley (1979). Muslim babies must be bathed as soon as possible after birth, and a male relative should whisper the call to prayer in the baby's ear. Among Hindus the father or another male relative should place honey or ghee on the baby's tongue. In some families this should be done before the father sees the child's face. Certain words from the *Guru Granth Sahab* should be whispered in the ear of a Sikh baby.

Traditionally a mother should have a forty days' rest to recuperate from the birth. During this time she will be excused from many of her household duties, including cooking. She will be encouraged to eat 'hot' foods if she is breast-feeding. After forty days she will have a purifying bath, accompanied by prayers, and then resume her normal duties (Henley 1979).

(b) Infant feeding

Breast-feeding is accepted practice in the Indian subcontinent, but is disappointingly uncommon among Asian mothers in the United Kingdom (Goel *et al.* 1978; Williams *et al.* 1985). This is probably due to a variety of reasons, including a belief that bottle-feeding is modern and somehow superior, concerns about privacy and modesty, and communication difficulties with health professionals who could provide support in hospital and at home in the critical early days and weeks, when problems often arise. The attitudes of husbands and other family members can also be very influential. In a sample of 206 Asian children in Glasgow Goel *et al.* (1978) found that nearly 80 per cent were bottle-fed. Most mothers did not wish to breast-feed, because of wrong information or misconceptions about British infant-feeding practices.

There is a belief amongst many Hindus and Sikh mothers that colostrum is harmful, resulting in breast-feeding's being delayed for two or three days until the milk 'comes in'. This should not be interpreted as indicating a desire not to breast-feed at all. With encouragement and support and the use of glucose feeds, lactation can be established while still respecting women's cultural beliefs.

Breast-feeding is regarded as a 'cold' condition by some mothers (see Chapter 8), and therefore needs to be balanced by the addition of 'hot' foods to the mother's diet.

Because Asian babies, especially those of Hindu mothers, tend to be 'light for dates', it is important not to be over-concerned about 'catching up', and not to encourage complementary feeds which may result in suppression of lactation.

In the Indian subcontinent weaning tends to occur at a much later stage than in Britain, often after the child is one or two years old. Consequently careful explanation is required by health professionals, so that Asian mothers may understand the reasons for recommending earlier weaning. It is also important, where appropriate, to suggest foods which are compatible with traditional practices (Karseras and Hopkins 1987). This allows mothers to introduce solids which are eaten by the rest of the family, saves time and effort, and avoids proprietary baby foods, which can be expensive and break religious dietary rules. For example, many proprietary baby foods contain meat extracts, which would not be acceptable to many Asians. Indeed, some artificial milk feeds, such as SMA, contain beef fat. Further details on these are given in Chapter 13.

(c) Family systems

The traditional extended family of the Indian subcontinent contrasts markedly with the British nuclear family, reflecting differing attitudes to roles, responsibilities, and authority. British health professionals must avoid imposing ethnocentric views of 'normal' family life on their Asian patients, and should learn to work with these different systems rather than against or despite them. Topics requiring particular sensitivity and understanding include moral responsibility and obligations, arranged marriages, and family honour.

In the Indian subcontinent pregnancy is often viewed as a high-risk activity, and women are accorded special treatment before and after the birth, and encouraged to rescind many of their everyday responsibilities. Adhering to such customs can be difficult in Britain, since many women may have to go out to work when pregnant, and may not enjoy extended-family support networks. Indeed, Asian women can be caught between two cultures, and the period of child-bearing and rearing can be particularly traumatic. This is a time of life when many women, irrespective of their ethnic background, feel particularly vulnerable. For Asian women, especially, problems of communication, isolation, loneliness, and cultural conflicts can be compounded by feelings of guilt and inadequacy.

A powerful description of such problems is contained in Amrit Wilson's book *Finding a voice: Asian women in Britain* (1978). It begins with a poem, *The Prisoner*, by Amiya Rao, which describes the life of a Bengali woman as related by her sari 'shut up tight in a cheap tin trunk, hidden under a mountain of musty mattresses and torn quilts cast away in the kitchen's sooty corner':

> Days have passed become months become years
> Alone in the darkening shadow sits she musing
> —Life is nothing only tears—
> 'You are right', whispers the sari, all in tatters,
> —Life is nothing only tears'.

Those wishing to learn more about Asian family life are referred to Ballard (1979) and Henley (1979).

Women as carers

The burden of caring for sick, handicapped, or elderly individuals tends to fall disproportionately on women. The added responsibilities of the extended family may place extra pressures on the Asian female carer.

The attitudes of many Asians towards mental and physical handicap are similar to those held in Britain over fifty years ago—guilt and shame (Henley 1979). Instead of accepting medical, physiological, and biological reasons for the child's condition, the parents and members of the family may believe that the handicap is due to bad *karma* (actions and deeds in previous lives). Accepting the child is not usually a problem; it is the guilt feelings that have to be worked through

(Ahmed and Watt 1986). Instead of leaving the fate of such children in the 'hands of God', parents may need much support and encouragement to take positive action in planning the future of their child. Most Asian families show particular care and devotion to handicapped members, and may be resistant to any suggestions of institutional or even respite care.

Handicap is a perception of disability relative to expectations, and therefore is strongly culture-based. As Pearson (1983) has pointed out 'similar conditions and disabilities may be perceived, accepted, and coped with in very different ways as the cultural context varies. This has implications for detection and assessment. Most official developmental milestones relate to white middle-class values . . . and assessments are invariably carried out in English, although it may not be the language spoken in the child's home'. Enlisting the help of a health worker with a working knowledge of Asian languages can avoid errors and under-assessment of developmental progress, especially in the area of language development.

Several studies have found that Asian families have limited understanding of their child's handicap, and inadequate knowledge of available services (Powell and Perkins 1984; Watson 1984; Gulliford 1984). Gulliford also found that Bangladeshi families of children with severe mental handicaps were more deprived and more socially isolated and lacking in social support than white families. As with other services, language can be a major barrier to utilization, and is not simply overcome by using interpreters—'families desperately need a named person who speaks their own language' (Powell and Perkins 1984). One such scheme in Tower Hamlets has involved employing a full-time Bangladeshi worker trained in counselling and child mangement skills as a Parent Adviser (Davis and Choudhury 1988). This individual provides mothers with: someone to talk to, who will listen; social and psychological support; information; someone to accompany them out of the house; child management and developmental advice; referral to other professionals; and social contacts outside the family. She also facilitates other professionals' work with the families by interpreting and explaining on their behalf, and she mediates between family members. The authors concluded that the need for specialist medical, social, thereapeutic, and educational skills is very much secondary to the need to facilitate people's own resources, provide them with general support, and treat them with respect.

Although Britain's Asians are relatively young compared with the indigenous population, the numbers of elderly requiring care and support will grow steadily over the coming years. In Asian families as with the majority population, the main responsibility for caring rests with women.

A recent survey carried out on behalf of the DHSS as part of the General Household Survey 1985 (Green 1988) reported that:

- One in five households contains a carer.
- Two out of three carers look after an elderly person with a physical disability.
- Fifty per cent of carers look after parents or parents-in-law.

• Women are more likely to carry the main responsibility for caring, and to provide personal care, for example bathing.

Donaldson's survey of Leicester's elderly Asians (1986) found that 82 per cent lived in a household with two or more generations. This suggests that the majority of Asian elderly are cared for within the family.

It cannot be assumed, however, that the extended family can always cope with this caring. Recent reports (Glendinning 1982; Moledina 1987) question 'the widely accepted myth' that the self-supporting extended family exists in the form it did in East Africa or the Indian subcontinent.

Socio-economic conditions, such as small houses or women working outside the home, may make it difficult for children to adopt their traditional responsibilities towards their parents, particularly as dependence increases.

There is now a growing body of information regarding the role and needs of informal carers for the elderly within the total population. Much of this information refers to the 'unremitting burden of care' (Anderson 1987), and identifies many of the main needs of carers—recognition of their work, planned respite care, and information about disabilities and services. A network of support groups is spreading throughout the country, and aims to provide advice, information, and support for carers for the elderly.

There is, however, minimal information regarding the extent and nature of informal caring within ethnic minority populations, and in particular about the needs of these carers. Indeed it is possible that the support systems available may be inappropriate or unacceptable to both Asian elders and their carers. Donaldson (1986) found that almost half of the Asian elderly interviewed were unwilling to consider residential care in the situation of the family's being unable to cope. There is evidence that knowledge and use of services is low within the Asian community. A survey of caring facilities for the elderly in Birmingham found a very low usage of community nursing services among Asians (Badger *et al.* 1989). Lack of a shared language makes many day-care and home-help services inappropriate for Asian clients; Asian meals are not always available from the meals-on-wheels service.

The outcome of this is that many of the statutory forms of support which have a direct impact on the lives of carers are inaccessible to Asian carers. In common with white carers, Asian carers need to have a choice about whether to care, and to have information about and access to support if needed. Lack of awareness or misconceptions of cultural factors and religious beliefs on the part of health professionals and lack of information in their preferred language compound the difficulties for Asian carers.

There is no doubt that Asian families want to care for their elderly; but it cannot be assumed that they are always able to care for them.

Clearly policies regarding the care of the elderly need to be orientated towards the family and not the individual alone. Information regarding the caring role and needs of carers within the Asian community, and their attitudes towards support systems both professional and voluntary, will facilitate the planning and delivery of appropriate services. It may also encourage the development of innovative forms of support which would be acceptable to Asian elders and their carers.

Health education

Since women are often the main carers in families, health education materials are commonly directed at them. The issues discussed in this section, however, apply equally to men.

Great sensitivity is required in preparing health education materials and developing programmes for ethnic minorities—it is not merely a matter of translating leaflets into minority languages. Health education is no longer seen simply as a means of 'experts' giving information to the masses, but is increasingly taking on the role of enabling individuals to make more informed choices about their health and health care. This necessitates basing materials on the expressed needs of ethnic minority communities, and not solely on the opinions of 'experts' from the majority community. It is also important to consider differences in health beliefs and attitudes towards service provision, topics which are covered in more detail in Chapter 3.

An attempt was made to evaluate the perceived health-education needs of London's Asian and Afro-Caribbean communities in 1979 (Webb 1982). This was based on monitoring telephone calls received over six months from listeners to two of Radio London's weekly ethnic minority programmes. Individuals were encouraged to ring in after the programmes to consult in confidence with Asian and Afro-Caribbean volunteer health professionals speaking the appropriate language. Interestingly, 60 per cent of the calls were made by men, and the most frequently mentioned concerns were: asthma, hay fever, and breathlessness (13 per cent of all questions); family planning, fertility, infertility and psycho-sexual problems (11 per cent); diabetes (11 per cent); general nutrition and slimming (8 per cent); mental health problems (8 per cent); homoeopathic/herbal treatments (7 per cent); and skin complaints (7 per cent). This list contrasts with the health needs expressed in the medical literature—sickle-cell anaemia, rickets, tuberculosis, and low-birth-weight babies.

The emphasis of current health-education campaigns is more towards community-developed approaches, which demand time, effort, and commitment. They require sensitivity, willingness to listen and to take direction from non-professionals, willingness to learn and to give up one's authority and the security of one's status, and willingness to give up preconceptions and dearly-held beliefs and cherished procedures (Mares *et al.* 1985). Such an approach can avoid the danger to well-intentioned campaigns of being seen as derogatory, racist, or victim-blaming.

Mares *et al.* (1985) have summarized the key elements of successful health education programmes:

- Out-reach work.
- The involvement of health educators from, and of, the community.
- An informal, flexible, and equal, but supportive, relationship between workers and clients.
- Using word-of-mouth networks to inform potential clients of the existence of the service and what it can offer.
- Offering individuals the help, support, and information they request, rather than imposing ideas of what they need.
- Building community support networks stemming from health-related matters.
- Accompanying, supporting, and acting as advocates for individuals in their contacts with the health service and health workers.

With increasing realization of the needs of ethnic minority communities, a number of booklets, leaflets, and videotapes have been produced in different languages. A selection of these, with sources, is described in Appendix 1. Detailed advice on the preparation of written and translated materials is readily available (Mares 1982), dealing with issues such as content, readability, layout, illustrations, and typeface. Examples of different Asian languages and scripts are shown in Fig. 10.1.

Finally, over the years a number of voluntary, self-help, and support groups have developed throughout the country. These are listed with other useful addresses in Appendices 2 and 3, and others relating to specific diseases are described at the end of individual chapters. Appropriate use of such groups can enable the general practitioner to reinforce and extend the advice and support offered to Asian women and their families.

Conclusion

Many health problems suffered by women occur in both sexes, but there are some which are unique to women. Likewise, many health problems suffered by Asian women affect all females, but there are some which are unique to Asians. Moreover, women's health is influenced by numerous factors, many of which are determined by their roles within the family and within society, which in turn are culture-based. Over the past decade or so the predominately male medical profession has become more aware of women's special needs and, hopefully, more sensitive to these. A similar understanding of the life-experiences and social circumstances of Asian women should enable doctors and planners to provide sensitive and appropriate services for this important group.

Patterns of culture and social behaviour are often easy to see from the outside, but may not, to people who know the whole picture from the inside, seem at all accurate. Furthermore you cannot treat individuals on the basis of generalisations about their culture, but you have to know the culture in order to understand the individual brought up within it.

(Henley 1979)

Cervical Smear Test Factsheet

સરવાઇકલ સ્મીયર ટેસ્ટ ની માહિતી પત્રીકા

(Gujarati)

ਬੱਚੇ ਦਾਨੀ ਦਾ ਟੈਂਸਟ । ਸਚਾਈ ਪੱਤੂ

(Punjabi)

सरवाइकल सीअर टेस्ट विवरण पत्र

(Hindi)

بچے دانی کے دہانے کا معائینہ

(Urdu)

স্যারভিকাল স্মিয়ার টেষ্ট

(Bengali)

Fig. 10.1 Examples of different Asian languages and scripts.

References

Ahmed, G. and Watt, S. (1986). Understanding Asian women in pregnancy and confinement. *Midwives' Chronicle and Nursing Notes*, **99**, 98–101.

Anderson, R. (1987). The unremitting burden on carers. *British Medical Journal*, **294**, 73–4.

Badger, F., Cameron, E., Evers, H., Atkin, K., and Griffiths, R. (1989). Why don't general practitioners refer their disabled Asian patients to district nurses? *Health Trends*, **21**, 31–2.

Baker, M. R., Bandaranayake, R. and Schweiger, M. S. (1984). Difference in rate of uptake of immunisation among ethnic groups. *British Medical Journal*, **288**, 1075–8.

Balarajan, R., Bulusu, L., Adelstein, A. M. and Shukla, V. (1984). Patterns of mortality among migrants to England and Wales from the Indian subcontinent. *British Medical Journal*, **289**, 1185–7.

Ballard, C. (1979). Conflict, continuity and change: second generation South Asians. In *Minority families in Britain: support and stress*, (ed. V. S. Khan) pp. 109–129. Macmillan/SSRC, London.

Beard, P. (1982). Contraception in ethnic minority groups in Bedford. *Health Visitor*, **55**, 417–21.

Bhopal, R. S. and Samim, A. R. (1988). Immunisation uptake of Glasgow Asian children: paradoxical benefit of communication barriers? *Community Medicine*, **10**, 215–20.

Bhugra, D. and Cordle, C. (1986). Sexual dysfunction in Asian couples. *British Medical Journal*, **292**, 111–2.

Bone, M. (1973). *Family planning services in England and Wales*. HMSO, London.

Bone, M. (1978). *The family planning services: changes and effects*: a survey carried out on behalf of the DHSS. HMSO, London.

Brown, C. (1984). *Black and white Britain: the third PSI survey*. Heinemann Educational, London.

Cartwright, A. (1976). *How many children?*, pp. 139–44. Routledge and Kegan Paul, London.

Christopher, E. (1986). Sexual dysfunction in Asian couples. *British Medical Journal*, **292**, 341.

Christopher, E. (1987) *Sexuality and birth control in social and community work*, pp. 234–54. Tavistock, London.

Davis, H. and Choudhury, P. A. (1988). Helping Bangladeshi families: Tower Hamlets parent adviser scheme. *Mental Handicap*, **16**, 48–51.

Donaldson, L. J. (1986). Health and social status of elderly Asians: a community survey. *British Medical Journal*, **293**, 1079–82.

Donaldson, L. J. and Clayton, D. G. (1984). Occurrence of cancer in Asians and non-Asians. *Journal of Epidemiology and Community Health*, **38**, 203–7.

Dunnell, K. (1979). *Family formation 1976*. HMSO, London.

Fuller, J. (1987). Contraceptive services for ethnic minorities. *British Medical Journal*, **295**, 1365.

Glendinning, F. (ed.) (1982). *The ethnic elderly: cause for concern*, **Unit 16:3** in Ethnic minorities and social community work E354. Open University, Milton Keynes.

Goel, K. M., House, F. and Shanks, R. A. (1978). Infant feeding practice among immigrants in Glasgow. *British Medical Journal*, **2**, 1181–3.

Green, H. (1988). *Informal carers; General Household Survey 1985*, Series GHS No. 15, supplement A. HMSO, London.

Gulliford, F. (1984). *A comparison study of the experiences and service needs of Bangladeshi and white families with severely handicapped children*. Unpublished dissertation for the Diploma in Clinical Psychology. British psychological Society, Leicester.

Hansard, Commons (1988). **Volume 125**, No. 70, column 140 (12.1.88).

Henley, A. (1979). *Asian patients in hospital and at home*. King's Fund, London.

Henley, A. (1983). *Asians in Britain. Caring for Hindus and their families: religious aspects of care*. DHSS/King's Fund, London.

Karseras, P. and Hopkins, E. (1987). *British Asians—health in the community*. Wiley, Chichester.

Mares, P. (1982). *The Vietnamese in Britain*. Health Education Council/National Extension College, Cambridge.

Mares, P., Henley, A. and Baxter, C. (1985). *Health care in multiracial Britain*. Health Education Council/National Extension College, Cambridge.

Marmot, M. G., Adelstein, A. M. and Bulusu, L. (1984*a*). Lessons from the study of immigrant mortality. *Lancet*, **i**, 1455–7.

Marmot, M. G., Adelstein, A. M. and Bulusu, L. (1984*b*). *Immigrant mortality in England and Wales 1970–78*, Studies on Medical and Population Subjects No. 47. HMSO, London.

Matheson, L. M., Dunnigan, M. G., Hole, D. and Gillis, C. R. (1985). Incidence of colo-rectal, breast and lung cancer in a Scottish Asian population. *Health Bulletin*, **43**, 245–9.

McAvoy, B. R. (1989). *Attitudes to and use of contraception and cervical cytology services amongst Asian women*. Thesis submitted for degree of Doctor of Medicine, Leicester University.

McAvoy, B. R. and Raza, R. (1988). Asian women: (i) Contraceptive knowledge, attitudes and usage. (ii) Contraceptive services and cervical cytology. *Health Trends*, **20**, 11–17.

Moledina, S. (1987) Caring for Asian elders. *Carelink*, **1**, 3–4.

OPCS (Office of Population Censuses and Surveys) (1985). Social Survey Division. *General Household Survey, 1983*. HMSO, London.

OPCS (Office of Population Censuses and Surveys) (1987). Births by birthplace of mother, 1986: local authority areas, OPCS monitor **FMI 87/3**. OPCS, London.

Pandya, S. K. (1988). Yearning for baby boys. *British Medical Journal*, **296**, 1312.

Parkin, D. M., Stjernsward, J. and Muir, C. S. (1984). Estimates of the worldwide frequency of twelve major cancers. *Bulletin of the World Health Organization*, **62**, 163–192.

Pearson, M. (1983). Racism and myths surrounding 'Asian handicap'. *Radical Community Medicine*, **14**, 33–5.

Petrakis, N. K., Ernster, V. L. and King, M. C. (1982). Breast. In *Cancer epidemiology and prevention*, (ed. D. Schottenfeld and J. F. Fraumeni), pp. 855–70. W. B. Saunders, Philadelphia.

Potter, J. F., Dawkins, D. M., Pandha, H. S. and Beevers, D. G. (1983). Breast cancer in blacks, Asians and whites in Birmingham. *Postgraduate Medical Journal*, **59**, 661–3.

Potter, J. F., Dawkins, D. M., Pandha, H. S. and Beevers, D. G. (1984). Cancer in blacks, whites and Asians in a British hospital. *Journal of the Royal College of Physicians*, **18**, 231–5.

Powell, M. and Perkins, E. (1984). Asian families with a pre-school handicapped child—a study. *Mental Handicap*, **12**, 50–2.

Rashid, J. (1983). Contraceptive use among Asian women. *British Journal of Family Planning*, **8**, 132–5.

Schonland, M., and Bradshaw, E. (1968). Cancer in the Natal African and Indian 1964–66. *International Journal of Cancer*, **3**, 304–16.

Waterhouse, J., Muir, C., Correa, P., Powell, J. and Davis, W. (1976). *Cancer incidence in five continents, Vol. III*, IARC Scientific Publications, No. 15. International Agency for Research on Cancer, Lyon.

Watson, E. (1984). Health of infants and use of health services by mothers of different ethnic groups in East London. *Community Medicine*, **6**, 127–35.

Webb, P. A. (1982). Ethnic Health Project, 1979/80. *Journal of the Royal Society of Health*, **102**, 29–34.

Williams, S. A., Fairpo, C. G., Howell, V., Duckworth, C. and Ahmed, I. (1985). Some Asian communities in the UK and their culture. *British Dental Journal*, **91**, 1244–5.

Wilson, A. (1978). *Finding a voice: Asian women in Britain*. Virago, London.

Zaklama, M. S. (1984). The Asian community in Leicester and the family planning services. *Biology and Society*, **1**, 63–9.

Appendix 1

Health education materials for Asians (all are multilingual)

Health Education for Ethnic Minorities. Resource list prepared by the Health Education Authority, July 1987 (address in Appendix 3). Includes books, bibliographies, resource lists, pamphlets, leaflets, posters, charts, notices, films, videos, slides, tapes, and packs.

Community Information (Asian Languages) Directory. Directory of leaflets on health, housing, social services, etc., produced by the Commission for Racial Equality (address in Appendix 3) and the National Association of Citizens' Advice Bureaux.

Directory of Information Material in Non-Asian Languages, produced by Migrant Services Unit of the London Voluntary Services Council, 68 Charlton Street, London NW1 1JR.

Leaflets on pregnancy, breast-feeding, children's diet, food hygiene, vitamin D, immunization, and maternal and child health clinics, available from the Health Education Authority.

A range of training materials including posters, leaflets, and videotapes available through the Asian Mother and Baby Campaign (address in Appendix 2).

Antenatal language kit: to teach English for pregnancy. Written by Judith Nesbitt and published by the Commission for Racial Equality (1979). This describes how to set up and run a course, and contains detailed teaching notes and useful illustrations.

Contraceptive methods leaflets available from the Family Planning Information Service, 27–35 Mortimer Street, London W1N 7RJ. Telephone 01-636-7866. Several Health Authority Health Education Units also produce their own leaflets on contraception and cervical cytology.

Booklet and videotape on the cervical smear test available from Leicestershire Health Authority Health Education Video Unit, Clinical Sciences Building, Leicester Royal Infirmary, PO Box 65, Leicester LE2 7LX. Telephone 0533-550461.

Leaflets on contraceptive methods, cervical cancer, and abnormal smears available from Women's Health information Centre, 52 Featherstone Street, London EC1 8RT. Telephone 01-251-6580.

Booklet on cervical smears and breast self-examination available from Women's Cancer Control Campaign, 1 South Audley Street, London W1Y 5DQ. Telephone 01-499-7532.

Leaflet on the cervical smear cancer campaign available from Sylvia Sheridan, Community Liaison Officer, TV-am, Hawley Crescent, London NW1 8EF. Telephone 01-267-4300.

Leaflets on AIDS available from BBC Local Radio Studios and the British Medical Association, Tavistock House, Tavistock Square, London WC1H 9JR. Telephone 01-387-4499 and from HELP! Office, Thames Television, 149 Tottenham Court Road, London W1P 9LL. Telephone 01-387-9494.

Videotapes on Asian diabetic diet and organ transplantation available from Leicester Health Authority, Health Education Video Unit, Clinical Sciences Building, Leicester Royal Infirmary, PO Box 65, Leicester LE2 7LX. Telephone 0533-550461.

Patient information audiotapes on Depoprovera available from Upjohn Ltd., Fleming Way, Crawley, Sussex RU10 2NJ. Telephone 0293-31133.

Prevention of heart disease leaflet available from Wolverhampton Health Authority Education Department, Brierley Lane, Bilston, West Midlands WV14 8TU.

Action on Asian Coronary Heart Disease videotape available from Concord Video, 201 Felixstowe Road, Ipswich IP3 9BJ.

Question and answers leaflet on eczema available from the National Eczema Society, Tavistock House East, Tavistock Square, London WC1H 9SR. Telephone 01-388-4097.

Leaflet on patient rights available from the Association of Community Health Councils for England and Wales, Mark Lemon Suite, Barclay's Bank Chambers, 254 Seven Sisters Road, London N4 2HZ. Telephone 01-272-5459/5450.

Appendix 2

Voluntary, self-help, and support groups for Asians

Asian Women's Network
London Women's Centre
4 Wild Court
London W2B 5AV
Telephone 01-831-6838

Asian Mother and Baby Campaign
c/o Ms Veena Bahl
Room A505

Alexander Fleming House
Department of Health
Elephant and Castle
London SE1 6BY
Telephone 01-407-5522 Extension 6834.

Asian Women's Resource Centre
27 Southley Street
London SW4 7QF
Telephone 01-274-8854/737-5901

Community Health Group for Ethnic Minorities
London   —13 Macclesfield Street
                    London W1V 7UL
                    Telephone 01-439-8765

Manchester—30 Warwick House
                    Central Avenue
                    Levenshulme
                    Manchester M19 2FF

National Association for Teachers of English as a
Second Language to Adults
Spring Grove Centre
Thornbury Road
Isleworth
Middlesex TW7 4UG
Telephone 01-568-3697 extension 123

Pakistan Women's Welfare Association
20 Blackstock Road
London N4 2DW
Telephone 01-226-4927

Bhamini Akhoonjee
Asian Women's Group
Newham MIND
55 Woodgrange Road
Forest Gate
London E7 0EL
Telephone 01-555-9070

Appendix 3

Other useful addresses
Commission for Racial Equality
10–12 Allington Street
London SE1E 5EU
Telephone 01-828-7022

Health Education Authority
Hamilton House
Mabledon Place
London WC1H 9TX
Telephone 01-631-0930

Hindu Centre
39 Grafton Terrace
London NW5

Muslim information Services
233 Seven Sisters Road
London N4 2DA

National Extension College Trust Ltd
18 Brooklands Avenue
Cambridge CB2 2HN
Telephone 0223-316644

Supreme Council of Sikhs
162 Great West Road
Hounslow
Middlesex

National Health Service Training Authority
St Bartholomew's Court
18 Christmas Street
Bristol BS5 5BT
Telephone 0272-291029
Incorporating Training in Health and Race, an inservice and external training unit to provide consultancy services, training, and resources to health professionals and organizations.

Women's Health Information Centre and Women's Reproductive
Rights Information Centre
52-59 Featherstone Street
London EC1Y 8RT
Telephone 01-251-6580

The Association of Linkworkers
16 Maythorne Avenue
Staincliffe Estate
Batley
West Yorkshire WF17 7DL
Telephone 0924-444540

11 Obstetrics

John MacVicar

Introduction

To be able to provide adequate and efficient medical services to a particular community it is essential to know the groups who make up that community, and the medical and social problems which are prevalent. As mentioned in other chapters, Asians are not a homogeneous group. Comparing the Hindu from Gujarat with the Sikh from the Punjab would be as inappropriate as comparing the English to the Dutch. This is especially so in obstetric practice.

Many of the comments in this chapter are based on experience in Leicestershire, where there are 70 000 Asians, of whom over 60 per cent are Hindu; and of these over half are vegetarians. The data relate to this specific group, and will vary depending on the ethnic group studied.

Communication

In many areas in the country, where there is a high proportion of Asians, more than half the women do not speak English. The ability to converse in English is often related to the degree of integration. Asian women who work, and whose husbands encourage them to mix freely, are able to express themselves in English much better than those, for example many of the Bengali women, who are not encouraged to leave the family environment and do not work other than within the confines of their home.

All patients have difficulty in understanding medical terminology, so that it must be remembered that familiarity with everyday language is unlikely to equip an Asian woman to understand phrases such as 'alpha-feto-protein', 'amniocentesis', 'pelvic examination', or even 'urinary symptoms'. A recent study (Blatchford 1986) confirmed that as many as 80 per cent of Asian women did not understand such terms. Little wonder, then, that the patient does not get the best a service can offer, through lack of understanding. She may be very fearful, and experience a feeling of isolation when coming to a surgery or clinic. If the doctor becomes irritated at being unable to communicate this will only lead to an intensification of these feelings.

Improving communication

The provision of classes in basic English, frequently run concurrently with antenatal classes, is one common approach to providing the Asian woman in pregnancy with greater English-language skills. Unfortunately, it is often the case that women who attend these classes are those who are already well integrated, whereas those who actually would benefit most do not make use of them.

Interpreters are usually available within a hospital setting, mainly coming from the nursing or ancillary staff. The interpreter may speak only one of five or six different languages, which gives rise to difficulty in having available an interpreter with the appropriate language skills at the right time. Attempts to establish clinics exclusively for women in different racial or language groups, in order that interpreters may more readily be made available, are however unlikely to gain widespread acceptance, because, through the process of segregation, they all too easily raise the spectre of racial discrimination.

The concept of the Asian 'link worker', initially funded on an experimental basis with support from the Save the Children Fund and the DHSS, is a more recent development. Link workers, since they must speak English and one other Asian language, are intended to help not only communication between the pregnant Asian patient and the medical services, but also to play a part in health education. Contact is established during pregnancy, and advice given regarding various aspects of care antenatally, with scope to provide guidance on babycare and contraception following delivery. One of the obvious problems of the scheme is the recruitment of link workers with appropriate skills in communication and health education, given the poor renumeration offered for the posts. It may take some time before the precise role of the link worker is identified, but preliminary impressions based on experience in Leicestershire (Mason, in press) are disappointing. Their use has chiefly been as interpreters—not surprisingly, being of most benefit to those patients who did not speak English. The health-education dimension of the posts seems to have been less successful, with most value being gained by those who already speak English and can take advantage of readily available literature. Many Asian women will be registered with an Asian doctor, who can speak their native tongue and can appreciate their particular cultural background. While this may help with the element of shared antenatal care provided in general practice, it is not of immediate benefit to hospital-based services. On the other hand, even the Asian general practitioner may not find it easy to converse with a patient in Bengali if he speaks only Hindi.

A proportion of Asian women especially, those of the Muslim faith, do not find it easy to speak to or be examined by a male doctor, especially when the more intimate examinations necessary in obstetrics and gynaecology require to be performed. A small investigation carried out by the author some years ago with Asian women of different groups attending for booking at the Leicester Royal Maternity Hospital indicated that most women preferred to be examined by a male who could communicate in the appropriate language, rather than a female doctor who could not. This seemed true even if the doctor was a female Asian, but could not speak the necessary dialect.

Social, religious, and dietary considerations in Asian women

A high proportion of pregnant Asian women will never have been employed outside the home, and domestic responsibilities may entail looking after an ageing extended family. This will undoubtedly involve them in considerable physical exertion, even in the late stages of pregnancy. While it is often the custom in India for the pregnant patient to go back to her own 'family circle' during pregnancy and lead a 'spoiled' existence, in the Asian community in Britain this often cannot take place. The patient with morning sickness hardly wants to prepare food for herself, far less be involved in the preparation of food for a large household. Little wonder that hyperemesis gravidarum is more frequently found in Asian women, especially if recently married.

In regions of high unemployment, the Asian male may find it difficult to get work unless he has some specialist training. Those Asian women who are used to working outside the home, on the other hand, can more readily find employment in the textile or knitwear industry, and may become the sole bread-winner in the family. Naturally, during pregnancy they are reluctant to stop work, usually carrying on until late in pregnancy; and this will be combined with heavy domestic responsibilities. It has been found in such groups of women, especially those with a poor socio-economic background to begin with, that the perinatal mortality maybe as high as three times that which would normally be expected (see Tables 11.1 and 11.2).

Table 11.1 *Risk factors in pregnant Asian women known at first clinic visit*

	%
Age over 36	361
Height under 150 cm	210
Manual worker	200

(Risk as a percentage with 100 being average)
Source: Leicestershire Perinatal Mortality Study: unpublished findings

Dietary habits may affect the health of the mother in pregnancy, thought it is agreed universally that actual diet in pregnancy has little effect on the outcome for the fetus, and that too-specific dietary interventions may do more harm than good. The relationship between the higher perinatal mortality found in Hindu vegetarian mothers in Leicester (MacVicar 1982) compared with complications found in similar groups in Harrow in London (Haines *et al.* 1982) is a reflection of socio-economic conditions not only at the present time but also historically. Moreover, patients who are vegetarian must find the diet relatively expensive if they have to keep to more than 2000 KCal or 60 g protein, which is the minimum recommended in pregnancy. As well as general considerations, the practitioner concerned with obstetric care should also be aware of the religious group to which the patient belongs. Religious beliefs may have a bearing on whether antenatal investigations for fetal abnormality should be pursued, especially if termination of pregnancy could be the suggested end result.

Table 11.2 *Risk factors in perinatal deaths, work, and dietary habits Leicestershire 1978–83*

	Vegetarian	Non-vegetarian	Total
Working	320	170	210
Not working	170	100	110
Total	240	130	150

(Risk as a percentage with 100 being average)
Source: Leicestershire Perinatal Mortality Study: unpublished findings

The Asian woman's first pregnancy is often the early result of an arranged marriage. In any culture to adjust to pregnancy and a marriage may take some time. Added to this the Asian woman and/or her husband may be in a completely strange environment, and the misery of a concomitant of pregnancy such as morning sickness may prove the 'last straw' to the already depressed patient.

Care prior to pregnancy

Pre-pregnancy counselling in the Asian community does not meet with any more success than it does in others. Exceptions are insulin-dependent diabetics, who because they have regular review of their diabetic state receive advice regarding good control prior to conception. This may reduce the risk of fetal abnormality, especially if the glycosylated haemoglobin is kept below 8 per cent. Successful obstetric outcome in mothers with diabetes is ensured by good control both immediately before and in the first three months of pregnancy.

Patients with a family history of congenital abnormality, especially if there is also parental consanguinity, should be referred for genetic counselling prior to pregnancy. This is not always readily accepted, because of religious beliefs which may make any form of family limitation undesirable. Counselling regarding screening for fetal abnormality in early pregnancy may also prove unacceptable should it lead to second-trimester termination of pregnancy. Asians who do not find first-trimester termination of pregnancy so difficult to come to terms with from a religious point of view will welcome the introduction of chorion villus sampling. This may ensure termination of pregnancy by suction curettage at a time in pregnancy which is more acceptable to the patient, and does not offend her religious beliefs.

More detailed discussion on different inherited diseases can be found in Chapter 12.

Care during pregnancy

The Asian woman embarking on a pregnancy may well have several advantages over many of her non-Asian sisters. Usually, she does not smoke, does not drink alcohol, and is married. First pregnancies usually occur at a slightly older age in the Asian woman in this country, compared to those occurring in the Indian subcontinent itself. Unfortunately, these potential advantages can be dissipated if the Asian woman is not aware of the benefits of early attendance at an antenatal clinic.

'But I am only half-way through my pregnancy' is frequently the answer when the patient is asked why she has not attended for antenatal care at a stage earlier than twenty weeks; perhaps not surprisingly for someone who has been brought up in a society where the advantages of antenatal care often cannot be fully appreciated. If an Asian woman in pregnancy adopts the behaviour of her mother, aunts, or sisters, she may not appreciate the significance of the fact that they had their pregnancies in a different environment and with different medical services. Nevertheless, it is the experience of those involved with antenatal care that once Asian mothers have attended an appropriate clinic, compliance and further attendance are good. There are a few exceptions, and, for example, those who return to their country of origin for an extended holiday when pregnant will sometimes be the patients who have been found to have a raised serum alpha-feto-protein level; but now further investigations are impossible. This illustration re-emphasizes the importance of good understanding and communication on the part of the doctors and patients, and the need for the doctor to be aware of traditional cultural beliefs and attitudes and for the patient to comprehend the nature and framework of modern obstetric care.

Two key objectives of health-education programmes aimed at Asian women who are, or may become, pregnant are: firstly, to encourage them to come early for care (if possible before three months); and, secondly, to emphasize the importance of continuity of care. It is well known that in any group of women late attendance for antenatal care and defaulting from clinic appointments are associated with a higher than expected perinatal mortality. Dissemination of information by leaflets in all the Asian languages helps; but a face-to-face transmission of the health-education message through either doctors, health workers, or link workers is also very important. A shift in pattern of first referral to antenatal clinics in Leicestershire was found after a clinic was sited within an area where Asian families predominated. It was hoped that the close proximity to the patient's home would encourage her to come earlier for antenatal care. In this respect, the clinic was a failure, and after a few months had to close (MacVicar 1983). Strangely, however, it was not without its benefits, since it seemed to impress on the local general practitioners and their patients the need to come early to hospital antenatal clinics, even if these clinics were not so geographically convenient. A similar outlying clinic started in a socially deprived area (entirely non-Asian) proved a great success, and continues to serve that community (MacVicar 1984). These experiences illustrate the necessity for medical services to adapt to the needs of the population served. The change in pattern of first attendance at antenatal clinics between the Asian and non-Asian patients is seen in Figs. 11.1 and 11.2. If anything the Asian patient now comes earlier than her non-Asian counterpart.

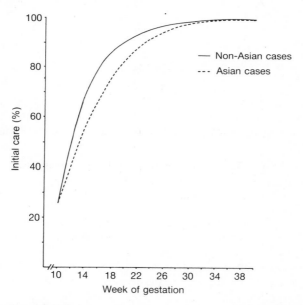

Fig. 11.1 Timing of initial antenatal care by week of gestation in Asian and non-Asian women in Leicestershire 1976–1979.
Source: Leicestershire Perinatal Mortality Study: unpublished findings.

The medical reasons for early attendance at an antenatal clinic are similar to those in any population. Probably as many as 30 per cent of women have some doubt about the date of their last menstrual period, and a clinical check to see if the uterine size corresponds to the dates given is of much more value early on in pregnancy, especially before sixteen weeks. The expected date of delivery can be further clarified by the use of ultrasound to estimate maturity; and thus by dates, clinical examination, and ultrasound an accurate expected date of delivery is calculated. This is of considerable importance in assessing

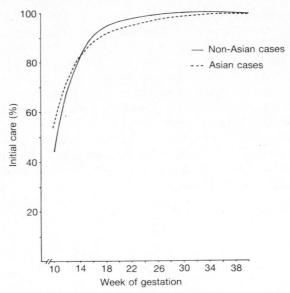

Fig. 11.2   Timing of initial antenatal care by week of gestation in Asian and non-Asian women in Leicestershire 1980–85.
Source: Leicestershire Perinatal Mortality Study: unpublished findings.

the correct time for taking serum alpha-feto-protein, the assessment of growth retardation, should this be suspected later, and the timing of delivery, should pregnancy complications make it necessary.

Screening for fetal abnormality

The estimation of the serum alpha-feto-protein level at sixteen weeks of pregnancy is particularly important, since there may be up to twice the number of babies with neural tube defects in the Asian population as in the indigenous population (MacVicar 1982). However, a full explanation as to why the test is being carried out is essential, because the patient may not, for religious reasons, wish to contemplate termination of pregnancy. Should the serum alpha-feto-protein level be raised the test must be repeated, and if possible a detailed ultrasound scan must be carried out by someone with sufficient expertise to be able as far as possible to exclude a neural tube defect in the fetus. Other abnormalities may be detected at this time in pregnancy by examination of the liquor obtained by amniocentesis at sixteen weeks of pregnancy. As far as chromosomal abnormality and certain other abnormalities referred to in Chapter 12 are concerned amniocentesis may be replaced in the future by chorionic villus sampling (CVS). In order to make use of this latter technique the patient has to go to her general practitioner by about eight weeks of pregnancy, and then be given urgent referral to the nearest centre undertaking CVS. Uncommonly in the Asian mother, should both the parents carry the thalassaemia trait, the baby may suffer from thalassaemia major. A diagnosis can be made by CVS, but if this is impractical a fetoscopy is carried out at sixteen weeks and fetal blood is taken from the cord vessels to ascertain whether the baby is affected or not. Ultrasound is used to diagnose certain cardiac defects in the fetus, but this is usually only appropriate where there is a previous history of a lesion, and the pick-up is comparatively small. Since termination of a pregnancy for fetal abnormality is by choice done before twenty-two weeks of pregnancy it is clear that considerable time is necessary to get all the investigations carried out, and consequently the earlier the patient comes to the antenatal clinic the better.

Antenatal complications

Anaemia is not uncommon in the Asian mother during the antenatal period, especially if she is a vegetarian. It is usually due to an iron deficiency, the consequence of an inadequate diet, so that insufficient iron stores are available to support the increased haematopoiesis and the demands of the fetus. Even if the patient appears not to be anaemic on the basis of a satisfactory haemoglobin level (more than 11 g/dl), it is wise to check the MCV, which, if below 80 fl, signals the possibility of iron deficiency and a fall in haemoglobin to come, if not corrected by iron supplements. Because of the number of vegetarians in the Asian community folic acid deficiency is not commonly found, and may appear only if severe iron-deficiency anaemia is corrected with iron therapy alone without accompanying folic acid. Vitamin B_{12} levels are not infrequently low, especially in vegetarians, but unless these are associated with anaemia, it is not an indication for giving injections of vitamin B_{12}. However, such women have to be followed up in case there is a continuing fall in the vitamin B_{12} levels even after the pregnancy is over.

When the Asian patient is found to be anaemic other complications should be considered. These include the presence of infection, particularly of the urinary tract, which may require treatment before there is an adequate response to iron therapy. Tuberculosis, in particular a pulmonary lesion, should be excluded, as should chronic malaria, especially if the patient is newly arrived in this country or has recently returned from the Indian subcontinent or Africa after a holiday. Intestinal helminths may also cause anaemia owing to small but significant erosions in the gut. The identification of the worms, usually easily seen on microscopic examination of the stools, enables the diagnosis to be confirmed.

The Asian patient with a beta-thalassaemia trait may have a haemoglobin level of about 8–10 g/dl, and no amount of iron therapy will improve this level. In fact, iron therapy may cause a degree of haemosiderosis, and should be avoided if the MCV is over 85 fl. It is important that folic acid supplements are maintained. Should the haemoglobin level be as low as 8.0 g/dl when the patient goes into labour it is worthwhile having two units of blood cross-matched, in case there is undue blood-loss at delivery.

It has been suggested that all pregnant Asian mothers should receive vitamin D supplementation during pregnancy to anticipate the presence of subclinical deficiency, which may affect the fetus later. In the latter, deficiency of vitamin D interferes with growth, and possibly with dentition. It should be remembered that osteomalacia is found infrequently, and reports regarding the value of vitamin D supplements for pregnant Asians have been conflicting. Only rarely does it seem really necessary; but there may be advantages to giving multivite tablets or calciferol to patients who are obviously undernourished, since this therapy is cheap and will certainly do no harm if calciferol dosage is less than 500 i.u. per day. Estimation of vitamin D and calciferol levels in the mother are expensive and can be unreliable.

Hypertensive disease is the commonest complication found in pregnancy in Britain. Pre-eclampsia seems to be more a disease of the Caucasian, since it is met with much less frequently in Asian, Negro, and Chinese racial groups (Doll and Hanington 1961). However, eclampsia may be more frequently encountered in mothers of African origin, which some workers (Doll and Hanington 1961) have postulated is due to differences in arterial response to pregnancy. This concept is interesting, and fits with clinical experience, since in the Asian mother in this country hypertension or pre-eclampsia is certainly not as common as in the Caucasian mother, but when it does occur it is often of the fulminating type. There is also evidence that fetal loss is more common in the Asian mother than in the Caucasian when there is a rise in blood-pressure during pregnancy, whatever the cause. It is obvious, therefore, that an increase in the level of blood-pressure and the appearance of oedema or proteinuria require further investigation and prompt admission to hospital.

During the antenatal period Asian mothers are admitted to hospital more frequently than others. The reason for admission may be 'pain', more often than not abdominal, and must be considered to be due either to premature labour or to a urinary tract infection. Many practitioners are aware that pain is a common generalized symptom in the Asian female—pregnant or not. If there are no obvious localizing signs or evidence of an organic lesion, mention of 'pain' by an Asian woman may be a general expression of concern and worry either related to her pregnancy or her social environment. It is unfortunate that when communication is poor, and 'pain' is repeatedly referred to, the doctor is liable to ignore it or make a misdiagnosis when the symptom is genuine and a serious organic lesion exists.

During the antenatal period the Asian baby *in utero* often feels small, and the possibility of intra-uterine growth-retardation must be considered. Since in some groups of Asians, such as those in parts of Birmingham, fetal death appears to occur in the two weeks before delivery (Settatree *et al.* 1982), it seems reasonable to suspect that these babies may be growth-retarded, and that death is due to placental insufficiency. This has caused many Asian mothers to be subjected to intensive fetal and placental function-monitoring, especially in later pregnancy, and studies derived from this process have yielded interesting data. Excretion of urinary oestriols seem to be lower than would be expected in a Caucasian mother at the same stage in pregnancy, and lower levels of human placental lactogen (HPL) are found in the maternal serum. Similarly, in studies of fetal growth based on ultrasound examinations, the growth of the Asian baby seemed to lag behind the level which would be expected in a Caucasian. However, many Asian babies, though small compared with the average baby in this country, show no signs of being small for gestational age after delivery. Suggestions have been made that tables should be constructed for the Asian population relating oestriol secretion, HPL, and ultrasound growth to different stages in pregnancy for the Asian population. With the total Asian population being so heterogeneous it would be very difficult to obtain meaningful data for each subgroup. It is probably sufficient to use the present tables, such as the Aberdeen data (Thomson *et al.* 1968), for the local population, since the study of the trend between one test and another is what is of most significance; but it should be appreciated, when interpreting results, that the values for the Asian mothers will be lower.

Intra-uterine growth retardation is not the only cause of sudden death *in utero* late in pregnancy. At one time it was thought that the Asian patient in pregnancy was more liable to develop gestational diabetes. However, extensive investigations have shown that, though in pregnancy the Asian mother finds some difficulty in coping with the alteration in carbohydrate metabolism, there is no evidence to suggest an increase in true diabetes or even gestational diabetes in this group of women. However, the possibility of diabetes must be considered if the patient has had a previous unexplained stillbirth or early neonatal death.

There is little justification in withholding induction of labour around term in a patient where intra-uterine growth regardation is suspected. Cardiotocography (CTG) on alternate days may help to reassure the clinician that all is well if there is doubt on dates or induction is liable to be unsuccessful. The use of fetal movement charts may be misleading. Unless the patient understands how to keep such a chart it can lead to unnecessary anxiety if she is given one. Too often bizarre charts are presented, and the patient does not appreciate the significance of movements decreasing, or even ceasing altogether. Whatever happens antenatally, the fetus of the Asian mother must be adequately monitored in labour.

Care during labour

Several factors must be taken into account when labour and delivery is planned in the Asian patient. During the antenatal period she should be encouraged to attend 'preparation for labour' classes; but, as pointed out previously, whether as a result of shyness or of poor communication these are seldom utilized, especially by those who really need them.

Problems of multiparity may occur in certain Muslim groups, especially those from Bengal.

There are important differences in height between the different groups of Asian mothers. In Leicester the shortest and lightest mothers are from the Hindu community, who come originally from Gujarat. They are on average 10–15 cm shorter than the British mother and 10 kg lighter. Within the Asian community the heaviest and tallest mothers are Sikhs who come from the Punjab. Fortunately, although the Hindu mothers are small, their babies are correspondingly smaller than the average baby born in this country. Some workers have suggested that this difference is about 300 g when compared with Caucasian babies born at a similar gestation. Centile birth weights calculated for Aberdeen in the United Kingdom (Thomson *et al.* 1968) can be used for all races, with a 300 g subtraction for Asians. From experience in Leicester it is obvious that birthweights differ considerably even within the Asian community, as well as in the indigenous population (Table 11.3). It is interesting that almost 60 per cent of the Hindu mothers in Leicestershire produce babies who are under 3000 g whereas more than half of other Asian mothers produce babies heavier than this. Fifteen per cent of Hindu babies weigh less than 2500 g. It is also interesting that generally these babies do well in terms of survival. On the other hand when the Bengali mother, who usually produces babies bigger than the Hindu, delivers a baby under 2500 g it does not have as good a chance of survival. This would seem to indicate that the size of the Hindu baby is closer to the norm for that ethnic group, as compared to the Bengali baby, which is lighter than it should be, and possibly suffering from growth-retardation.

Table 11.3 *Breakdown of birthweights in different ethnic and religious groups in Leicestershire 1976–81*

	Hindu (%)	Muslim (%)	Bengali (%)	Sikh (%)	All births in Leicester Royal Infirmary (%)
1500–2000	1.4	0.7	0.5	0.6	1.8*
2001–2500	13.9	9.0	13.5	8.8	5.8
2501–3000	44.1	38.1	31.3	32.6	22.0
3001–3500	31.5	35.8	42.7	39.7	37.4
3501–4000	8.2	14.0	9.2	15.5	24.9
4001+	0.9	2.4	2.7	2.7	8.1

* High figure due to referrals especially for area neonatal intensive care unit

Despite the height of the patient, should her pelvis be clinically adequate, it is always worth allowing her (at least in a first pregnancy) to have a trial of labour. However, despite a successful outcome during a first labour, if the baby is small it should not be taken for granted that the patient will not run into trouble with cephalopelvic disproportion in a subsequent pregnancy, should the baby be bigger or the head in a different position.

It has been shown that death of the fetus during labour is more common in the Asian mother than in the Caucasian (Clarke *et al.* 1988). This may be due to the fetus being compromised in some way before labour starts, so that the stress of labour is the final insult. As indicated above, this has led to suggestions of earlier delivery by inducing labour at about thirty-eight weeks, or at least at term. There must always be a good indication for induction of labour; and in our present state of knowledge there are no proven reasons for this action in all patients; but careful antenatal CTG monitoring is essential, possibly twice a week. Monitoring fetal well-being during labour, both with CTG and fetal scalp pH, is essential, and early recourse to Caesarean section is advised if there is evidence of fetal distress. The second stage of labour may be shortened by the use of forceps. This will naturally increase the incidence of operative delivery in the Asian mother (Table 11.4). It should not be overlooked that fetal distress in labour can be due to a fetal abnormality, and so an ultrasound scan or an X-ray should be taken before Caesarean section is performed, provided time is available.

Table 11.4 *Instrumental delivery rates for Asians and non-Asians at Leicester Royal Infirmary 1980*

	Asian	Non-Asian
Forceps	21.4%	17.5%
LUSCS	20.3%	11.4%

Because the Asian patient tends to be smaller, and since the fetus withstands labour poorly, forceps delivery should not be undertaken lightly, and the attendant should be satisfied that delivery can be easily accomplished before embarking on such a procedure. Caesarean section, even in the second stage of labour, is preferable to a difficult forceps delivery. It is appropriate to carry out the forceps delivery in theatre, with the patient prepared for Caesarean section, if there is any doubt regarding vaginal delivery.

With regard to the length of labour itself studies carried out in an Asian population in London detected no difference in the total length of active labour, but considered that the length of the latent phase of labour may be somewhat increased (Duignan *et al.* 1975). A low threshold of pain, which makes the early contractions in labour more upsetting for the patient, may account for this. Fear of the unknown plays a part in any patient unprepared for labour. This state of affairs may continue until the mothers are adequately prepared antenatally for labour. The degree of pain experienced early in labour increases the need for epidural anaesthesia, and this subsequently increases the operative delivery rate. Another London study (Studd *et al.* 1982) noted that the rate of Caesarean section in the Asian patient was almost double that in the Caucasian. However, as in Leicester (Table 11.4), this may have been related to the particular groups of Asians and Caucasians under review.

Nevertheless, it must be appreciated that the Asian mother in labour requires careful monitoring, and does have an increased risk of operative delivery. The need for booking for delivery in a specialist unit is obvious.

Perinatal mortality

The perinatal mortality rate may reflect the quality of medical care for a patient. If this is the case national data on perinatal mortality for ethnic groups would indicate that the quality of care for the Asian mother is considerably poorer than that for the Caucasian (see Chapter 6). Fig. 11.3 shows the difference in perinatal mortality in Leicestershire between Asians and non-Asians. Only in 1986 has the rate been similar. It is almost certain that further variations between the rates will occur. Adverse perinatal mortality rates probably exist throughout the country, and local initiatives should be used in order to identify these and the possible reasons for them. The causes of perinatal deaths have been simplified by Wigglesworth (1980) into more or less four main groups: those due to congenital malformations; those where death takes place *in utero* prior to labour; those due to asphyxia in labour; and those where the baby dies of immaturity.

A study of the causes of perinatal death in the Asian mother compared to the Caucasian in Leicestershire is illuminating (Table 11.5). Deaths from immaturity are not over-represented. The preponderance in the Leicestershire Asian population of Hindus, who, as indicated above, have a higher proportion of smaller babies compared to other religious groups, may be relevant in that these are not truly babies who are small for gestational age, but rather are babies who are normal for maternal size.

Because of the slightly increased risk of congenital malformation, any Asian community should have adequate facilities for screening in early pregnancy. Needless to say this may be even more important where there is intermarriage. The advantage of chorionic villus sampling, especially for those in whom first trimester abortions are more readily accepted, has been emphasized. Conditions such as Down's syndrome and other chromosomal abnormalities, haemoglobino-pathies, and some sex-linked disorders, such as muscular dystrophies and certain inborn errors of metabolism, can all be diagnosed by this method. Because of the increased number of neural tube defects found in certain groups of Asian patients, screening for serum alpha-feto-protein at sixteen weeks, and scanning with ultrasound at seventeen to eighteen weeks if indicated, is also to be recom-mended. Steps taken to reduce the incidence of deaths as a result of labour

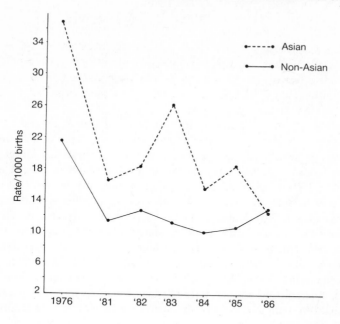

Fig. 11.3 Perinatal mortality rates in Asian and non-Asians in Leicestershire 1976–86.
Source: Leicestershire Perinatal Mortality Study: unpublished findings.

Table 11.5 *Causes of perinatal mortality in non-Asians and Asians in Leicestershire 1976–1982*

	Non-Asian	Asian
Congenital malformations	23.2	24.9
Asphyxia in labour	14.4	17.0
Macerated stillbirth	34.9	36.4
Immaturity	27.4	21.7

Source: Leicestershire Perinatal Mortality Study: unpublished findings

have already been referred to. Fetal death *in utero* remains the major factor in perinatal mortality in all women in this country (Table 11.5).

Perinatal mortality-risk factors

Risk factors for perinatal deaths have been identified within the Leicestershire Asian population, many of which are almost certainly relevant to other Asian mothers. These factors may indicate the patients most in need of careful monitoring, especially if there is a logistical problem in monitoring all pregnancies (Table 11.1).

If the patient is over the age of thirty-five years and Asian she runs more than three times the average risk of a perinatal death. This is not necessarily related to high parity, but may be biased by the comparatively larger number of Bengali women who have their babies at a more advanced age. A maternal height under 150 cm requires careful attention, not only in terms of the pure mechanics of a small pelvis, but also because such patients frequently have experienced poor socio-economic conditions from an early age, which in itself is an adverse factor. Inaccurate as the standards for determining socio-economic status in Great Britain may be, it is well-nigh impossible to apply them to the Asian immigrant community, since many have obviously altered their social and financial status since immigration. As in any group, couples where the husband is unemployed and the wife has never worked must be considered as at high risk. As indicated previously, if the Asian mother is working during pregnancy she may run twice the normal risk of a perinatal death, and this increases to a threefold risk if she is vegetarian or if her husband is unemployed. Mothers who do not work have only a slightly increased risk (Table 11.2). There must be good medical care and adequate social support for those couples who require, for financial reasons, that the wife continues in manual work until late in pregnancy.

Prior-to-labour events can also be pin-pointed which carry with them a substantial degree of risk to the baby (Table 11.6). One of these is the presence of pre-eclampsia, which raises the chance of perinatal death in the Asian mother seven times.

This is possibly related to the effect of pre-eclampsia on the mother, which, although less frequently encountered, has more serious effects when it occurs. Similarly there is a fourfold risk if the patient has had vaginal bleeding during her pregnancy, from whatever cause. This is little different from what is found in other women. It is important to check the gain in weight during pregnancy in the Asian mother, since a poor weight-gain may often indicate poor growth of the baby, with consequent risk of the baby's withstanding the stress of labour badly. Such poor weight-increase seems more relevant to the Asian mother than the Caucasian. If any of these complications is present at the onset of labour it is obvious that unless continuous monitoring of the fetus indicates a healthy fetus the patient should be delivered by Caesarean section. Another interesting factor associated with an increased risk to the baby is the patient's having had repeated hospital admissions, and having spent more than a total of seven days in hospital during her pregnancy, for whatever reason.

Table 11.6   *Risk factors in pregnant Asian women known at onset of labour 1976–85*

Pre-eclampsia	701
Antepartum bleeding	392
Poor weight gain	333
More than 7 days in hospital	574

Source: Leicestershire Perinatal Mortality Study: unpublished findings

Postnatal care

It is disappointing that breast-feeding, which is the usual practice in the East, is not universally practised by Asian mothers in this country. The mother-in-law is not uncommonly the person who undermines the young mother's attempts to establish breast-feeding. She may believe that Western society does not encourage breast-feeding, and that the daughter-in-law should follow the pattern of the country she lives in, especially if problems arise (for further discussion see Chapter 10). Asian patients seem to suffer considerably more pain than Caucasian mothers, both in terms of after-pains and pain from perineal sutures. This is frequently associated with an unwillingness on the part of the patient to become mobile and to look after her own baby. Early mobilization is in contrast to the treatment of the newly delivered mother in the Indian subcontinent, where she is often surrounded by the extended family, and scarcely needs to do anything either for herself or for her new baby. Unfortunately, the association of immobility and venous thrombosis remains pertinent.

Hospitals in this country must seem strange to many Asian patients. Limitation of visiting stops the extended family getting together. A degree of insecurity added to a sense of depressive isolation and combined with postnatal blues may have adverse effects on the young Asian mother, especially if the offspring is female. Hospital meals may also cause her concern, in case they consist of food forbidden by her religious beliefs. The immediate postpartum period is the time to discuss family planning and further pregnancies. At least one in three Asian mothers has had an abdominal or instrumental vaginal delivery, and the chance of a similar happening in a subsequent pregnancy must be explored and explained.

Contraceptive advice is important, and the mother should be made aware of the options open to her. The husbands may be less well motivated. The use of link workers and interpreters, especially if the discussion is in the presence of a female doctor, is often very helpful. More detailed discussion takes place elsewhere regarding contraception (chapter 10).

It must be appreciated that the reaction of the Asian mother should she have a perinatal death may be different to that of her non-Asian counterpart. This is illustrated by the non-Asian mother's question 'What did they do wrong?'; whereas the grieving Asian mother very often asks 'What did I do wrong?'. The Asian mother appears to have an excessive grief-reaction, but is usually sustained by the many relatives who come to surround her at this time. What is most important is to attempt to give an explanation for the unfortunate event, and to suggest what can be done in the future to avoid a recurrence. The couple must be reassured of their own adequacy. This is difficult enough when communication is good, and simple terms are understood; but to try to do this through an interpreter may be difficult, if not impossible. The doctor must realize that the couple involved may be under great pressure to replace the lost child, especially if it was a son. Also the mother may imagine that she will have to adhere to various religious rituals if she is to have a successful pregnancy. It is often helpful to try to see the couple, with an interpreter present, six to eight weeks after delivery. This is no different from what should happen with all patients who have lost a baby; but it is often omitted when difficulty is experienced in communication. It is also an appropriate time to reiterate the advice regarding early attendance during a subsequent pregnancy.

It is to be hoped that many of the problems referred to in this chapter will be much reduced in the second generation of Asian women who experience their pregnancies in Britain.

Conclusion

The Asian communities in this country are as variable as the parts of Africa and the Indian subcontinent they originate from. This means that medical care may have to vary, depending on the particular group to whom the services are given. Communication between doctor and patient may be a particular problem, and initiatives should be started in each locality to try to improve this.

The Asian pregnant patient may have a completely different outlook and environment to her non-Asian sister, and services must respond accordingly. The need to continue work, especially manual work, if she is the sole breadwinner, can be of serious consequence to the mother and to her baby. Pregnancy complications such as anaemia are found more commonly in the pregnant Asian mother, and fetal distress is not unusual during labour. A higher incidence of operative delivery exists in this group of patients, and the perinatal mortality rate tends to be greater than that of the indigenous population.

In general, but with some notable exceptions, family size and spacing in the Asian community closely resemble the non-Asian pattern.

With further adaptation within the community, with improvement in communication, and with better socio-economic conditions, after one or two generations obstetric problems peculiar to the Asian mother should diminish considerably.

References

Blatchford, H. (1986). *Health knowledge in pregnancy. A comparison between British Caucasian and Asian women.* Thesis submitted for degree of Bachelor of Science in Medical Science. Leicester University.

Clarke, M., Clayton, D. G., Mason, E. S., and MacVicar, J. (1988). Asian mothers' risk factor for perinatal death—the same or different? A ten-year review of Leicestershire perinatal deaths. *British Medical Journal*, **297**, 384–7.

Doll, R. and Hanington E. (1961). International survey of eclampsia and pre-eclampsia 1958–59: epidemiological aspects. *Pathologia and Microbiologia (Basle)*, **24**, 531–541.

Duignan, N. M., Studd, J. W. W., and Hughes, A. O. (1975). Characteristics of normal labour in different racial groups. *British Journal of Obstetrics and Gynaecology*, **82**, 593–601.

Haines, A. P., McFayden, I. R., Campbell-Brown, M., North, W. R. S., and Abraham, R. (1982). Birthweight and complications of pregnancy in an Asian population. In *Obstetric problems in the Asian community in Britain* (ed. I. R. McFayden and J. MacVicar), pp. 119–126. Royal College of Obstetricians and Gynaecologists, London.

MacVicar, J. (1982). The effect of race on perinatal mortality. In *Progress in Obstetrics and Gynaecology* (ed. J. Studd) **Vol. I**, pp. 92–104. Churchill Livingstone, Edinburgh.

MacVicar, J. (1983). Cutting Asian death toll at birth. *Current Practice*, **14**, 16–17.

MacVicar, J. (1984). In *Perinatal Notes (the newsletter of the Leicestershire Perinatal Survey)*, **No. 1**, 3–4.

Mason, E. S. (In press). Asian mother and baby campaign (the Leicestershire experience). (*Journal of the Royal Society of Health.*)

Settatree, R. S., Terry, P. B., Mathews, P. M., and Condie, R. G. (1982). Asian stillbirths in West Birmingham. In *Obstetric problems of the Asian community in Britain*, (ed. I. R. McFayden and J. MacVicar), pp. 47–54. Royal College of Obstetricians and Gynaecologists, London.

Studd, J. W. W., Tuck, S. M., Cardozo, L. D., and Gibb, D. M. F. (1982). Labour in patients of different racial groups. In *Obstetric problems of the Asian Community in Britain.*, (ed. I. R. MacFayden and J. MacVicar), pp. 57–65. Royal College of Obstetricians and Gynaecologists, London.

Thomson, A. M., Billeqicz, W. Z., and Hytten, F. E. (1968). The assessment of fetal growth. *Journal of Obstetrics and Gynaecology of the British Commonwealth*, **75**, 903–16.

Wigglesworth, J. S. (1980). Monitoring perinatal mortality: a pathophysiological approach. *Lancet*, **ii**, 684–6.

Further reading

Barron, S. L. and Vessey, M. P. (1966). Birthweight of infants born to immigrant women. *British Journal of Preventative and Social Medicine*, **20**, 127–34.

Benny, P. S., MacVicar, J., Parkin E. N., and Montague, W. (1980). Carbohydrate profiles in two groups of mothers with differing perinatal mortality. *Journal of Obstetrics and Gynaecology*, **1**, 20–23.

Campbell, D. M. and Gillmer, M. D. G. (ed.) (1982). *Nutrition in pregnancy*. Proceedings of the Tenth Study Group of the Royal College of Obstetricians and Gynaecologists. RCOG, London.

Clarke, M. and Clayton, D. (1981). The design and interpretation of case-control studies of perinatal mortality. *American Journal of Epidemiology*, **133**, 636–45.

McFadyen, I. R. and MacVicar, J. (ed.) (1982). *Obstetric problems of the Asian community in Britain*, A Scientific Meeting of the Royal College of Obstetricians and Gynaecologists. RCOG, London.

Meire H. B. and Farrant, P. (1981). Ultrasound demonstration of an unusual fetal growth pattern in Indians. *British Journal of Obstetrics and Gynaecology*, **88**, 260–63.

Model, B. (1987). Prenatal diagnosis of the haemoglobinopathies. In *Advanced medicine* (ed. R. E. Pounder and P. L. Chiodini), pp. 171–87. Baillière Tindall, London.

Rodeck, C. H., Morsman, J. M., Nicolaides, K. H., McKenzie, C., Gosden, C. M. and Gosden, J. R (1983). A single operator technique for first trimester chorion biopsy. *Lancet*, ii, 1340–41.

Rodeck, C. H. (1984). Obstetric techniques in prenatal diagnosis. In *Prenatal diagnosis* (ed. C. H. Rodeck and Ҁ. H. Nicholaides), pp. 15–28. Royal College of Obstetricians and Gynaecologists, London.

Terry, P. B., Condie R. G., and Settatree, R. S. (1980). Analysis of ethnic differences in perinatal statistics. *British Medical Journal*, **281**, 1307–8.

Terry, P. B. and Condie, R. G. (1981). Ethnic differences in perinatal mortality. *Postgraduate Medical Journal*, **57**, 790–91.

Wharton, B. A., Smalley, C., Millns, C., Nirmal, J., Bissenden, J. G., and Scott, P. H. (1980). The Asian mother and her baby at Sorrento. In *Topics in Perinatal Medicine*, (ed. B. A. Wharton), pp. 141–51. Pitman Medical, Tunbridge Wells.

Young, I. D., Rickett, A. B., and Clarke, M. (1986). Genetic analysis of malformations causing perinatal mortality. *Journal of Medical Genetics*, **23**, 58–63.

Useful booklets and agencies

Association for Spina Bifida and Hydrocephalus
22 Upper Woburn Place, London, WC1H 0EP

Compassionate Friends (for bereaved parents)
5 Lower Clifton Hill, Clifton, Bristol, BF8 1BT

Down's Children Association
4 Oxford Street, London, W1N 9FL

Health Education Authority Pregnancy Book. Also small booklets in various Asian languages, for example: Are you pregnant? Taking care of yourself and baby. A healthy pregnancy: some helpful advice on breast feeding. Published by and obtainable from: Health Education Authority, Hamilton House, Mabledon Place, London WC1H 9TX.

Stillbirth and Neo-natal Death Society
Argyle House, 29–31 Euston Road, London NW1 2SD

The Spastics Society
12 Park Crescent, London, W1N 4EQ

Asian women's groups, with person to contact

UK Asian Women's Conference
19 Wykeham Road, London, NW4 2TB
- Tara Kothari, 19 Wykeham Road, London, NW4 2TB
- Sudershan Abrol, 180 Plantsbrook Road, Walmley, Sutton Coldfield, Birmingham
- Sneh Shah, 29 Cornfield Road, Bushey, Hertfordshire, WD2 3TB
- Lata Kumaraswarmi, 8 Loughton Avenue, Witherington, Manchester

Patidar Samaj
253 Balham High Road, Tooting Bec, London SW17

Sangham
235/237 West Hendon Broadway, London, NW9
- Usha Bhatt, Chairman

National Congress of Gujaratis
- Prabhaben Amin, 67 Downs Road, Epsom, KT18 5JT

Ismaili Women's Organization
- Salma Giga, 6 The Four Tubs, Bushey Heath, Herts, WD2 3SJ
- Zainul Lalji, 265 Lauderdale Mansions, Lauderdale Road, London, W9

Leicester Asian Ladies' Circle
- Gulshan Ahmed, Chairperson, 1 Eastwood Road, Leicester, LE2 8DD
- Mira Trivedi, Vice-Chairperson, 29 Rushford Drive, Leicester, LE4 7UF

Joint Council for the Welfare of Immigrants
44 Theobalds Road, London, WC1

Community Health Groups for Ethnic Minorities
28 Churchfield Road, London, W3 6EB

Ms Veena Bahl, Advisor on Ethnic Minority Health
Room A505
Alexander Fleming House
Department of Health
Elephant and Castle, London SE1 6BY

12 Hereditary disorders

Ian Young

Introduction

The post-war years have witnessed a revolution in health care and patterns of disease in the United Kingdom. The introduction of antibiotics, coupled with improved living standards and social amenities, have ensured that the great majority of British children grow up with reasonable prospects of fulfilling the traditional Biblical remit by surviving to at least their seventieth birthday. The virtual eradication of formerly endemic disorders, such as rickets and tuberculosis, has switched attention to the relatively large residue of conditions in which inheritance plays a role. Thus, while there is no evidence to suggest that inherited diseases are becoming more common, there is increasing awareness that their relative contribution to morbidity and mortality is rising. Recent studies indicate that in childhood approximately 40 per cent of all hospital admissions are related to congenital malformations and/or inherited disease. In adult life roughly one in ten of the population suffers from a chronic disabling disorder, such as diabetes or schizophrenia, in which genetic factors are implicated.

The study of inherited disease has received an enormous boost over the last few years as a consequence of dramatic and very exciting developments in molecular biology. Insight has been gained into the basic pathology of many of the more common and serious single-gene disorders, opening up the possibility of carrier-detection and prenatal diagnosis. This applies to a host of conditions such as polycystic kidney disease, Huntington's chorea, cystic fibrosis, and Duchenne muscular dytrophy, in all of which the basic defect at the protein biochemical level was, until recently, largely unknown. Molecular biology has also helped unravel some of the secrets of the inherited cancer syndromes, and provided evidence for underlying somatic change in DNA in many acquired forms of neoplasia.

The arrival in the UK since the war of large numbers of Asian immigrants has provided a new challenge for health-care services, not least for those dealing with inherited disease. There is certainly nothing to suggest that the Asian community harbours more or less 'bad' genes than any other ethnic group, but it would not be too surprising if a different range of disorders were encountered, and the practice of consanguineous marriage in some Asian subgroups might be expected to increase the incidence of rare autosomal recessive conditions. At the scientific level there are many problems associated with the identification and study of genetic disorders in the Asian community. These include the obvious difficulties of communication, gaining confidence, and avoiding any suggestion that one particular race is genetically superior or inferior to another. Then there are the more subtle problems associated with disentangling the complex interaction of nature and nurture. Despite these obstacles much useful information has emerged over the last few years, and certain particular problems have been identified. It is hoped that the outline presented below will prove of practical value to the general practitioner encountering Asian families, by highlighting particular problems which have been noted, and considering how these might best be approached.

The spectrum of disease

It is conventional to classify inherited disorders under three headings.

(a) Chromosomal

These conditions arise as a result of loss or gain of chromosomal material. Chromosomes obtained from cultured lymphocytes or any other source of dividing cells (amniocytes, trophoblast, fibroblasts) can be studied under the light microscope. Essentially any rearrangement of the autosomes which is unbalanced, thereby resulting in excess or loss of chromosome material, will lead to physical and developmental abnormalities. These may be so severe as to be almost invariably lethal (for example, triploidy, trisomy 13 and 18), or may be relatively mild, and compatible with normal or near-normal survival (for example, Down's syndrome or trisomy 21). Abnormalities of the sex chromosomes such as Klinefelter's syndrome (XXY), Turner's syndrome (XO), and the XYY syndrome, are usually less serious than autosomal abnormalities in their phenotypic effects. Approximately one in two hundred of all newborn babies has a chromosome abnormality.

(b) Mendelian

At the latest count over 4000 traits or diseases showing single-gene inheritance have been identified in man (McKusick 1988). Of these 59 per cent are autosomal dominant, 34 per cent are autosomal recessive, and the remaining 7 per cent show sex-linked inheritance. Most of these disorders are extremely rare, but others, such as familial hypercholesterolaemia (1 in 500), sickle-cell disease (1 in 40 in some Afro-Caribbeans), and red-green colour-blindness (1 in 10 males) are relatively common. Several autosomal recessive disorders show quite striking differences in incidence in different ethnic communities. Well known examples with a high frequency include the aforementioned sickle-cell disease in Afro-Caribbeans, Tay–Sachs disease in Ashkenazi Jews, cystic fibrosis in western European Caucasians, and thalassaemia in Greek Cypriots. Other examples are summarized in Table 12.1. Thalassaemia is also common in Asian immigrants, and is discussed later in this chapter.

Table 12.1   *Inherited disorders showing a high incidence in certain ethnic groups*

Ethnic group	Disease
Afrikaners	Sclerosteosis
	Variegate porphyria
Amish	Cartilage-hair hypoplasia
	Ellis–Van Creveld syndrome
Ashkenazi Jews	Familial dysautonomia
	Gaucher's disease
Eskimos	Congenital adrenal hyperplasia
	Pseudo-cholinesterase deficiency
Finns	Aspartylglycosaminuria
	Congenital nephrosis
Norwegians	Alpha-1-antitrypsin deficiency

In these ethnic groups the high incidence of particular inherited disorders can be explained on the basis of a founder-effect in a relatively small 'isolated' community. In contrast the high incidence of cystic fibrosis in Caucasians, thalassaemia in Indians, and sickle-cell in Afro-Caribbeans can be much more plausibly explained by heterozygote advantage.

(c) Multifactorial

This rather unsatisfactory term embraces a large number of common malformations and acquired disorders of later life which are believed to result from the interaction of an underlying genetic predisposition controlled by many genes (polygenic) with ill-defined environmental trigger factors. Malformations believed to be inherited in this fashion include neural tube defects (anencephaly, encephalocele, and spina bifida), non-syndromal cleft lip and palate, talipes, and congenital dislocation of the hip. Disorders of later life include schizophrenia, glaucoma, epilepsy, and possibly coronary artery disease. Until recently research effort has been concentrated on the identification of possible aetiological environmental factors, but recent advances in molecular biology have prompted a search for relevant genetic polymorphisms—which is beginning to bear fruit for coronary artery disease, bipolar affective disorders and schizophrenia.

The Asian community in the UK

The evident heterogeneity of the British Asian community, which is described in other chapters in this book, and the factors which underlie it, are things which must also be taken account of in any genetic study.

Asians in Bradford, the majority of whom originate from Pakistan and are of the Muslim faith, show a high incidence of consanguineous marriage. In contrast, the majority Asian population of Leicester, Gujarati Hindus, rarely if ever marry close blood-relatives. Nevertheless, even within the relatively small city of Leicester, the diversity which is found in almost every British Asian community makes the interpretation of any genetic survey very difficult, and emphasizes the importance of avoiding sweeping conclusions.

Consanguineous marriage

Social aspects

Marriage between close relatives is common in many parts of the world, particularly the middle East and the Indian subcontinent. In parts of southern India, in which over 50 per cent of marriages are between maternal uncle and niece or between first cousins, consanguineous marriage has been practised on a large scale for over two thousand years. In contrast, consanguineous marriage in the populaces of Northern India, with the exception of the Muslim community, is uncommon.

The reasons for these differences are complex and steeped in history. First there is the very strong influence of tradition and custom, which could not be challenged in the south by the regulation of consanguineous marriages (*sapinda*) which prevailed in Northern India. Then there are the many social benefits which derive from consanguineous marriage. These include: the importance attached to finding a suitable and congenial marital partner, which is often regarded as a major parental responsibility; the limitation of the amount of dowry given; the importance of keeping property within the family; and the maintenance of large areas of agricultural land as a single large unit.

For immigrants to the United Kingdom who have a strong tradition of consanguineous marriage, these factors are compounded by the restricted choice of marital partner available in a small ethnic minority. In a study of the Muslim community in Bradford, of 101 consecutive pregnancies observed, 70 per cent were to some consanguineous relationship (Darr and Modell 1988). This compares with a figure of around 50 per cent noted recently in Lahore in Pakistan. Thus for this particular community the frequency of close consanguineous marriage appears to be increasing. A similar trend is probably occurring in other British centres in which Pakistani immigrants have settled, such as Luton, Rochdale, and parts of London.

Genetic aspects

The social and family benefits conveyed by consanguineous alliances may far outweigh any possible deleterious genetic effects. On general principles marriage between close relatives is likely to increase the incidence of autosomal recessive disorders seen in offspring. This is based on the knowledge that most humans carry at least one disadvantageous recessive gene, which by definition does not cause any problems in the heterozygous (carrier) state. Problems only occur when two individuals carrying the same recessive gene marry, in which case there will be one chance in four that any child will inherit two copies of the abnormal gene (one from each parent), and therefore be homozygous and affected. Intuitively it can be seen that related individuals are at increased risk of carrying the same recessive gene by descent from a common ancestor when compared with unrelated members of an outbreeding population.

However, there has been considerable controversy over the possible effects of consanguineous marriage in Southern India, where it has been argued that the long-term practice of consanguineous inbreeding will have led to the loss of deleterious genes in the gene pool through the death of affected homozygotes over the millennia; the 'bad' genes will have been 'bred out'. In contrast consanguineous marriage in Pakistan dates back only a few hundred years, to the popular adoption of Islam, so that a noticeable reduction in the incidence of autosomal recessive disorders might not yet be apparent. This debate continues in Southern India, where at least one recent study has concluded that long-term inbreeding has not resulted in the loss of serious recessive genes from the gene pool (Devi *et al.* 1987).

As far as the United Kingdom is concerned this is largely of academic interest, since immigration from Southern India is uncommon. Among the British Muslim community there is good evidence that consanguineous marriage is genetically disadvantageous. This is based on studies of perinatal mortality (Young and Clarke 1987; Chitty and Winter 1988) and epidemiological surveys of sensorineural deafness, retinitis pigmentosa, and severe idiopathic mental retardation (Bundey 1987). In all of these surveys the Pakistani Muslim communities are disproportionately represented.

Practical aspects

When any couple, Asian or otherwise, wishes to know of possible risks associated with consanguineous marriage, four steps are necessary to fully assess the situation and counsel the family.

- The precise genetic relationship of the two individuals must be estabished.
- Tactful enquiry should be made to determine whether anyone in the extended family has, or has had, an inherited disease.
- Risks of abnormality in future offspring must be calculated.
- Information concerning these risks and how they may be modified has to be conveyed to the couple.

Clearly this exercise requires a sensitive and cautious approach. Any hint of condemnation or reproach is not only unacceptable medical practice, but will also almost certainly be counter-productive. Particular care is needed if the counselling process is to be extended to other members of the family.

Establishing the genetic relationship The careful and painstaking construction of a family pedigree is essential. From this it should be possible to pin-point the degree of relationship. This is defined on the basis of the proportion of genes shared—see Table 12.2. Some highly inbred family pedigrees may present major analytical problems. An example of such a situation is shown in Fig. 12.1. In this family the arrowed individuals seeking information are in fact double first cousins, who will share on average 25 per cent of their genes.

Table 12.2 *Genetic relationship and increased risk of abnormality in offspring*

Relationship	Proportion of genes shared	Increased risk of serious abnormality in offspring*
First degree		
Parents		
Children	½	30–50%
Sibs		
Second degree		
Uncles, aunts		
Nephews, nieces	¼	5–10%
Half-siblings		
Double first cousins		
Third degree		
First cousins		
Half-uncles, -aunts	⅛	3%
Half-nephews, -nieces		

*These figures are based on theoretical calculations and empirical studies.

The extended family history Tactful but persistent inquiry will usually clarify whether anyone in the extended family has had a genetic disorder, particularly one showing autosomal recessive inheritance. Such inquiry should be extended to include possible neonatal or childhood deaths, as well as information about disabled relatives in the country of origin.

Calculation of risk This can be relatively straightforward or remarkably complex. In a simple situation, such as when the presenting couple are first cousins with no history of relevant hereditary disease, empirical risks obtained from studies of the outcome in first-cousin marriages can be given. These generally correspond to the risk calculated on the basis that everyone carries one harmful autosomal recessive gene. Thus for first cousins the observed and calculated increased risk of abnormality is approximately three per cent (Table 12.2 and

Fig. 12.2). It should be stressed than this increased risk is not for a specific disorder but covers all possible autosomal recessive conditions. Given that over 1400 have been described, it is obviously impossible to screen for all of these.

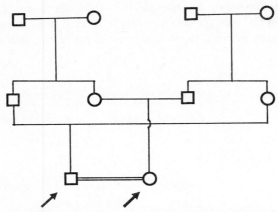

Fig. 12.1   A 'simple' example of a relatively complex pedigree. In this family the arrowed individuals are double first cousins.

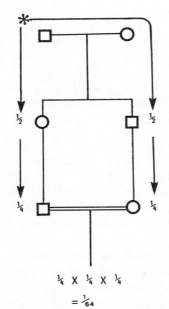

$$\tfrac{1}{4} \ \text{X} \ \tfrac{1}{4} \ \text{X} \ \tfrac{1}{4}$$

$$= \tfrac{1}{64}$$

Fig. 12.2   Derivation of the risk of homozygosity in the offspring of first cousins. This will be $\tfrac{1}{64}$ by common descent from grand-father and $\tfrac{1}{64}$ by common descent from grand-mother (not shown). Therefore total risk = $\tfrac{1}{32}$ = approximately three per cent.

If there is a relevant family history it should be possible to determine the specific risk for that disorder in a future child. Fig. 12.3 shows the pedigree of a family in which the shaded individual has a severe rare recessive condition. The likelihood for being a carrier is shown for other family members. (If the disorder in question is rare the general population carrier-risk is ignored, as are the

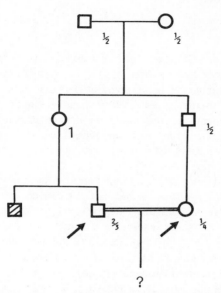

Fig. 12.3 The shaded individual has a rare autosomal recessive disorder. The likelihood for being carriers is shown for other family members. The risk of homozygosity in the offspring of the arrowed consultands $= \frac{2}{3} \times \frac{1}{4} \times \frac{1}{4} = \frac{1}{24}$.

risks for new mutations.) In Fig. 12.3, for the couple seeking advice (indicated by arrows) the risk for their first child being affected will be:

$$\frac{2}{3} \times \frac{1}{4} \times \frac{1}{4} = \frac{1}{24}.$$

If the couple arrowed in Fig. 12.3 already have one healthy child this makes it less likely on statistical grounds that they are both carriers. The new risk can be calculated by Bayesian methods, as shown in Table 12.3.

Thus the posterior or relative probability that both parents are carriers falls from $\frac{1}{6}$ to $\frac{3}{23}$ $[\frac{3}{24}/(\frac{3}{24} + \frac{5}{6})]$, and therefore the risk for having an affected child falls from $\frac{1}{24}$ (4 per cent) to $\frac{3}{92}$ (3 per cent).

Believe it or not, this is a relatively simple example of the sort of consanguinity problem which can present at a genetics clinic! Some highly inbred kindreds, perhaps manifesting more than one autosomal recessive disease, can generate formidable counselling problems.

Table 12.3

Probability	Both parents are carriers	Both parents not carriers
Prior	$\frac{1}{6}$	$\frac{5}{6}$
Conditional (1 normal child)	$\frac{3}{4}$	1
Joint	$\frac{3}{24}$	$\frac{5}{6}(=\frac{20}{24})$

Counselling the family   It cannot be overstressed that this requires considerable diplomacy and tact. First it is vital to gain the couple's confidence, and make it clear that no judgement is being made or personal opinion expressed. Information about risks should be conveyed with understanding and empathy. This is particularly pertinent if a consanguineous couple already have a child handicapped as a consequence of an autosomal recessive disorder, since it is desirable to convey information about risks without adding to the parents' already considerable burden of guilt.

Sometimes it may be possible to initiate appropriate carrier tests, for example with the haemoglobinopathies, to see if risks can be modified. Alternatively a discussion about prenatal diagnosis may be appropriate; but it should be remembered that prenatal diagnosis leading to termination in the second trimester is unacceptable to many Muslim couples. Given the sensitive nature of the issues involved, and the complexity of some of the calculations, a strong case can be made for referring consanguineous couples for expert advice. Genetics clinics are now held on a regular basis at most teaching hospitals in the United Kingdom.

Thalassaemia

The thalassaemias constitute a heterogeneous group of autosomal recessive disorders in which haemoglobin synthesis is impaired. Collectively they and sickle-cell disease are by far the commonest single-gene disorders in the world, affecting approximately 250 000 children a year. Recent reports estimate that up to four per cent of the world's population, about 190 million people, carry a haemoglobinopathy gene.

Why these disorders should be so common is far from clear, since in the homozygous state they are usually associated with severe ill-health. While there is good evidence to support the hypothesis that carriers of sickle-cell disease are at a biological advantage compared with non-carriers, because of relative immunity to *Plasmodium falciparum*, the evidence for a similar heterozygote advantage in thalassaemia carriers is not so convincing. This tends to be based on coincidence of geographical distribution of the disease and the parasite, rather than on direct laboratory demonstration of immunity.

Whatever the explanation, it is a fact that beta-thalassaemia is common in the Indian subcontinent, and this is reflected in the British Asian population also, in whom the incidence of carriers varies from three to six per cent (Modell 1987). Beta^0-thalassaemia, in which no globin chains are synthesized, is a severe, potentially life-threatening disorder, requiring extensive regular treatment with blood-transfusion and chelating agents. This life-long therapy is not only expensive, amounting to some £500 a year for each case, but is also unpleasant and frightening for a child, involving regular hospitalization and venesection.

Prenatal diagnosis

The serious nature of beta-thalassaemia has prompted major public education programmes in countries such as Cyprus, in which the incidence is very high. An integral component of these programmes is the availability of prenatal diagnosis.

Until recently this was based on second-trimester fetal blood-sampling, and careful study of haematological indices. Second-trimester prenatal diagnosis is far from being a satisfactory technique, even for those who find it ethically acceptable. Fetal blood-sampling conveys a two to five per cent risk of miscarriage. Termination can then only be carried out by induction of labour, usually with prostaglandins, at around the time when fetal movements are first being felt. This can be a long, painful, and extremely distressing experience. For many Asian couples, particularly Muslims, it is totally unacceptable.

The advent of first-trimester prenatal diagnosis for beta-thalassaemia has radically altered what until recently has been rather a gloomy picture. The timely coincidental development of chorionic villus sampling and molecular techniques for studying globin genes has ensured that at least eight per cent of couples who have had a baby with beta-thalassaemia now have the option of reliable first-trimester prenatal diagnosis. This is particularly relevant for the Muslim community.

Several important points should be stressed concerning these techniques.

- Chorionic villus sampling is still a relatively novel procedure, so that experience tends to be greatest in those centres which have pioneered it. It is not yet universally available.
- Preliminary results suggest that the increased risk of miscarriage associated with chorionic villus sampling may be as high as three per cent.
- Beta-thalassaemia is caused by a very large number (in excess of forty at the latest count) of different molecular defects, including nonsense mutations, frameshift mutations, RNA-processing mutations, and deletions. Thus it is absolutely critical that careful family studies are undertaken, preferably well in advance of pregnancy. This will usually involve analysis of DNA extracted from 5–10 ml of blood from parents and their affected child/children.

- If the affected child has perished, it may be possible to evaluate the family by studying haematological indices and DNA from the healthy siblings, parents, and grand-parents.
- Beta-thalassaemia can have different clinical effects depending on the nature of the molecular defect and on interaction with other haemoglobinopathies. Obviously the likely clinical outcome may have a strong influence on parental attitudes to pregnancy intervention.

It will be apparent from the above that the prenatal diagnosis of beta-thalassaemia is a complex undertaking, raising sensitive ethical issues, and requiring close collaboration between obstetrics and haematological and molecular-diagnostic services. Nevertheless it does offer parents of a severely ill child the option of avoiding a recurrence. Increasingly couples of all religious persuasions and ethnic backgrounds are making use of this facility (Old *et al*. 1986).

General population screening

In a community with a high incidence of beta-thalassaemia a strong case can be made for offering a population-screening programme. Carriers can be detected by relatively simple haematological tests (reduced mean red-cell haemoglobin and raised Hb A2) so that if two carriers marry they can be alerted to the one in four risk of having an affected child. Programmes of this nature have been spectacularly successful in countries such as Sardinia and Cyprus, resulting in a dramatic decline in the number of births of affected homozygotes.

It has been suggested that similar programmes could and should be initiated for the British Asian communities. For example in a city such as Leicester, in which approximately 1500 babies of Asian descent, principally Gujarati, are born annually, it would be possible to offer screening at the antenatal clinic. Of the 1500 mothers presenting annually, approximately 90 (six per cent) would have beta-thalassaemia trait (=carriers). The husbands of these women could then be screened. On average five or six would be carriers. This small number of couples could then be offered prenatal diagnosis. If this offer were taken up this would result in the 'prevention' of one to two cases of homozygous beta-thalassaemia every year.

It will be readily apparent that a screening programme of this nature will pose considerable logistic problems, with the need for communication, counselling, and co-ordination paramount. Almost inevitably the time factor involved will mean that only second-trimester termination could be offered. Thus a pre-pregnancy population-screening programme conducted with the support of local community and religious leaders would seem more appropriate. This has been welcomed by the Greek Cypriot community in London.

Nevertheless screening for beta-thalassaemia trait in the Asian population is likely to be a contentious issue. Meticulous care will have to be taken to avoid any hint of racism. A large-scale public education programme will be necessary to explain at length the clinical and genetic aspects of the disease. The possibility of effective therapy with bone-marrow transplantation serves to illustrate the complexity of the moral issues which will undoubtedly arise. Without question this is a nettle which will have to be grasped if public-health services are to respond appropriately to one of the major challenges presented by the growing Asian population in the United Kingdom.

Neural tube defects

Neural tube defects (NTDs) are second only to congenital heart disease in the incidence table of congenital malformations. They include a number of severe and sometimes lethal malformations such as anencephaly, encephalocele, myelocele, meningocele, and meningomyelocele. Collectively, these disorders are often referred to by the general public as 'spina bifida', although in medical circles this term tends to be reserved for lumbo-sacral lesions.

For various reasons which are far from clear the incidence of NTDs has declined in the UK and elsewhere over the last ten to fifteen years. This cannot be explained solely by the introduction of prenatal diagnostic screening programmes, but probably also has resulted from subtle changes in diet and/or working environment, reflecting causal factors which are not yet understood. Nevertheless these disorders remain a major source of morbidity and mortality in infancy, accounting for approximately 10–15 per cent of deaths occurring in the perinatal period. In parts of the UK having a Celtic population the incidence of these conditions reached almost epidemic proportions in the so-called 'swinging sixties'. In certain areas of South Wales an incidence of over one per cent was recorded. The overall incidence in the United Kingdom at present is estimated to be around two to three for every thousand births. There is a marked gradient of increasing incidence, moving from the prosperous south-east to the poorer western parts of the country with high Celtic populations.

The underlying cause of NTDs remains unknown. They are said to show multifactorial inheritance, implying interaction between a genetic predisposition and environmental factors. Family studies certainly support the concept that genetic factors are implicated; but the environmental 'trigger' agents are poorly understood. Recent attention has centred on diet, and in particular vitamin intake. This is discussed later in this section.

Neural tube defects in Asians

There is good evidence that the incidence of NTDs, particularly anencephaly, is high in Northern India in both the Sikh and Hindu populations (Verma 1978). A high incidence in Sikh immigrants has also been noted in Canada (Baird 1983). Similar observations have been made in British studies, both in

Birmingham (Leck 1984) and in Leicester, where the incidence of NTDs in the Asian population during the years 1976–80 was 2.74 per 1000, as compared with the non-Asian incidence of 1.6 per 1000 deliveries (Dhariwal 1982).

Overall the incidence of NTDs in British Asians is probably lower than in their country of origin, but higher than for the indigenous British population. This is in keeping with the observation that ethnic differences for NTDs are influenced considerably by migration, pointing to a major environmental aetiological contribution (Leck 1969).

Recurrence risks

As far as the author is aware no studies have been undertaken aimed specifically at deriving empiric recurrence risks for neural tube defects in the British Asian population. Thus at present the best that can be achieved is to provide information obtained from large surveys carried out in various parts of the United Kingdom. Average risk figures for relatives derived from these studies are given in Table 12.4. Thus parents who have had one affected child can be offered a recurrence risk of five per cent, two affected children ten to twelve per cent and so on.

Table 12.4   *Recurrence risks for neural tube defects*

Affected relative	Recurrence risk
One sibling	5%
Two siblings	10–12%
Parent	4%
Aunt, uncle	
Nephew, niece	2%
Half-sibling	
Cousin	
Great uncle or	
aunt	1%

These risks are applicable in high-incidence areas, and are thus likely to be appropriate for the British Asian community.

There is some evidence that these risks may be slightly greater when the affected individual is related through the matrilineal line, and correspondingly lower when through the patrilineal line. There is also evidence for the British population that social class may influence the risk of recurrence (higher social class—lower recurrence risk). Until confirmatory evidence in support of these observations is available for the Asian communities it would seem reasonable to counsel on the basis of the risks quoted in Table 12.4.

Prenatal screening and diagnosis

The association between neural tube defects and raised alpha-feto-protein (alpha-FP) in both amniotic fluid and maternal serum was first recognized in 1972. Unfortunately the distribution curves of serum alpha-FP levels in normal pregnancies and in those with an open NTD overlap, so that serum alpha-FP screening, usually undertaken at sixteen weeks into pregnancy, is far from being a perfect test. Even in ideal situations, assuming complete patient co-operation, no more than 70 per cent of open neural tube defects will be detected, so that there is a high false negative rate. False positive results may also be obtained as a result of incorrect gestational assessment, multiple pregnancy, threatened miscarriage, congenital nephrosis, or other open defects, such as exomphalos.

Most Regional Health Authorities in the United Kingdom offer a pregnancy screening programme based on maternal serum alpha-FP assay. Abnormal results, usually defined as being above an arbitrary cut-off point such as the 97th centile, or 2.5 times the median, are investigated by a repeat blood-test and ultrasonography. Only a small proportion (around 5–10 per cent) of these pregnancies will be affected. Some Regions have abandoned screening programmes, because of their low and falling incidence of NTDs and the anxiety generated by the test.

For pregnancies in which there is a high index of suspicion based on serum alpha-FP result or family history, two approaches to specific diagnosis can be utilized. The first, careful second-trimester ultrasonography, is a very sensitive technique in skilled hands, and is likely to detect all but the smallest defects. As far as is known ultrasonography is entirely risk-free. In contrast the second approach, amniocentesis, carries a small risk, of around one per cent, of causing a miscarriage, and may also entail a small risk of inducing deformations such as talipes and dislocation of the hip, although this is a subject of dispute. Amniotic fluid alpha-FP levels from pregnancies with an open NTD show much clearer distinction from normal than is the case with serum alpha-FP. In the small number of equivocal cases which occur, ultrasonography and acetylcholinesterase electrophoresis band-patterns (looking for CNS-derived bands) may resolve the crucial issue of whether the fetus is or is not affected.

Periconceptional vitamin supplementation

Supportive evidence that periconceptional vitamin supplementation may prevent the development of an NTD comes from two sources. The most widely quoted is the United Kingdom multicentre study which indicated that Pregnavite Forte F taken before and during early pregnancy appeared to significantly reduce the risk of recurrence for mothers who already had an affected child (Smithells *et al.* 1981). This study was criticized on the grounds that study and control groups were not balanced for parameters such as social class, and that there was a disproportionately large number of controls from one particular centre.

The results of the second study were announced after re-questioning mothers about compliance. One mother changed her response, thus allowing statistical significance to be achieved. This study concluded that folic acid supplementation (4 mg per day) 'might be an effective method of primary prevention of neural tube defects' (Laurence *et al.* 1981).

The results of these studies generated considerable controversy, which remains unresolved. The Medical Research Council launched a major national trial, using four different vitamin regimes to try to establish efficacy and safety. The results of this study are keenly awaited, and are likely to remain so for some time, since many mothers, prompted by publicity in the press, have preferred to take Pregnavite Forte F rather than enter a trial. At the time of writing the Government has just announced its intention to return Pregnavite Forte F to the approved list for NHS prescribing, so that poorer families will not be disadvantaged in any way.

Until the situation about the role of vitamin supplementation is clearer, the author's practice is to offer families at increased risk of having a baby with an NTD the option of joining the trial or of supplementation with Pregnavite Forte F. This should commence at least one month prior to conception, and continue until the date of the second missed period. If both of these offers are declined, then encouragement to eat a well-balanced vitamin-rich diet seems a safe and non-controversial alternative.

There is no information about the possible role of vitamin supplementation for preventing NTDs in Asian mothers. Until data emerge to the contrary, it would seem entirely reasonable not to distinguish in any way between ethnic groups. Careful study of the dietary characteristics of Asian mothers who have had a baby with an NTD could provide important insights into the aetiology of these common and seriously handicapping disorders.

Attitudes to genetic counselling

Given the broad spectrum of cultural and religious backgrounds present in the British Asian community, it would not be too surprising if Asian patients at genetics clinics showed diverse attitudes to the emotive and sensitive issues raised. For some patients there is a stigma associated with any suggestion that their genes may be anything but perfect, so a discussion of inherited disease in the family may have to be handled with great delicacy. As has been mentioned previously, this applies particularly when considering possible risks associated with consanguineous marriage.

Communication and attendance at a genetics clinic may themselves pose major problems. Many Asian families work long hours, and find it very difficult to find adequate cover for absence from work. Wives rarely attend on their own. It may not be clear to the family why they have been referred, so that there is little incentive to attend. Once at the clinic language problems may arise, and knowledge of the extended family in the country of origin may be limited. When the first group of Asian families referred to the Leicestershire genetics clinic was interviewed retrospectively about their experiences there, the responses were generally favourable, but there were complaints about communication and the importance of interpreters. Natural politeness may make it difficult for Asian patients to express dissatisfaction. Families appreciated receiving a summary letter following their consultation, claiming that this enhanced their understanding and recall of the information given.

During this retrospective survey the families were invited to express their views about sensitive issues such as termination of pregnancy on genetic grounds. Their responses are indicated in Table 12.5, and reveal important differences between the subgroups. Of the 16 Hindu and Sikh families, 15 would consider termination in the first trimester and 13 in the second trimester. In contrast only 5 of the 11 Muslim families would consider termination in the first trimester, and 3 in the second. The suggestion of AID (artificial insemination by donor) was universally unacceptable; and one Muslim couple had found the subject offensive when it had been mentioned at the clinic.

Table 12.5 *Attitudes of Asian familes to genetic termination and consanguineous marriage*

	Would consider termination		Is consanguineous marriage bad?		
	1st trimester	2nd trimester	Yes	No	Don't know
Hindu/Sikh					
$n = 16$	15	13	3	0	13
Muslim					
$n = 11$	5	3	1	7	3

Asked whether they believed parental consanguinity to be potentially hazardous to the genetic well-being of future offspring, three of the Hindu/Sikh families believed that it was, while the other thirteen had no firm opinion. The responses of the Muslim families were strikingly different. Seven did not believe that parental consanguinity was potentially hazardous, and made the very reasonable point that many other relatives had married cousins and then had normal children, so that the fact that they themselves had had an abnormal child could not be due to consanguinity!

The overriding impression gained from this survey was that Asian families are receptive to genetic information, and are usually influenced by it. It appears that termination on genetic grounds is generally acceptable to those of the Hindu faith but less often to Muslims, although there is a suggestion that this attitude may change in response to realization of the gravity of conditions such as homozygous beta-thalassaemia, and the development of first-trimester prenatal diagnosis.

Conclusion

The Asian community in the United Kingdom is very heterogeneous, with diverse origins in the Asian subcontinent. There is no evidence to indicate that individuals of Asian origin are more or less genetically fit than those of any other ethnic group, but, as is the case for every population ever studied, certain particular problems have emerged.

There is a high incidence of consanguineous marriage in some Asian populations, chiefly in Southern India and in the Muslim communities of Pakistan and Bangladesh. In theory parental consanguinity would be expected to result in an increase in autosomal recessive disorders, and this has been borne out in British studies. The social benefits of consanguinity may far outweigh any possible genetic disadvantages, so that great tact should be exercised when counselling consanguineous Asian couples.

Approximately three to six per cent of Pakistani Muslims and Gujaratis are carriers of beta-thalassaemia. In the homozygous state this is a severe, and potentially life-threatening, disorder. Carrier detection can be achieved by relatively simple haematological tests (FBC, MCH, HbA2), so that population screening is possible in theory. Prenatal diagnosis, using chorionic villus sampling and new molecular genetic techniques, can now be achieved in the first trimester for most couples with an affected child.

The incidence of neural tube defects is high in British Asians compared to that in the indigenous population. The reasons for this are unknown. Recurrence risks are well established, as are prenatal diagnostic screening programmes in most parts of the United Kingdom. Specific prenatal diagnosis can be achieved in over 90 per cent of cases of open neural tube defect, using amniocentesis and/or second trimester ultrasonography. Periconceptional vitamin therapy may provide effective prophylaxis.

Asian families are becoming increasingly responsive to the utilization of genetic and prenatal diagnostic services. This has important implications for health-care planning in terms of management and prevention. The study of inherited disease in the British Asian community will continue to provide insight into the evolutionary aspects and molecular mechanisms of chronic disease, while presenting at the primary-care level a major challenge for the National Health Service.

References

Baird, P. A. (1983). Neural tube defects in the Sikhs. *American Journal of Medical Genetics*, **16**, 49–56.

Bundey, S. (1988). The Birmingham birth study. *Biology and Society*, **5**, 13–15.

Chitty, L. and Winter, R. (1988). A perinatal study in the North-West Thames region. *Biology and Society*, **5**, 15–17.

Darr, A. and Modell, B. (1988). The frequency of consanguineous marriage among British Pakistanis. *Journal of Medical Genetics*, **25**, 186–90.

Devi, A. R. R., Rao, N. A., and Bittles, A. H. (1987). Inbreeding and the incidence of childhood genetic disorders in Karnataka, South India. *Journal of Medical Genetics*, **24**, 362–5.

Dhariwal, H. S. (1982). Leicestershire—decline in perinatal mortality. In *Obstetric problems of the Asian community in Britain*, (ed. I. R. McFadyen and J. MacVicar), pp. 101–7. Royal College of Obstetricians and Gynaecologists, London.

Laurence, K. M., James, N., Miller, M. H., Tennant, G. B. and Campbell, H. (1981). Double-blind randomised controlled trial of folate treatment before conception to prevent recurrence of neural tube defects. *British Medical Journal*, **282**, 1509–11.

Leck, I. (1969). Ethnic differences in the incidence of malformations following migration. *British Journal of Preventive and Social Medicine*, **23**, 166–73.

Leck, I. (1984). The geographical distribution of neural tube defects and oral clefts. *British Medical Bulletin*, **40**, 390–95.

McKusick, V. A. (1988). *Mendelian inheritance in man* (8th edn.) John Hopkins University Press, Baltimore.

Modell, B. (1987). Prenatal diagnosis of the haemoglobinopathies. In *Advanced Medicine*, **23**, (ed. R. E. Pounder and P. L. Chiodini), pp. 171–87. Baillière Tindall, London.

Old, J. M., Fitches, A., Heath, C., Thein, S. L., Weatherall, D. J., Warren, R. *et al.* (1986). First-trimester fetal diagnosis for haemoglobinopathies: report on 200 cases. *Lancet*, **ii**, 763–7.

Smithells, R. W., Sheppard, S., Schorah, C. J., Seller, M. J., Nevin, N. C., Harris, R., *et al.* (1981). Apparent prevention of neural tube defects by periconceptional vitamin supplementation. *Archives of Disease in Childhood*, **56**, 911–18.

Verma, I. C. (1978). High frequency of neural-tube defects in North India. *Lancet*, **i**, 879–80.

Young, I. D., and Clarke, M. (1987). Lethal malformations and perinatal mortality: a 10 year review with comparison of ethnic differences. *British Medical Journal*, **295**, 89–91.

13 Paediatrics

John Black

Introduction

Despite the presence here of large Asian communities for over thirty years, relatively little attention had been given to documenting the special needs of this growing part of the childhood population of the United Kingdom until Arthurton (1972), working in Bradford, described the work of a paediatrician with Asian children. Six years later Lobo (1978), who came from India himself, and was working in the Luton and Dunstable area, published a much fuller account in *Children of immigrants in Britain, their health and social problems'*, and Alix Henley (1979) gave a comprehensive description of the beliefs, customs, and needs of Asian patients more generally. More recently the 'Stop Rickets' (1981) and the 'Asian Mother and Baby' (1984) campaigns, run jointly by the Department of Health and Social Security and the Save the Children Fund, have done much to improve knowledge among Asian families of what is available, and to heighten awareness among British health-workers of the needs of the Asian community. The linkworker scheme which was set up as part of the 'Asian Mother and Baby' campaign has been of special value. Community workers have also been appointed to some hospitals to act as 'advocates' for the Asians, and to help patients and hospital staff to understand each other (Winkler and Yung 1981).

This chapter will describe the special needs of Asian children in the UK, with particular reference to their emotional and psychological problems. The commoner genetically determined conditions, nutritional disorders, and infections will also be considered.

Recent work

The first comprehensive survey of the growth patterns of Asian children in the United Kingdom was published by Rona and Chinn in 1986, using a language-based classification for speakers of Urdu, Gujarati, and Punjabi; the number of Bengali speakers was too small for statistical analysis. The Urdu and Punjabi groups differed little from the white population, but the Gujarati children were significantly shorter than the children in the other two Asian groups. The authors concluded that 'generalisations from findings in one ethnic group to another in England are not appropriate'. Kamboh and Ferrell (1986) examined the population frequencies for the possession of the protein GC1F allele in different parts of the world. This protein has an increased affinity for vitamin D_3 in comparison to other related proteins, and is probably important in the transport of vitamin D_3 from the skin to the target organs. Kamboh and Ferrell found that there was a high population-frequency for GC1F in most dark-skinned races and in the Chinese and Japanese, and suggested that the possession of this characteristic might be selectively favoured in dark-skinned races. However in the Indian communities examined the frequency of GC1F was no higher than in Europeans; this may explain, in part, why Asian children in the UK develop rickets more frequently than Afro-Caribbean children.

In spite of recent increased interest in the health needs and the diseases of the Asian community progress has been very slow. Ehrardt (1986), in Bradford, found that a higher proportion of Asian children suffered from iron deficiency than did white children, and Williams *et al.* (1985), in Leeds and Bradford, found that the majority of Asian mothers were bottle-feeding their babies, and that two-thirds of the children were still using a bottle containing sweetened drinks up to the age of four or five years.

The teaching of medical students about the cultural aspects of Asian communities in the UK remains very inadequate. Poulton and Rylance (1986) found that in eleven out of twenty-three medical schools in England there was no direct teaching of this subject, and that over half the junior hospital doctors in Birmingham had received no formal training and had done no specific reading about it.

The importance of the child

An Asian family's first contact with the health services is often through an ill child, and the way in which a doctor or other health professional deals with this situation may influence permanently the family's attitude to the health services in the UK. Most of the genetically determined conditions which occur in Asians first become apparent in infancy or childhood, and those infections which are seen more frequently in Asian families are often acquired in childhood. Finally, a child's symptoms may be a signal that the family is under stress, or that one or more of the adults is emotionally disturbed, with adverse effects upon the rest of the family.

Cultural attitudes to illness

The concepts of preventive medicine and follow-up visits are unfamiliar to people from the Indian subcontinent (ISC) where, in general, illness is regarded as an isolated event, and is treated as such.

Doctors who grumble about non-attendance at follow-up appointments need to appreciate this attitude. Also, it is difficult, and sometimes dangerous, for an Asian woman, unaccompanied by an adult male, to take her child through the streets to attend a surgery or outpatient appointment. If her husband is working he may only be available after his return from work, at a time when most surgeries and clinics have finished. In addition, the husband may be reluctant to take time off work for frequent visits to the doctor, for fear of losing his job; unscrupulous employers who know or suspect that the man is an illegal immigrant may exploit this situation with long hours, poor working conditions, and low pay. These factors may explain the popularity of the Accident and Emergency Department of the local hospital.

Unfamiliarity with the common illnesses in the UK, such as recurrent upper respiratory infections, may cause the parents to be unduly concerned by conditions which the indigenous population have come to accept; one way of explaining this to parents is to point out that by coming to the UK they have exchanged recurrent upper respiratory infections for recurrent gastrointestinal ones, and that the climatic conditions are responsible for the difference.

Religious prohibitions on certain foods

Certain foods are prohibited within the different religious groups (see chapter 8). Accurate information should be available to advise on which food products are acceptable and which are not. For infants and children this situation arises when advising on which baby milk or weaning food to choose. Some of the commonly available baby milks, and information on their composition, are given in Table 13.1. If an Asian mother is in doubt about a product or drug she may apparently accept the advice, but not give the suspect substance to her child.

Death and bereavement

The usual customs in the Hindu, Sikh, and Islamic communities are described below, but the formalities are often simplified for stillbirths, and for the death of very young children. If the family does not know of a priest or religious leader of their faith, the hospital should be able to give them the name of someone in the district, and also the name of an undertaker familiar with the necessary customs and procedures. Hospitals in an area with a sizeable Asian community should have a list of suitable names. The hospital staff, especially the nurses, should help bereaved parents to find their way through the bureaucratic procedures associated with death certification and registration, and cremation; sometimes the hospital chaplain takes on this responsibility, unless a priest or religious leader has been appointed to the hospital in a post equivalent to hospital chaplain. A general rule for nursing staff is that jewellery and objects of possible religious significance should not be removed from the body without the parents' permission.

Table 13.1 *Composition of some commonly used baby milks*

	Acceptability to: Muslims	Hindus and Sikhs	Remarks
Whey-based modified milks			
Gold cap SMA (Wyeth)	No*	No	Contains beef
Premium (Cow & Gate)	Yes	Yes	fat
Osterfeed (Farley)	Yes	Yes	
Apramil (Milupa)	Yes	Yes	
Modified cow's milk formulae			
SMA White cap (Wyeth)	No*	No	Contains beef
Baby Milk 'Plus' (Cow & Gate)	Yes	Yes	fat
Ostermilk Complete (Farley)	Yes	Yes	
Progress (Wyeth) for use after age of 6 months	Yes	Yes	
Preterm or low-birth-weight formulae			
SMA Low Birth Weight Formula (Wyeth)	No*	No	Contains beef
Prenatalac (Cow & Gate)	Yes	Yes	fat
Osterprem (Farley)	Yes	Yes	
Nanatal (Cow & Gate)	Yes	Yes	
Pre-Apramil (Milupa)	Yes	Yes	

*Halal fat would be accepted, but in this instance it would not be *halal*.

(a) Hinduism When death is imminent, the patient is given holy water from the River Ganges (Ganga) to drink, and the family or priest reads from one of their holy books. Non-Hindus should wear gloves when touching the body. With the exception of stillbirths and children under the age of four years, who are buried, all Hindus are cremated. From the spiritual point of view a stillborn child is not regarded as in any way different from a child who has been born alive and has died. The period of mourning is for ten to sixteen days, and ends with a special ceremony. Necropsies are not generally approved of, but if required by a coroner are accepted, provided that the reasons for the examination are fully explained.

(b) Sikhism When a person is close to death the relatives or a *Granthi* (reader from the Sikh *gurdwara* or temple) pray at the bedside and read from their holy book, the *Guru Granth Sahb*. Sikhs have no objection to non-Sikhs touching the dead body. Sikhs are cremated, except for stillbirths and young children, who are buried. The mourning period usually lasts for ten to thirteen days.

Though there is no prohibition against necropsy, relatives from rural Punjab, where necropsies would be unusual, may find the procedure difficult to accept.

(c) Islam   The family pray at the bedside of the dying person, whose head must be turned towards Mecca *(Makka)*. Non-Muslims should wear gloves when touching the body. Muslims are buried, and are never cremated; most local authorities provide a special area for Muslim burials. Necropsies, other than those required by a coroner, are not permitted; no organs can be permanently removed from the body during a necropsy. There are no special formalities for stillbirths and young children; the undertaker or the hospital is usually asked to make the necessary arrangements.

Counselling the bereaved parents

There appears to be no great demand for these services, but it is difficult to discover a mother's feelings, since any discussion is usually conducted by the father. However, in spite of linguistic and cultural differences, many Asian mothers have been helped by bereavement counsellors, usually through the Stillbirth and Neonatal Death Society (SANDS), whose address is given at the end of this chapter. Further details on terminal care and bereavement are given in Chapter 18.

The consultation

It is essential that the parents should feel at ease in the consulting room or surgery; parental anxiety is readily transmitted to the child. Receptionists, records clerks, nurses, and doctors should be able to pronounce Asian names and know the correct form of address. Hospitals and practices with a large Asian community should be able to call upon suitable interpreters; except in an emergency, children should not be expected to act as interpreters, as this is embarrassing to the child and to the parents. There is no excuse for failing to obtain a proper history on linguistic grounds, except in an emergency. A record should be made of the family's first language, and of other languages spoken. In some hospitals there are community liaison workers for the appropriate ethnic groups, who are able to help parents or patients with their problems and represent their point of view. Further details are given in Chapter 5.

Family history

In addition to the usual family history, details, including their state of health, should be requested about other adults and children living in the same household, as this is important when considering social problems and cross-infection, particularly with tuberculosis. Normally the father, as head of the family, speaks for his wife and child, and it may take a number of visits before the mother's story can be obtained.

The child's history

A necessary preliminary is to record the child's place of birth, the date of departure from the country of origin, the date of entry into the UK, and the dates of any visits to their home country, especially the date of return from the last visit. Details of any illness and treatment received while away from this country should be requested. Where appropriate, and this is in most cases, information about any malaria prophylaxis during the last visit should be obtained.

The clinical examination

Asian women and girls do not expect to have to undress completely for a clinical examination, but are prepared to expose one part of their body at a time. Asian girls, and Muslims in particular, should be examined by a woman; where this is not possible, as in an emergency, the father or accompanying male relative should be asked to give his permission for the examination to be done by a man. In non-urgent situations, it may be necessary to arrange for a second visit at which a woman doctor can examine the patient. Rectal examinations are regarded as deeply offensive, and no drugs should be given rectally unless it is absolutely essential. When it is necessary to do a rectal examination or to insert a proctoscope or sigmoidoscope, the importance of the examination should be carefully explained.

When prescribing treatment which is to be continued for some time, the various methods of obtaining a repeat prescription should be explained, and an instruction sheet should be given, where appropriate, in one of the languages spoken by the parents.

Diagnostic difficulties in the clinical examination

In children with dark skins, it may be difficult to assess anaemia, jaundice, or central cyanosis. Anaemia and cyanosis can be estimated by looking at the tongue and oral mucous membranes, and jaundice by examining the sclerae, or, in babies, by blanching the palate or gum margins by light pressure with a spoon or spatula. Rashes may be difficult to recognize in Asian children; if measles is suspected, Koplick's spots may often be detected on the buccal mucosa even when the skin rash has appeared; in malnourished children measles may be a severe illness, sometimes with a haemorrhagic rash or severe diarrhoea. In infants and young children, *surma* may be applied round the eyes, partly for the cosmetic effect, and partly to prevent eye infections. Some preparations of *surma* contain lead sulphide, which exposes the child to the risk of lead poisoning. Though non-toxic preparations are easily available and the sale of lead-containing *surma* is prohibited in the UK, it is sometimes imported by individuals.

Some important clinical problems

(a) Emotional and psychological disorders

In both adults and children emotional or psychological disturbances may present to the doctor in the form of symptoms with an apparently physical basis—somatization: headaches, backache, limb pains, and 'fever' are common symptoms. Even when it seems most unlikely that any physical disease is present, it may be necessary to arrange an organically orientated investigation, such as a blood-count or X-ray, or otherwise the parents may feel that their child's symptoms are not being taken seriously. It may be some time before the parents can be convinced that the child's problem is an emotional or psychological one, usually with its origin in the home or at school. There may be difficulty in getting the parents to accept a referral to a child psychiatrist, and a diagnosis of untreatable mental handicap or actual psychiatric illness is often resisted or resented.

(b) Emotional or psychological disorders in the parents and their effect on the child

Difficulties in adaptation to life in the UK may be exacerbated by humiliating or insensitive treatment at the point of entry to the UK, and subsequently by racial prejudice or harassment, and difficulty in obtaining adequate housing or a satisfactory job. The young married woman may feel isolated, without the support of the extended family. In many instances, however, a family joins an already established relative, or finds accommodation in an area where there are members of their own community, often with their own shops and religious centres.

Difficulties in adaptation to life in the UK may cause insecurity, over-anxiety, depression, or paranoid feelings. Unusual or disturbed behaviour in parents may cause feeding difficulty or sleep disturbance in the infant, and enuresis, encopresis, food refusal, school phobia, or other behaviour disorders in the older child. Parental anxiety may cause repeated requests for hospital referral or second opinions. A common complaint, usually about a boy, is that he is 'not growing'; this is rarely true, but the parents are really saying that they want their child to grow up big and strong, and able to cope with a physically and socially hostile environment. Family separation may also cause difficulties, and these are exacerbated by past and present policies on immigration, which may cause a delay of years before a family can be reunited. Children may arrive in the UK to find a father whom they do not know and who does not know them. The reunited parents may produce children at an advanced age, when they are more rigid towards child-rearing than are young parents. The children may develop behaviour disorders as a result of these stresses.

(c) School problems

Learning difficulties due to poor English are less frequent than formerly; most schools with many children of ethnic minority groups in their area have special reception classes for those with 'English as the second language'. Older children, recently arrived in the UK, may have great difficulty at school, particularly in an area which is not used to helping non-English speakers. Even if they do speak English their accent may be mocked and imitated. Inability to live up to parental expectations is not uncommon, as Asian parents, particularly those from East Africa, are anxious that their children should do well at school. Poor school progress may be due to illegal juvenile employment, often in back-street factories (Mahmood 1987), which is connived at by the parents, who need the extra money. Racial bullying in school can cause great distress. Any of these problems may result in school refusal, truanting, elective mutism, or other behaviour disorders.

(d) The child's difficulties in adaptation

Children, like adults, may have difficulty in adapting to a multicultural society. Adolescence, in any society, is often a time of conflict and emotional turmoil. Asian teenagers in particular may find it hard to establish their own identity, and to resolve the conflicts between the traditional Asian way of life and that of the British (white) community; this can be particularly difficult for a girl, who is expected to be a dutiful daughter at home, and at the same time would like to go to discos with her friends. An arranged marriage may prove very distressing to a girl who has established her own social circle outside the home. As do their white counterparts, Asian parents often disapprove of their children forming an attachment to someone of a different ethnic group, or of a different religion. If unresolved, these conflicts may present as psychosomatic complaints such as headache, backache, or abdominal pain, or the 'periodic syndrome'; more extreme reactions include absconding from home, or suicidal attempts, usually by means of a drug overdose.

(e) Physical abuse

Physical abuse is not confined to any particular ethnic group or social class, and Asian families are not immune. A recent survey of 14 238 births in the Surrey area, concerned with the potential for child abuse (Browne and Saqi 1988), demonstrated that the proportion of Asian families in the group considered to be at 'high risk' (two per cent) was the same as their representative proportion in the birth population as a whole (two per cent). Asian families therefore have about the same chance of physically abusing their children as other families. This is confirmed by the fact that three per cent of abusing parents in the Surrey Area are from the Asian community (Browne, personal communication). This may be because physical chastisement as a disciplinary measure, that is as a punishment, is probably accepted among Asian parents as widely as among British ones. Child abuse should only be considered when there is clear evidence of physical injury. It should be pointed out, however, that the Mongolian blue spot is sometimes mistaken for a bruise.

(f) Sexual abuse

As with physical abuse, sexual abuse is probably as common in Asian as in other families. However, child abuse is a complex field, which is still not understood, so that it would be unwise to draw firm conclusions about its occurrence in Asian families.

The antenatal period

Screening during the antenatal period

(a) Beta-thalassaemia   Asian mothers (and in most clinics, all non-white women and all those of Mediterranean or Aegean origin) should be screened for the heterozygous carrier state (thalassaemia minor). If positive, the husband should also be tested. If both are positive they should be advised of the one in four risk that a child of any pregnancy could have the severe homozygous form (thalassaemia major); at the same time they should be told that a prenatal test on the fetus can detect whether it is homozygous or not. There is, of course, little point in subjecting the mother and fetus to the risks of chorionic villus biopsy or blood-sampling by fetoscopy if there is no prospect of a termination being accepted.

(b) Rubella   There is evidence (Peckham *et al.* 1983) that many Asian mothers in the UK have not been immunized against rubella; the non-immune women are most likely to be those who were born in the ISC and came to this country to get married. All Asian women should be tested for rubella antibodies in the antenatal period; non-immune women, if exposed to infection during pregnancy, should be offered immunoglobulin or a termination, and immunization a few days after delivery.

(c) Hepatitis B (HBV)   Between three and ten per cent of Asian women are infective carriers of HBV; and all should be screened antenatally. Those whose blood contains the surface antigen (HBsAg) should be screened by hepatitis

B virus DNA analysis, which is the most sensitive indicator of infectivity. If the mother is known to be a carrier the infant is likely to be infected during delivery, rather than transplacentally. At birth maternal blood should be wiped from the infant's skin, and the stomach should be aspirated to remove swallowed maternal blood. As soon after birth as possible, and in any case within 48 hours of delivery, 10 mcg (0.5 ml) of specific hepatitis B immunoglobulin should be given intramuscularly, and at the same time, or within 48 hours, 10 mcg (0.5 ml) of hepatitis B vaccine should be given intramuscularly at a different site. A second dose of the vaccine is given one month later, and a third dose six months after the first dose.

(d) Hepatitis Non-A Non-B (NANB)   At present the diagnosis of NANB hepatitis is one of exclusion, with negative tests for active hepatitis A and B, B with delta, cytomegalovirus, and EB virus. The main risk of acquiring NANB hepatitis in Asian adults and children is on a visit to Nepal, Bangladesh, or Northern India, especially Kashmir. In children and adults in the United Kingdom the risk is from transfusion of blood and blood-products. The incubation period is usually around forty days. Chronic liver disease, which may be asymptomatic, has been described, but many cases are 'sporadic', with no evidence as to the route of infection; this form is the commonest cause of acute fulminant hepatic failure in children in the UK. In the ISC and parts of the Soviet Union epidemics of water-borne NANB hepatitis have occurred in which there is a clinical resemblance to hepatitis A. In one epidemic in the Kashmir Valley (Khuroo 1980) there was a predilection for severe, sometimes fulminant, infections in women in the third trimester of pregnancy (Khuroo *et al.* 1981). There is a risk of infection of the newborn, though the route is not known; infants at risk from maternal infection should be given the same prophylaxis as from HBV infection, but the degree of protection is unknown. Infected infants may develop a chronic asymptomatic carrier-state, or fulminant hepatic failure. The enteral forms do not appear to progress to chronic liver disease, and there is no evidence that Asian women in the UK are chronic carriers of the water-borne form of NANB hepatitis. Immune globulin does not seem to protect against any of the NANB agents.

Nutrition in pregnancy

(a) Iron deficiency   Iron deficiency is common in Asian women before and during pregnancy; this is due to vegetarian diets poor in iron-containing foods (mainly in Hindus and some Sikhs), or to poor socio-economic circumstances, as in the Bangladeshi (Bengali) community. In strict vegetarians, folic-acid deficiency may also develop. Deficiency of either of these substances may impair fetal growth, and maternal iron deficiency combined with pregnancies at short intervals may reduce the iron stores of the newborn.

(b) Vitamin D deficiency (see Table 13.2)   Adolescent rickets may cause pelvic deformity and a contracted outlet. Severe deficiency of vitamin D during pregnancy causes osteomalacia, which may result in fetal or neonatal rickets, and hypocalcaemic fits.

The perinatal period

Perinatal mortality

A number of studies have shown that the perinatal mortality rate (PMR) in Asians is higher than in the white population. In Birmingham (Terry *et al.* 1983) the PMRs of the Indian and Pakistani communities were compared. The Indian mothers were in a low-risk group for age and parity, while in the Pakistani group there was a high proportion of grand multiparae and women over the age of thirty-five years. The relatively high PMR in the Indian community was due mainly to late stillbirths and bowel atresias, while in the Pakistanis the main contribution to the high PMR was an excess of multiple malformations, and chromosomal abnormalities presumably associated with advanced maternal age. It was also thought that the malformations in the Pakistani infants might be related to the high rate of parental consanguinity, since 55 per cent of the marriages were between first cousins; whereas only two per cent of the Indian marriages were between first cousins, a rate only slightly greater than that of the white population (for discussion on consanguineous marriage see p. 223 Chapter 12). There was no explanation for the high rates of stillbirth and bowel atresias in the Indian group.

Birth-weight

Chetcuti *et al.* (1985) compared the birth-weights and lengths of the newborns in Leicester in the Hindu, Sikh, and Muslim communities with those of the white population. On average the Asian babies were lighter and smaller than the white babies, but the Sikh babies most nearly approached the measurements of the white infants. The Sikh mothers were somewhat taller, and significantly heavier, than the Hindu and Muslim mothers. Whether these findings were due to differences in maternal diet, or to other biological or genetic factors is not clear. Preterm birth did not seem to be unduly frequent in the Asian communities.

Breast-feeding

Many Asian mothers believe the colostrum is harmful to the infant, and are reluctant to breast-feed during the first few days after delivery. This belief should be respected, and not construed as a refusal to breast-feed. In view of the high incidence of maternal vitamin D deficiency it is important that vitamin supple-

Table 13.2 *Causes of vitamin D deficiency rickets in Asian children*

Fetus	Newborn	Infant to toddler	Preschool	Adolescents	All ages
Maternal D-deficiency (non-use of vitamin supplements during pregnancy, vegetarian diet (Hindus), lack of exposure to sunlight (Muslims)	As for fetus	Prolonged breast-feeding by D-deficient mother. Use of unfortified cow's milk, use of unfortified weaning foods. Non-use of vitamin drops.	Vegetarian diet (Hindus). Non-use of vitamin drops	Vegetarian diet (Hindus), lack of exposure to sunlight (Muslims)	Reduced formation of vitamin D_3 in pigmented skin

ments should be given to the infant from the age of one month, or earlier if the mother has osteomalacia.

Infancy

Artificial feeding and weaning diets

The use of ordinary ('doorstep') cow's milk should be discouraged, as it contains negligible quantities of vitamin D and iron. All the usually available baby milks are fortified with vitamin D and with small quantities of iron, though probably in amounts insufficient to prevent iron deficiency anaemia completely. If artificial milks are used, they should be continued as the main source of milk until the age of one year. A list of milks which are acceptable and not acceptable to the various Asian groups is given in Table 13.1.

Many Asian mothers, being uncertain about the type and origin of meat-containing weaning foods, play safe and use carbohydrate-based sweet dessert foods, which contain very little iron, but with a few exceptions now contain added vitamin D.

Immunizations

BCG should be offered for all Asian newborns. Provided that a clear explanation of their purpose is given, acceptance of the routine immunization programmes is usually good, and Asian mothers seem to have, in most cases, escaped the fears about pertussis immunization. All Asian children should have their BCG status and tuberculin reactions checked, if this has not been done at school.

Vitamin and iron supplements: see under *Vitamin D deficiency rickets* and *Iron deficiency*, pp. 232 and 231.

Circumcision

Circumcision is performed on all male Muslim infants, usually in the first few days after birth; but in Bangladeshi families it may not be done until the age of eight. Though there is no provision for ritual circumcision to be done under the National Health Service, some paediatric surgeons are prepared to do the operation under the NHS, on the grounds that they would prefer to do the operation themselves rather than spend time in tidying up circumcisions which have gone wrong owing to a shortage of skilled ritual operators in the UK.

Genetically determined conditions

Consanguineous marriage

The frequency of first- or second-cousin marriages in the Asian community varies greatly. Consanguineous marriages are common in the Pakistanis, and also among the Bangladeshis, but in the Indian communities in the UK (Hindus and Sikhs) they are only slightly more common than in the indigenous population. However, there are parts of South India (Andhra Pradesh, Karnataka, Kerala, and Tamil Nadu) where such marriages are quite common; but these areas have not contributed greatly to the Indian communities in the UK. In Birmingham Terry and his colleagues (1983) found that 55 per cent of Pakistani marriages were between first cousins, but only 2 per cent of those in the Indian community.

The influence of parental consanguinity upon the pattern of disease in a particular community has been much debated. The following points are generally agreed:

(a) The custom should not be condemned by 'outsiders' on moral or eugenic grounds, since this is presumptuous and intolerant.

(b) It is clear that a consanguineous marriage, particularly between first cousins, increases the chance that each parent is carrying the same gene for some rare recessively determined condition. As a result some conditions, such as the rare inborn errors of metabolism, are commoner in consanguineous marriages than in unrelated ones.

(c) When advising parents who are first cousins about the risk of having a child with a genetically determined condition of clinical importance, they should be told that, though the risk is increased, it is still a genetically acceptable one. However, if a relative or a relative's child is known to have a clinically serious recessive condition, the risk is increased that the related couple may produce children with the same condition; the advice of a clinical geneticist should be obtained.

(d) When consanguineous parents, who are clinically well, have produced a child who is homozygous for a known recessive, the risk for subsequent children is the same at each pregnancy (one in four), and is identical to the risk of unrelated parents who are heterozygous carriers of a recessive gene.

(e) The real difficulty arises when a severely malformed or handicapped child is born to parents who are first or second cousins, and the condition cannot be fitted into any known syndrome, and the chromosomes are normal. When only one child has the condition the parents should be referred to a clinical geneticist or a dysmorphologist to make certain that a rare autosomal recessive condition has not been missed. Nevertheless there are always recessively determined syndromes which have not been previously described, and there are certain clinical combinations, such as mental retardation and polydactyly, which carry an empirically increased risk of recurrence in the absence of a syndrome diagnosis. If the malformation is one that could be recognized by ultrasound, or other non-invasive investigation, in a subsequent pregnancy, the parents should be encouraged to have the appropriate investigation done. The logical outcome of the detection of the condition prenatally would, of course, be a termination if the condition is untreatable and severely handicapping. Obviously, if the condition has appeared in more than one child, and there is no recurring environmental factor likely to affect the fetus, then a recessive mode of inheritance should be assumed, and the parents advised accordingly. Detailed advice on genetic counselling is given in Chapter 12.

Some common genetically determined disorders

(a) Beta-thalassaemia   Antenatal testing and genetic counselling have already been described. The anaemia of homozygous beta-thalassaemia does not develop until between six months and one year, when the infant presents with pallor, lethargy, and hepatosplenomegaly. Affected children should be referred to a paediatrician or haematologist with a special interest in the condition. Modell (personal communication) gives the incidence of beta-thalassaemia trait in Asians in Britain as follows: Pakistanis, 6–6.5 per cent (Sindis, 10 per cent), Gujaratis, 6–15 per cent, Sikhs and other north Indians, 3–3.5 per cent, Bangladeshis, 1–2 per cent; the incidence of thalassaemia major in the Pakistani community in Britain is 1 in 500 live births.

(b) Other haemoglobinopathies   Haemoglobin D-thalassaemia and haemoglobin E-thalassaemia are clinically similar to homozygous beta-thalassaemia. Haemoglobin D-thalassaemia is seen mainly in children from North India and Pakistan, while HbE-thalassaemia is more common in those from Bangladesh and India east of the Brahmaputra. Though sickle-cell disease occurs in central India (Kar *et al.* 1986) and in isolated hill tribes in South India and elsewhere, these are not areas from which much migration into the UK has occurred. Sickle-cell anaemia in India appears to be less severe than in the 'African' variety.

(c) Glucose-6 phosphate dehydrogenase (G-6-PD) deficiency   The incidence of this condition in the Asian communities in the UK has not been fully investigated, but it rarely presents serious problems. Choubisa *et al.* (1987) found 4 per cent of schoolchildren in Udaipur (Rajasthan) to be deficient in G-6-PD, but offered no evidence as to its clinical importance or the degree of enzyme deficiency. Modell (personal communication) gives an overall incidence of about 7 per cent hemizygous males in the ISC. Nevertheless the possibility of G-6-PD deficiency should be considered in an Asian infant with an unexplained haemolytic anaemia in the early neonatal period, and in any sudden haemolytic anaemia in other age-groups. Further details are given in Chapter 12.

(d) Other genetically determined conditions (i) *Metabolic disorders.* There is little doubt that in consanguineous marriages rare metabolic disorders occur more frequently than in unrelated marriages, and this is certainly true of the Pakistani community.

(ii) *Multiple malformations and other severe or lethal conditions.* As in the metabolic disorders, recessively determined syndromes occur relatively frequently in Asian families, particularly in first-cousin marriages. The difficulties which arise when the condition cannot be assigned to any recognized syndromes are discussed under consanguineous marriages (Chapter 12) and p. 223.

(e) Chromosomal disorders As already mentioned, there appears to be an excess of mothers of over thirty-five years in the Pakistani community, when compared with the Indian mothers. The reasons for this difference are unclear, since there is no reason to suppose that prolonged separation of husband and wife, owing to immigration procedures, would affect one group more than another.

Acquired diseases

Asian infants are liable to be exposed to a wider variety of infectious diseases than are white infants, as there is a greater probability of an infective adult in the household; and many Asian families, including the children, make frequent visits to the ISC, where infection may be acquired. Details of some of the infections which can affect Asian children are shown in Table 13.3.

(a) Protozoal infections

(i) Malaria Asian families visiting the ISC do not always take adequate malaria prophylaxis, and many take none at all. Those intending to visit their home country should be strongly advised to take proguanil (paludrine) and chloroquine; this should include children of all ages. Prophylaxis is sometimes not given to infants, in the mistaken belief that the drugs are too toxic for them; a generally accepted dosage scheme is given in Table 13.4. Infection is almost always with *Plasmodium vivax* (benign tertian (BT) malaria) or *Plasmodium falciparum* (malignant tertian (MT) malaria). Symptoms commonly developed within six weeks of return to the UK, and malaria should be considered in any febrile child who has recently returned from the ISC. Febrile fits may occur in the preschool child with BT malaria. When malaria is suspected, thick and thin blood-films should be taken at four-hourly intervals irrespective of the presence or absence of spikes of fever. MT malaria may present in a variety of ways, and is a potentially fatal condition. There may be little or no fever, or there may be hyperpyrexia; another manifestation is diarrhoea and shock; cerebral malaria may cause fits, coma, confusional states, hemiplegia, or a meningitis-like picture.

Table 13.3   *Common infections in Asian children*

Infecting agent	Acquired in ISC	Acquired in UK
Bacterial		
Shigellosis	Yes	Yes
Salmonellosis (including typhoid)	Yes	Yes
Tuberculosis, pulmonary	Yes	Yes
Tuberculosis, non-pulmonary	Yes	Rarely
Tuberculosis, meningeal and miliary	Yes	Yes
Viral		
Hepatitis A	Yes	Yes
Hepatitis B	Yes	Yes
Hepatitis Non-A Non-B	Yes	No, except perhaps perinatally
Rotavirus	Yes	Yes
Protozoal		
Amoebiasis	Yes	No
Giardiasis	Yes	Yes
Leishmaniasis	Yes	No
Malaria	Yes	No
Helminthic		
Hookworm (*Ankylostoma duodenale*)	Yes	No
Roundworm (*Ascaris lumbricoides*)	Yes	Yes
Strongyloides stercoralis	Yes	Very rarely (Sprott *et al.* 1987)
Tapeworms (beef and pork)	Yes	Yes
Whip-worm (*Trichuris trichiura*)	Yes	No

Congenital malaria is sometimes seen in the UK when the mother is infected with either *Plasmodium vivax* or *P. falciparum*. The usual age of onset is four to six weeks, with fever, irritability, anorexia, jaundice, and hepatosplenomegaly. Occasionally congenital malaria may mimic neonatal hepatitis, with obstructive jaundice (Davenport 1986). Further details on malaria are given in Chapter 15.

(ii) Leishmaniasis   Leishmaniasis occurs mainly in northern and eastern India, in Bangladesh, and in Pakistan. There are two forms, the systemic form (*kala-azar*), with fever, wasting, and hepatosplenomegaly, and the cutaneous form, which presents either as a raised, crusted lesion (the usual form) or as a lupoid

Table 13.4 *Dosage scale for malaria prophylaxis*

Age	Chloroquine and proguanil (proportion of adult dose)
0–5 weeks	⅛
6 weeks–5 months	¼
6 months–1 year	¼
1–5 years (5–20 kg)	½
6–12 years (20–40 kg)	¾
12 years (> 40 kg)	Adult

form. Any child suspected of having either form of Leishmaniasis should be transferred to a specialist in tropical diseases.

(iii) Giardiasis   See Table 13.5.

(iv) Amoebiasis   See Table 13.5.

(b) Gastrointestinal infections (Infective diarrhoea: important features, Table 13.5)

(i) Gastroenteritis   Infantile gastroenteritis affects mainly families in poor socio-economic circumstances. Traditionally, and quite correctly, Asian parents regard infantile gastroenteritis as a serious disease, and therefore may take their children to the Accident and Emergency Department of the local hospital. The use of oral rehydration solutions (ORS) has improved and simplified the treatment of gastroenteritis, but successful management requires a proper understanding of the use of ORS at home, and instruction leaflets should be supplied in the appropriate Asian languages. Rotavirus is the commonest infecting agent in East London (Khan *et al.* 1986), where there is a large Bangladeshi population.

(ii) Shigellosis   *Shigella* infections are common in children who are taking an adult diet; or they may be acquired from an infected adult at home, or during a visit to the ISC. In young children there may be a septicaemic illness, or a febrile convulsion may occur at the onset. In about 25 per cent of cases there is watery diarrhoea alone, without blood or mucus.

(iii) Salmonellosis (non-typhoid)   The mode of infection is similar to that in shigellosis. The usual symptoms are abdominal pain and diarrhoea, occasionally

Table 13.5. *Infective diarrhoea: important features*

Infecting agent	Clinical presentation	Incubation period	Epidemiology	Immediate treatment
Rotavirus	Acute watery diarrhoea; vomiting common; dehydration in severe cases	24–72 hours	Mainly in infants and young children. Worldwide distribution	Oral rehydration solution.
Shigellae	Loose watery stool usually with blood and mucus; fever and abdominal pain common	36–72 hours	Rare in infancy. Otherwise all age groups	Oral rehydration solution; cotrimoxazole
Salmonellae (non-typhoid)	Nausea, vomiting and abdominal pain, fever; loose stools with flecks of blood and mucus	8–36 hours	Age groups as for Shigellae; outbreaks from infected food common	Oral rehydration solution
Salmonellae (typhoid)	Fever, lethargy, meningism, or stupor are more common in children than gastrointestinal symptoms	10–14 days (5–21)	All age groups may be infected, commonly from a faecal carrier or infected food	Chloramphenicol or amoxycillin
Giardia lamblia	Abdominal distension, watery diarrhoea (*no blood*), crampy abdominal pain	1–3 weeks	Young children particularly, but all age groups, except infants, affected	Metronidazole or tinidazole
Entamoeba histolytica	Abdominal discomfort. Stools with blood and mucus; occasionally acute onset as in shigellosis (both infections may co-exist)	2–6 weeks	All age groups, infants very rarely	Metronidazole or tinidazole
Malaria (*Pl. falciparum*)	Cholera-like picture with shock (but see also Ch. 15 for other clinical syndromes)	6 weeks	All age groups	I.V. rehydration, parenteral chlorquine or quinine
Measles	Profuse rash, sometimes haemorrhagic. Diarrhoea only in malnourished children		Only non-immune children; newborn if mother non-immune	Oral rehydration solution or I.V. rehydration

with flecks of blood. A septicaemic illness with splenomegaly may mimic miliary tuberculosis.

(iv) Typhoid infections The infection may be acquired from a carrier in the home, or during a visit to the ISC. Systemic symptoms such as high fever and apathy, or meningism, may be more common in children than are gastrointestinal symptoms. Further details are given in Chapter 15.

(v) Giardiasis This is often a family infection, or may be acquired in the ISC. Symptoms in children may be more acute than in adults, with nausea or vomiting at the onset, followed by crampy abdominal pain and watery diarrhoea.

(vi) Amoebiasis This cannot be acquired in the UK. Amoebiasis should be suspected in any diarrhoea of insidious onset, with blood and mucus mixed with a loose stool. The identification of the motile amoebae, containing red blood-cells, from a stool or from an ulcer in the rectum or colon, requires warm stage microscopy and someone with the necessary experience. For hepatic amoebiasis see below.

(c) Hepatic infections

(i) Hepatitis A infection (infective hepatitis, HAV) More than one child in the family may be infected. Anicteric cases are common in the preschool child. The infection is commonly acquired on a visit to the ISC.

(ii) Hepatitis B (HBV) Infection may be acquired during delivery, within the family, or from the use of infected syringes, especially in the ISC. There is a wide spectrum of disease; in infancy there may be a chronic carrier-state or chronic hepatitis; acute liver failure may occur in malnourished children. In the older child, there may be hepatic cirrhosis, and in adult life a primary carcinoma of the liver.

(iii) Non-A non-B hepatitis (NANB), see p. 219. Sporadic NANB hepatitis is the commonest cause of fulminant hepatic failure in children. A liver graft, if required, has a survival rate of greater than 50 per cent in this group of cases, with an otherwise very poor prognosis.

(iv) Amoebic hepatitis Multiple abscesses are more common in children than in adults; infection may occur at any age from four weeks, with a peak incidence of three years. The liver is enlarged and tender, but jaundice is rare.

(d) Tuberculosis

(i) Pulmonary tuberculosis   Though BCG is given routinely to the newborn infant in many Asian countries and to Asian newborns in the UK, immunity may not persist into later childhood. The usual source of infection is an adult in the household, or a frequent visitor, and not necessarily a member of the immediate family. Asian children seem to develop the adult type of pulmonary tuberculosis, with cavitation or fibrosis, more frequently than do European children.

(ii) Non-pulmonary tuberculosis   All forms of non-pulmonary tuberculosis are seen, particularly in the older child. Infection in the UK is unlikely, and infected milk in the ISC is probably the commonest cause. Cerivical adenitis and abdominal tuberculosis are the most common forms seen. Abdominal tuberculosis should be suspected in a child with recurrent abdominal pain and loss in weight; an acute intestinal bleed is an occasional presenting symptom.

(iii) Miliary tuberculosis   Miliary tuberculosis is rare in British children, but is relatively common in Asian children. The diagnosis should be suspected in a child with lassitude, fever, and weight-loss; a moderate enlargement of the liver and spleen is usual; the miliary shadows in the lung fields may be very fine, and are easily missed.

(iv) Tuberculous meningitis   When there is an insidious onset, without hepato-splenomegaly, the indefinite symptoms of lethargy, irritability, and headache may be attributed to an emotional disorder, with disastrous results if the diagnosis is delayed. Further details are given in Chapter 15.

(e) Helminthic infections

(i) Hookworm (Ankylostoma duodenale)   Infection usually occurs in toddlers, but infants are occasionally infected. There are no intestinal symptoms, but in heavily infected children an iron-deficiency anaemia develops. The diagnosis is made by finding the ova in the stools; a test for faecal occult blood is usually positive.

(ii) Roundworm (Ascaris lumbricoides)   Children between one and five years are most commonly infected. There may be no symptoms at all, but in malnourished children nutrition is further impaired. In heavy infections there may be colicky abdominal pain or intestinal obstruction. The ova can be easily identified in the stool.

(iii) Strongyloides stercoralis, tapeworms, whip-worm   See Table 13.3, p. 228.

Nutritional disorders

(a) Iron-deficiency anaemia

A number of surveys have confirmed the frequency of iron-deficiency anaemia in Asian children. All groups appear to be affected; a vegetarian diet (Hindus and less commonly Sikhs) and poor socio-economic circumstances (Bangladeshis) are the commonest predisposing factors. In children whose anaemia appears to date from a visit to the ISC, hookworm infection should be considered. In infancy prolonged breast-feeding and the late introduction of carbohydrate-based weaning foods containing negligible amounts of iron may cause severe iron deficiency, and maternal iron deficiency and a low birth-weight may be contributory factors. The peak incidence for symptomatic iron-deficiency anaemia is around three years, with recurrent infections, lack of energy, poor appetite, and pallor; in severe cases, particularly under the age of one year, the liver and spleen may be moderately enlarged.

If a child is found to be anaemic, the rest of the family should have a full blood-count done. Treatment is simple; the cheapest form of iron therapy is Paediatric Ferrous Sulphate Mixture (BP), which should be given in the following dosage for three months:

up to 1 year,	5 ml three times daily;
1–6 years,	10 ml three times daily;
6–12 years,	15 ml three times daily.

The full dosage should be built up gradually over two or three weeks, starting with a quarter of the full dose. Iron preparations should be given after meals. There are numerous, and more expensive, iron preparations available.

In order to prevent a recurrence of the anaemia, dietary advice should be given to the whole family by someone familiar with Asian customs and dietary beliefs.

(b) Vitamin D deficiency rickets

The causes of vitamin D deficiency in Asian children are shown in Table 13.2.

(i) Fetal rickets   Fractures of the long bones, craniotabes.

(ii) Neonatal rickets   Hypocalcaemic fits, radiological evidence of rickets.

(iii) Infantile rickets   Bowing of the long bones, and enlargement of the metaphyses. In persistent crawlers, bowing of the forearm bones may occur. It is not always realized that active rickets is a painful condition, and may cause a toddler to stop walking, or delay or prevent a child from starting to walk.

(iv) Rickets in the school child   This is rarely severe, but the results of previous rickets may be seen at the examination on school entry. Bowing of the legs or knock-knees may be found.

(v) Adolescent rickets   This seems to be related to the adolescent growth spurt; it is commoner in girls than boys, and is particularly common in Muslim girls, owing to the lack of exposure of their limbs to sunlight. The symptoms of adolescent rickets are limb pains, backache, and lassitude; prolonged deficiency may cause pelvic deformity and a contracted pelvis.

If one child in the family is found to have rickets, the other children and the mother should also be examined. The family's diet should be reviewed by a dietitian familiar with Asian diets.

Prevention of rickets

All Asian children should take five drops of the 'government' vitamin drops from the age of one month to five years. There is a good case for resuming this prophylaxis in adolescent Asian girls. Stephens *et al.* (1981) have suggested giving a single oral dose of Ergocalciferol (2.5 mg., 100 000 units) during the autumn.

Diseases of uncertain aetiology

(a) Steroid-responsive (minimal-change) nephrotic syndrome

Two surveys have shown (Sharples *et al.* 1985; Feehally *et al.* 1985) that this condition is more common in the Asian community in the UK than in the indigenous population. The reason for this difference is not known.

(b) Indian childhood cirrhosis (ICC)

Though this condition is unlikely to be seen at all frequently in the UK, the features are worth mentioning, because of the diagnostic difficulty it may present, and the possibility of effective treatment in the early stages. ICC is a severe liver condition largely confined to the area round Pune (Poona) and Maharashtra. The peak incidence is between one and five years, with boys affected four times more often than girls. The onset is insidious, with fever, malaise, abdominal distension, and jaundice; there is a high mortality. Bhave and Pandit (1987) have shown that treatment with D-penicillamine may be effective in the early stages. A high intake of copper, from cooking vessels, is thought to be an aetiological factor, though Bhave *et al.* (1982) found an increased incidence in relation to parental consanguinity. On present evidence, therefore, children with ICC seen in the UK are likely to be below the age of five years, and to have spent their early years in India.

Common diagnostic problems

(a) Mongolian blue spot

This condition, with areas of bluish-black pigmentation in the sacrogluteal, scapular, and lumbar regions is present in 25 per cent of Indian babies (Singh 1986), and is presumably equally common in infants of Pakistani and Bangladeshi parentage. It is sometimes mistaken for the bruising of non-accidental injury, with unfortunate results for all concerned. In all racial groups, the pigmentation gradually disappears by the age of eighteen months to two years.

(b) Hepatosplenomegaly

This is a common problem in Asian children; it can be conveniently considered according to the degree of anaemia.

(i) Hepatosplenomegaly with slight or no anaemia   One needs to consider chronic malaria, *kala-azar*, (systemic Leishmaniasis), miliary tuberculosis, cirrhosis with portal hypertension, and, in the under-five age-group with an appropriate history, Indian childhood cirrhosis. In hepatosplenomegaly with lymphadenopathy, infectious mononucleosis is a possibility.

(ii) Hepatosplenomegaly with anaemia   If severe anaemia without lymphadenopathy is obvious clinically, homozygous beta-thalassaemia (thalassaemia major) should be suspected, with HbD-thalassaemia and HbE-thalassaemia less commonly; in any event the differential diagnosis will need to be made by a haematologist. Severe anaemia with lymphadenopathy suggests acute lymphatic leukaemia; in most cases there are petechiae due to thrombocytopenia. Severe iron-deficiency anaemia in children under one year may be accompanied by slight enlargement of the liver and spleen.

(c) Bizarre or inexplicable symptoms

Symptoms which do not fit in with the child's diagnosis, and cannot be attributed to toxic effects or side-effects of prescribed treatment, may be due to the use by the parents of medicines obtained from herbal shops or from practitioners of *Unani* or Ayurvedic medicine. Some of the oral preparations prescribed or bought over the counter may contain lead.

(d) Conditions which may be mistaken for psychosomatic or psychiatric disorders

  (i) *Adolescent rickets*: limb pains, and backache (see p. 232).
 (ii) *Cerebral malaria*: confusional state (see p. 225).
(iii) *Tuberculous meningitis*: headache and lassitude (see p. 230).
(iv) *Rabies* Most cases of rabies in the UK have been initially considered to be suffering from some type of behaviour disorder, even when there is a clear history of an animal bite before returning to the UK. Since active immunization, with passive immunization if thought necessary, is effective during the prolonged (one week to more than a year) incubation period, failure to consider rabies is a disastrous mistake.

Conclusion

Over the last thirty years our knowledge of the problems of Asian children in the UK has slowly increased, but many questions remain unanswered, and much work needs to be done. There have been no comprehensive studies of properly-defined Asian groups, starting in the perinatal period and continuing into adolescence. Further work is required on the causes of stillbirths and malformation in the Indian and Pakistani communities, and upon the results of consanguineous marriages. A study of the PMR in the Bangladeshi community should be done.

Teaching of medical students and nurses about Asian children (and adults) is still quite inadequate. There is also a need for cross-fertilization of ideas between paediatricians in the ISC and those in the UK.

Acknowledgements

I am grateful for the help of Dr Bernadette Modell on the incidence of the haemoglobinopathies in the Asian groups in Britain, to Dr Elizabeth Fagan on Non-A Non-B hepatitis, to Dr Michael Baraitser on the genetic aspects of consanguinity, and to Miss Sue Dyke on infant nutrition in the Asian communities.

References

Arthurton, M. W. (1972). Immigrant children and the day-to-day work of a paediatrician. *Archives of Disease in Childhood*; **47**, 126–30.

Bhave, S. and Pandit, A. (1987). D-penicillamine in the therapy of Indian childhood cirrhosis. *Indian Journal of Paediatrics*, **54**, 587–90.

Bhave, S. A., Pandit, A. N., Pradhan, A. W., Sidhaye, D. G., Kantarjian, A., Williams, A. *et al.* (1982). Liver disease in India. *Archives of Disease in Childhood*, **57**, 922–8.

Browne, K. D. and Saqi, S. (1988). Approaches to screening for child abuse and neglect. In *Early prediction and prevention of child abuse*, (ed. K. D. Browne, C. Davies and P. Stratton), pp. 57–85. Wiley, Chichester.

Chetcuti, P., Sinha, S. H., and Levene, M. I. (1985). Birth size in Indian ethnic subgroups born in Britain. *Archives of Disease in Childhood*, **60**, 868–70.

Choubisa, L., Pande, S., and Srivastave, Y. K. (1987). Incidence of abnormal haemoglobins and G-6PD deficiency in school children in Udaipur (Rajasthan), India. *Indian Journal of Tropical Medicine and Hygiene*, **90**, 215–16.

Davenport, M. (1986). Neonatal malaria and obstructive jaundice. *Archives of Disease in Childhood*, **61**, 515–16.

Ehrardt, P. (1986). Iron deficiency in young Bradford children of different ethnic groups. *British Medical Journal*, **292**, 90–93.

Feehally, J., Kendell, N. P., Swift, P. G. F., and Wallis, J. (1985). High incidence of minimal change nephrotic syndrome in Asians. *Archives of Disease in Childhood*, **60**, 1018–20.

Henley, A. (1979). *Asian patients in hospital and at home*. King's Fund, London.

Kamboh, M. I. and Ferrell, R. E. (1986). Ethnic variations in vitamin-D binding protein (GC). *Human Genetics*, **72**, 281–93.

Kar, B. C., Kulozik, A. E., Sirr, S., Sarapathy, R. K., Kulozik, M., Serjeant, B. E., and Serjeant, G. R. (1986). Sickle cell disease in Orissa State, India. *Lancet*, **ii**, 1198–1201.

Khan, S., Chong, S. K. F., Cullinan, T., and Walker-Smith, J. A. (1986). Gastroenteritis and its impact on nutrition in Asian and Caucasian infants in East London. In *Diarrhoea and malnutrition in childhood* (ed. J. A. Walker-Smith and A. S. McNeish), pp. 129–34. Butterworth, London.

Khuroo, M. S. (1980). Study of an epidemic of Non-A Non-B Hepatitis. *American Journal of Medicine*, **68**, 818–24.

Khuroo, M. S., Teli, M. R., Skidmore, S., Sofi, M. A., and Khuroo, M. I. (1981). Incidence and severity of viral hepatitis in pregnancy. *American Journal of Medicine*, **70**, 252–5.

Lobo, E. de H. (1978). *Children of immigrants in Britain, their health and social problems*. Hodder and Stoughton, London.

Mahmood, M. (1987). Scandal of Britain's illegal child labour. *Sunday Times*, April 5, p. 3.

Peckham, C. S., Tookey, P., Nelson, D. B., Coleman, J., and Morris, N. (1983). Ethnic minority women and congenital rubella. *British Medical Journal*, **287**, 129–30.

Poulton, J. and Rylance, G. W. (1986). Medical teaching of the cultural aspects of ethnic minorities; does it exist? *Medical Education*, **20**, 492–7.

Rona, R. J. and Chinn, S. (1986). National study of health and growth: social and biological factors associated with height of children from ethnic groups living in England. *Annals of Human Biology*, **13**, 453–71.

Sharples, P. M., Poulton, J., and White, R. H. R. (1985). Steroid responsive nephrotic syndrome is more common in Asians. *Archives of Disease in Childhood*, **60**, 1014–17.

Singh, T. (1986). A clinical study of Mongolian Spot. *Journal of Obstetrics and Gynaecology of India*, **36**, 994–5.

Sprott, V., Selby, C. D., Ispahani, P. and Toghill, P. J. (1987). Indigenous strongyloidiasis in Nottingham. *British Medical Journal*, **294**, 741–2.

Stephens, W. P., Berry, J. L., Klimuk, P. S., and Mawer, E. B. (1981). Annual high-dose vitamin D prophylaxis in Asian immigrants. *Lancet*, **ii**, 1199–1201.

Terry, P. B., Condie, R. G., Matthew, P. M. and Bissenden, J. G. (1983). Ethnic differences in the distribution of congenital malformations. *Postgraduate Medical Journal*, **59**, 657–8.

Williams, S. A., Fairpo, C. G., Howell, V., Duckworth, C. and Ahmed, I. (1985). Some Asian communities in the U.K. and their culture. *British Dental Journal*, **159**, 139.

Winkler, F. and Yung, J. (1981). Advising Asian mothers. *Health and Social Services Journal*, **91**, 1244–5.

Further reading

Bangladeshis in Britain (1986). Volume 1: First report from the Home Affairs Committee. HMSO, London.

Black, J. (1985). The new paediatrics: child health in ethnic minorities. *British Medical Journal*, London.

Black, J. (1987). Broaden your mind about death and bereavement in certain ethnic groups in Britain. *British Medical Journal*, **295**, 536–9.

Fleming, A. F. (ed.) (1982). *Sickle cell disease*. Churchill Livingstone, Edinburgh.

Mares, P., Henley, A. and Baxter, C. (1985). *Health care in multiracial Britain*. Health Education Council and National Extension College Trust, Cambridge.

Perinatal and neonatal mortality. (1980). Second report for the Social Services Committee ('The Short report'). HMSO, London.

Weatherall, D. J. and Clegg, J. B. (1981). *Thalassaemia syndromes*. (3rd edn). Blackwell Scientific Publications, Oxford.

Useful address

Stillbirth and Neonatal Death Society, (SANDS), 28 Portland Place, London, W1. Telephone 01-436-5881.

14 Elderly Asians

Liam Donaldson and Marie Johnson

Introduction

Elderly Asian people, in keeping with other age-groups within the Asian communities of the United Kingdom, have been much less studied, as a population, than their non-Asian counterparts. Moreover many people from the majority population will have never had prolonged direct contact with elderly people from the Asian community.

It is in these circumstances, of paucity of research data and the absence of widespread direct experience on the part of the indigenous population, that quite stereotypic assumptions develop. For example, it is widely believed that old age is a greatly revered state within the Asian community, and hence an elderly person will enjoy the warmth, support, and care of an extended family, so that little priority needs to be given to policy-making to meet the needs of the elderly. It is reported that Asian-Americans—meaning people who migrated from the Pacific basin, particularly Japan, to America—have been subjected to a similar form of stereotyping, and viewed as a 'model minority' (Kitano 1969; Lum 1983).

Caring for elderly people may represent a cultural ideal held by the Asian population itself; but it may not be realized in practice in the elderly people's countries of origin (Harlan 1964). While it may also be the ideal shared by Asian people in the UK today, patterns of mobility and other factors will mean that it is unlikely always to be realized, and the contrast between this cultural ideal and the social reality may give rise to problems for elderly Asian people themselves, as well as leading to false assumptions among those who are responsible for providing services.

There is also the view that characteristics attributed to minority groups, such as strong kinship bonds, which are thought to be a cultural characteristic, may, where they are found, be a response to living in a hostile environment where kinship and other forms of mutual aid are reinforced because of reduced access to the rewards and services of the wider society (Colen and McNeely 1983).

In contrast to the roseate view of the extended Asian family, a body of literature has emerged which makes much of the potentially serious problems and disadvantages faced by people who are not only old, but also bear the additional burdens of discrimination which accompany non-white status (so called 'double jeopardy'); to this has been added the 'triple jeopardy' of perceived lack of access to services Norman (1985), and even the 'quadruple jeopardy' of being non-English-speaking (Lum 1983).

While it has been quite justifiably argued that studies of the health of the Asian population have placed too much emphasis on the differences from the majority population, rather than the similarities (Bhopal 1988), it would seem to be the case for Asian elderly people, more so than for other age-groups, that they have significantly different life-experiences from the indigenous elderly. They are, after all, a group who have experienced migration, marked cultural change, and racial prejudice. They are minority members of a minority group, often poor and politically weak. Much of the evidence on the effect of ageing on ethnic groups comes from American studies, which emphasize not just ethnicity *per se* but the over-representation of minority elderly people in the lower socio-economic groups. Thus, a report by the American National Council on Aging reported the five most prevalent chronic conditions of elderly people as arthritis, hearing impairment, visual impairment, hypertension, and heart conditions; and five conditions as the most common causes of death of old people: ischaemic heart disease, cerebrovascular disease, malignant neoplasms, infectious diseases, and diabetes.

> Although these conditions predominate among the aged as compared to younger people, they are not equally distributed among the aged population. There is some evidence to suggest that they are disproportionately higher among the aged in racial and ethnic minority groups. However, racial or ethnic group membership *per se* does not appear to be the determining factor. Rather, it is the disproportionate representation of minority aged in the lower socio-economic strata that appears to explain much of the variance in both health status and utilization of health care services. (Morrison 1983.)

Any consideration of the needs of elderly Asian people must address the fact that there has been reluctance, in some quarters, to plan and provide services for them, on the grounds that this would represent a positive discrimination that was somehow unfair to the majority of the elderly population. In answering this objection, it is important to remember that one of the key functions of the Welfare State is to identify sensitively and fairly groups of the population who have particular needs, and then to try to meet them. If those in the minority elderly population were to be offered access to services designed on the basis of the needs of the majority population, then they would only be being treated equally if their needs were the same as those of their majority-population counterparts: if their needs were different, it is likely that they would then be disadvantaged, because then their needs would not be being met. Moreover, reviewing and improving services for Asian elderly people should be seen as part of the effort to ensure that welfare services are sensitive to the needs of all of Britain's culturally diverse society:

> Indeed, one of the questions which the whole issue of care for older people with particular ethnic characteristics forces us to face is the appropriateness and efficiency of our services for *all* elderly people. (Norman 1985).

The size of the elderly Asian population

Difficulties in developing precise demographic estimates and projections for the Asian population have been discussed in detail in chapter 6. It is clear, however, that elderly people represent a relatively small proportion of the Asian population of the UK today, markedly so when compared with the elderly in the white population (Table 14.1).

Table 14.1 *Percentage of elderly people within different ethnic groups: Great Britain 1985*

Ethnic group	Percentage who were elderly*
White	19
Total non-white	3
West Indian or Guyanese	4
Indian	3
Pakistani	1
Bangladeshi	1
Chinese	4
African	1
Arab	2
Mixed	2
Other	4
Not stated	14
All ethnic groups	18

* Men aged 65 years or over and women aged 60 years and over
Source: OPCS 1986

Another factor of particular importance will be the point at which those Asians who were born in the UK start to form increasingly higher proportions of the elderly population. This will have a numerical impact, as the Asian population starts to resemble the age-structure of the white population; but it will also be of importance because this group is likely to have different life-experiences and cultural expectations from those of their parents and grandparents who migrated to the UK.

Assessing the needs of the elderly Asian patient

The general practitioner or other health-care professional who is providing advice or care for elderly Asian people should bear in mind a number of key points which are explored in more detail in the rest of the chapter.

- With few exceptions the illnesses and physical accompaniments of old age will be similar to those of the indigenous elderly.
- The Asian population is not culturally homogeneous, so establishing the cultural group to which the old person belongs will be fundamental in giving them the most appropriate help.
- Many elderly Asians, particularly women, have a poor ability to speak, read, or understand English.
- Old people will often be living in multigenerational households.
- Few elderly Asians will have knowledge of, or familiarity with, the full range of services, particularly those delivered by non-health-service agencies.
- Asian people are equipped with their own cultural understanding of illness, and have culturally shaped expectations of old age. These are significant in determining when they seek medical help, the type of help they look for, and their judgement of appropriate types of treatment and care.

Health problems of elderly Asian people

There has been criticism of studies of the health of Asian people which have concentrated on those conditions which are unusual in the majority population, but present in the Asian population. The effect is that a disproportionate amount of emphasis may be put on the possibility of Asian people suffering from these conditions. The fact is that the Asian population suffers many of the health problems which also affect the majority population, as has been described in more detail in Chapters 6 and 9.

The British data support the American findings quoted earlier on the similarity of minority and majority ethnic groups' health problems. While the greater incidence of some conditions such as tuberculosis or intra-hepatic bile-duct cancer among the Asian population cannot be ignored, their absolute frequency should mean there is not overemphasis on such illnesses among Asian people at the expense of the common causes of illness and death.

Ethnic diversity

The term 'Asian' has been adopted to refer to people resident in the UK who themselves originated, or whose parents and grandparents originated, from the Indian subcontinent. Use of this term by the majority population, social scientists, and caring professionals does tend to mask the ethnic diversity found among Asians living in the UK today. As is well demonstrated in other chapters of this book, Asian people are diverse in terms of language, religious affiliation, caste, class, and place of residence prior to migration to the UK. It is equally inappropriate when considering older members of the Asian community to regard them as a homogeneous, undifferentiated social group.

A study of blacks and Asians aged fifty-five and over carried out in Manchester and London gave information about Asians who migrated to the UK during the course of this century. Early arrivals were single Asian men, often seamen who settled here in the 1930s and 1940s, and often did not marry, and in their old age tend not to belong to extended households. During the late 1940s and 1950s many Asians migrated with their families to take up public-sector and industrial work. In the next two decades spouses, usually wives, of earlier immigrants came to this country. Another two categories of Asians who came to the UK during the 1970s were aged parents of people already settled here, and those Asians expelled from East Africa who arrived as refugees. It is from these people, with their very diverse life-experiences, that the elderly Asian population of today is drawn (Barker 1984).

In addition to the likelihood that their personal history prior to arriving in the UK will have been very diverse, elderly Asians' experience of life in this country may also be quite varied. For instance, living in contact with a group of people sharing the same ethnic identity may mean for the elderly person that there are local-level networks which provide support. On the other hand, if they are separated from other people sharing their ethnicity old people may lack such support and sources of information. Moreover, if Asians are a significant presence in a locality, service-providers may have, through direct experience, more awareness of the needs of elderly Asian people, and there may be local pressure-groups which have worked to ensure a more sensitive approach to assessing and providing for the needs of elderly people from the different ethnic groups.

Facility in English

Facility in language is made up of the skills of understanding the spoken language, and of reading, writing, and speaking it.

Ability in these skills varies across the elderly Asian population, and any one individual may have a differing degree of competence in the four skills. The first language of elderly Asian people will largely refect their country of origin and the religious group to which they belong. A description of the languages used by the Asian community as a whole is given in Chapter 1, and further details on fluency and literacy in Chapter 5.

In many health settings an elderly Asian person will have to rely on knowledge of written and spoken English. In a survey carried out in Leicester over one-fifth of people said they could speak English, but there was a marked difference between the sexes, as Table 14.2 shows.

In a range of everyday situations which called for a certain degree of fluency, in three out of six situations more than half the elderly Asian people interviewed felt they would have difficulty in communicating without an interpreter, while in the remaining situations this was so for a substantial minority (Table 14.3).

Table 14.2   *Percentage of elderly Asians in Leicester who said they could speak, read or write English*

English language	Men	Women	Both sexes
Spoken	37	2	21
Read	24	>1	13
Written	21	>1	11

Source: Donaldson and Odell 1986

Overall 35 per cent could not read in any language, and this proportion was much higher for women than men: 63 per cent compared to 11 per cent.

There is also evidence that older Asians, particularly women, are not able to read in their first language, and therefore, while providing health leaflets in Asian languages is to be encouraged, it should not be assumed that this solves

Table 14.3   *Elderly Asians' assessment of their own ability to use English in a range of 'everyday' situations*

Situation	Would be able to make themselves understood:			
	Easily (%)	With difficulty (%)	Only with interpreter (%)	TOTAL (*n* = 145) (%)
On a bus asking cost of fare	68	22	10	100
Asking for goods in English shops	64	27	9	100
Returning faulty goods to English shop	47	31	22	100
Telephoning to re-arrange out-patient appointment	43	23	34	100
Giving directions to an English person	52	31	17	100
Explaining a problem to a doctor	41	21	38	100

Source: Donaldson and Odell 1986

the problem of communicating information to the elderly population. Younger generations may read Asian-language leaflets for their older relatives; but audio cassettes or videos may in fact be a much more efficient way of reaching this population.

Household patterns

Acknowledging the problem of simply accepting the cultural stereotype of elderly people inevitably being cared for within the community, Asian people do tend to live in extended households (Table 14.4).

Table 14.4 *Household size by ethnic group of head of household: Great Britain 1985*

Ethnic group of head of house-hold	Household size (%)						All households (thousands; = 100%)	Average household size
	1	2	3	4	5	6 and over		
White	24	33	17	17	6	2	20 235	2.5
Total non-white	14	18	18	20	12	17	673	3.5
West Indian or Guyanese	19	25	19	18	10	9	195	3.0
Indian	5	12	21	26	15	21	178	4.0
Pakistani or Bangladeshi	7	7	10	17	16	44	106	4.9
Other non-white	23	23	19	19	10	7	194	2.9
Not stated	24	34	15	19	5	3	188	2.7
All ethnic groups	24	33	17	18	6	3	21 096	2.6

Source: OPCS 1986

The households that many elderly Asian people live in also tend to be multi-generational ones. In the Leicestershire survey nearly three-quarters of the people in the sample had four or more grown-up children alive, and over 70 per cent had at least one grown-up child living in the same household as themselves.

The most frequent household configuration for elderly Asian people seen in this study was multigenerational (Table 14.5)—usually the elderly person, their children, and their grandchildren. Of those who did not live in multigenerational households over three-quarters had children living elsewhere in the city, and over half, elsewhere in the UK. This pattern was common to the three main religious groups.

Table 14.5 *Composition of households in which a sample of Leicestershire elderly Asians lived*

Household composition	Percentage of old people (Numbers in brackets)	
Lived alone	5	(34)
One generation	13	(95)
Two generations	24	(173)
Three generations	55	(397)
Four generations	3	(26)
With non-relatives	—	(1)
All households	100	
(Total sample =)		(726)

Source: Donaldson and Odell 1986

This is in marked contrast to the type of household in which non-Asian people lived, shown in a comparable survey. About half of those aged seventy-five and over were living alone, 38 per cent with a spouse, and 12 per cent with a child.

Clearly living within a multigenerational household potentially provides considerable social support for an elderly person; but there may also be disadvantages in this situation, particularly as British domestic architecture is not on the whole designed for these types of domestic arrangement. For example, in the Leicester Survey 22 per cent of those old people interviewed shared a bedroom with someone else, most commonly a grandchild.

If a large family group lives in crowded conditions, the elderly person may be disadvantaged by surrendering living-space within the house to younger members; and for those elderly Asian people on low incomes, poor housing conditions may exacerbate chronic illness and disabilities acquired from a working life spent in low-paid jobs in unhealthy working conditions (Norman 1985).

Status within the household can be an important factor. In Leicester, elderly Asian women played a prominent role within the household in relation to domestic tasks; but elderly Asian men played relatively little part in these activities, although more than half helped with shopping. An important source of social contact is the range of involvement in activities outside the house, and while many people did spend time out of the house, quite a large minority did not (Table 14.6).

As might be expected, time spent outside the home was related to age, but,

Table 14.6 *Percentage of periods of the day spent out of the house by elderly Asians in Leicester over a one-week period*

| Period | Number spent out during week | | | | Total |
	0	1–2	3–4	5 or more	($n = 726$)
Mornings	32	15	15	38	100
Afternoons	48	14	15	23	100
Evenings	52	16	11	21	100

Source: Donaldson and Odell 1986

notwithstanding this effect, there was a striking difference between the sexes: for example, 45 per cent of elderly women had not been out on any morning during the previous week, compared with 13 per cent of elderly men. It is not uncommon for it to be understood that elderly Asian men will spend much of the day outside the house; and this can lead to them spending a great deal of unstructured time outdoors, even in bad weather.

While many elderly Asian people live in extended, multigenerational households, there are those who live independently or with others than their kinsfolk, for a variety of reasons. There are those referred to above who formed one of the early groups of migrants to this country, the single male seamen who led an independent, peripatetic life, and in their old age are settled in this country, often without close kinship ties. Those Asians who came to this country when they were expelled as refugees from East Africa often find themselves without the type of communal support they were familiar with in Africa (Norman 1985). Such people are sometimes lodgers with other families; and in this situation it cannot be assumed that they receive the support or have the high status within the domestic setting which is often considered as typical of Asian culture.

Knowledge and use of welfare services

Research has shown that Asians and other members of ethnic groups do tend to be registered with GPs. A study in 1981 of 2000 households (but one that excluded those over sixty years old) showed that 96 per cent of Asians were registered with a local GP, and the remaining 4 per cent with a GP elsewhere. Two-thirds of these people were registered with a GP of Asian origin, and a further 10 per cent at a practice with an Asian doctor (Johnson 1986).

The research also showed that Asians were likely to have visited their GP in the previous year, and more frequently than either whites or Afro-Caribbeans. This pattern was confirmed by a study of elderly people from similar ethnic groups in Birmingham (Blakemore 1982). It is not possible to be categorical about the reasons for the relatively frequent use of the GP service by Asian people, but among the relevant factors may be cultural expectations of the type of role the GP has, higher rates of disease and illness engendered by their socio-economic circumstances prior to migration and since arrival in the UK, and the stress which may be experienced by elderly people who have had to adjust to an alien society.

The figures for registration and use of the services do not in themselves demonstrate that elderly Asian people find their interaction with their GPS easy, even if the GPs are of Asian origin themselves. As has already been emphasized, the ethnic diversity of Asian Britons means that the patient and doctor may not necessarily have language, religion, or other characteristics in common. However, these data do underline that GPs have a major role in ensuring that elderly Asian people obtain appropriate care and facilities from the health and social services, because they are the representatives of the caring professions most likely to have frequent contact with older members of the Asian community.

While there have been initiatives to ensure uptake of community services by the Asian population, in general there seems to be a low utilization of the services provided by community-based NHS staff. Improving elderly Asians' use of these services is not simply a question of letting them know that they exist, but also ensuring that they are of an appropriate type; making sure, for instance, that full use is made of community nurses and health visitors from the Asian community, and approaching the community through the traditional meeting places, such as temples, mosques, and community centres. Utilizing the local institutions and networks set up by the Asian population is one of the most constructive ways of disseminating information about services currently available, and learning what the needs of the community are.

Consideration has to be given to setting up residential homes and day centres specifically for Asian elderly people. Facilities where the large majority of clients, residents, and staff are white, and where the sexes are mixed, may not be seen as an attractive option for an elderly person from the Asian community.

In response to the need for sheltered accommodation for elderly Asian people, and the perceived inappropriateness of most of the existing provision, a number of initiatives have been taken to provide housing for elderly Asians. Norman (1985) cites the ASRA (Asian Sheltered Residential Accommodation) initiatives in Wandsworth and Lambeth. Another London scheme is based in Southall, and provides homes for elderly men.

Outside London there are projects in Leeds, Birmingham, and Leicester. The ASRA organization in Leicester, active since 1980, has provided a variety of types of accommodation, including homes for frail people. In 1988 it had 85 flats in occupation, and 42 being developed; and ASRA Leicester's role has expanded to providing information to the whole Midlands area.

Improving the sensitivity of hospital-based services is very much the repsonsibility of the District Health Authorities; but GPs have to be aware of how potentially alienating hospital services are to elderly Asian people. Concerns about lack of signs in community languages and of opportunities for religious observances, about whether food will conform to religious dietary norms, and whether personal hygiene preferences will be respected, can all ensure that the perception of services is poor and uptake low. Being able to give reassurance and information about these aspects of the health service can have a strong influence on whether elderly Asian people take up the services and get the best out of them.

Cultural attitudes to illness and health care

Those writing on Asian attitudes to illness and health-care have tended to concentrate on the extent to which the systems of medicine in the Indian subcontinent, the *Tibe-Unani* and Ayurvedic systems, are used in this country. As is explained in more detail in Chapter 7, in the Indian subcontinent these two systems co-exist with homeopathy, which established itself well there, and with allopathic medicine. The *Tibe-Unani* and Ayurvedic systems take a holistic approach, and involve the understanding of personality, humours, and lifestyle in the causation and treatment of conditions. Practitioners called *hakims* (*Tibe-Unani*) and *vaids* (Ayurvedic) are trained in schools for traditional medicine, and are registered by the governments of India and Pakistan.

Reports vary on the extent to which *hakims* and *vaids* are active in the UK, and the amount of use made of them by British Asians. Mays (1981) quotes a report to the DHSS which suggests that traditional practitioners are to be found in all the main Asian communities in the UK, and that it is common for patients to consult both a traditional practitioner and a GP about their condition. Mays warns against 'a very real danger' of overlooking the possibility of drug interaction between drugs prescribed by GPs and by *vaids* or *hakims*. In contrast Johnson (1986) found that a majority of Asian respondents disagreed with the statement that there are many conditions for which traditional remedies are better than conventional medicine, and only 2 per cent of respondents in his survey had consulted a *hakim* or a *vaid* in the previous year. Bhopal (1986) similarly found a low rate of consultation of traditional healers in Glasgow, and his findings question the notion that there is significant danger in the use of traditional medicines; because, while there was quite widespread knowledge of the theory of the Asian health-care systems, and some use of the medicines, there was a degree of scepticism about their efficacy, and of alertness to the potential dangers of the metal-based remedies in particular.

The way in which Asian knowledge of traditional systems and medicine may be most significant to the GP is that these approaches are of a general, holistic nature, and predispose the patient to expect the practitioner to take an interest in their total condition, and to spend time and care over consultation. The fact that this type of approach is not axiomatic under the NHS may cause patients to doubt the efficacy of the treatment and remedies they are being prescribed.

Conclusion

The numbers of elderly Asian people are as yet small; but this will change as the structure of the Asian population begins to resemble that of the majority. As has also been demonstrated, the elderly Asian population not only shares many of the health problems of the elderly white population, but also shares the characteristic of being disenfranchised from services. Improving services for all elderly people should in some measure improve services for elderly Asian people. However it is important to be aware of the particular life-experiences and social situations of elderly Asian people, so that sensitively designed services can be provided, while not falling into the trap of operating merely at the level of myth and stereotype. It is proper to be alive to the particular problems that affect elderly Asian people, which can have a very direct influence on their health and the type of services they receive.

The overwhelming majority of health problems faced by ethnic minorties in Britain are different in degree, but not in kind, from those experienced by the rest of the population. Social factors contributing to ill-health, and the general health-care experience of the NHS, are often intensified for the ethnic minority users by racism and racial prejudice, cultural insensitivity and language differences (Pearson 1984).

Providing welfare services which are sensitive to cultural diversity, but do not treat the individual elderly person as a cultural stereotype, is one route to ensuring proper health care for all citizens.

References

Barker, J. (1984). *Black and Asian old people in Britain*. Age Concern Research Unit, London.

Blakemore, K. (1982). Health and illness among the elderly of minority ethnic groups living in Birmingham: some new findings. *Health Trends*, **14**, 69–72.

Bhopal, R. S. (1986). The inter-relationship of folk, traditional and western medicine within an Asian community in Britain. *Social Science and Medicine*, **22**, 99–105.

Bhopal, R. S. (1988). Health care for Asians: conflict in need, demand and provision. In *Equity: a prerequisite for health*, Proceedings of 1987 Summer Scientific Conference, pp. 52–6. Faculty of Community Medicine and WHO, London.

Colen, J. L. and McNeely, R. L. (1983). Minority aging and knowledge in the social professions. In *Aging in Minority Groups*, (ed. R. L. McNeely and J. L. Colen) p. 19. Sage, London.

Donaldson, L. J. and Odell, A. (1986). Health and social status of elderly Asians: a community survey. *British Medical Journal*, **293**, 1079–82.

Harlan, W. (1964). Social status of the aged in three Indian villages. *Vita Humana*, **7**, 239–52.

Johnson, M. (1986). Inner city residents, ethnic minorities and primary health care in the West Midlands. In *Health, Race and Ethnicity* (ed. T. Rothwell and D. Phillips), Croom Helm, London.

Elderly Asians and the NHS 249

Kitano, H. (1969). *Japanese Americans: the evolution of the subculture.* Prentice-Hall, New Jersey.

Lum, D. (1983). Asian-Americans and their aged. In *Aging in minority groups* (ed. R. L. McNeely and J. L. Colen, pp. 85–94. Sage, London.

Mays, N. (1981). The health needs of elderly Asians. *Geriatric Medicine*, **11**, 37–41.

Morrison, B. J. (1983). Physical health and the minority aged. In *Aging in minority groups*, (ed. R. L. McNeely and J. L. Colen), pp. 161–73. Sage, London.

Norman, A. (1985). *Triple jeopardy: growing old in a second homeland.* Centre for Policy on Aging, London.

OPCS (Office of Population Censuses and Surveys) (1986). *OPCS Monitor Reference LFS 86/2 Labour Force Survey 1985: ethnic group and country of birth.* HMSO, London.

Pearson, M. (1984). An insensitive service. In *Health Care UK 1984: an economic and social and policy audit.* (ed. A. Harrison and J. Gretton), pp. 122–4. CIPFA, London.

15 Infectious diseases

Karl Nicholson

Introduction

Asian immigrants and Asians born in this country develop the same infections as the indigenous white population. In addition, through travel and other connections overseas, they are at increased risk for diseases commonly found in the Third World, such as malaria or typhoid, which present shortly after overseas travel, and other conditions such as amoebic liver abscess and bilharzia, which may only become evident months or years after a period abroad. Certain infections such as hepatitis B and tuberculosis are also seen at a higher frequency among Asians—even those who never leave these shores.

The diagnosis and management of most acute infections in Asians is straightforward and can readily be carried out in general practice. Unfortunately the gravity of certain life-threatening conditions, notably *falciparum* malaria and meningococcal meningitis, are sometimes overlooked, especially early in their clinical course, and particularly when there are language barriers between the patient and practitioner. The increasing popularity of long-haul package holidays has resulted in holiday-makers, medical practitioners, tour operators, and airlines all becoming increasingly aware of imported medical conditions and of the importance of seeking medical guidance before travel overseas. In contrast, many Asian immigrants believe that travel to India or Africa is risk-free; and so the onus is on medical practitioners to educate their Asian patients about the hazards of travel at every opportunity (details on booklets and further sources of information are given at the end of the chapter).

This chapter considers the diagnosis and management of the more common or important infectious diseases and tropical infections, and also considers certain aspects of preventive medicine, including education, screening, and vaccination.

Infections of greater prevalence among Asians

Compared with their British compatriots, Asian immigrants and their British-born offspring are more commonly exposed to infections that are generally found overseas. Some, such as malaria and typhoid fever, declare themselves within a short period of the return from foreign travel, and are recognized by the astute practitioner. Other imported conditions may only become evident years after a period of residence in Africa or Asia, and may be diagnosed with difficulty for example, non-pulmonary tuberculosis, *vivax* malaria, and bilharzia.

(a) Tuberculosis

In certain parts of Britain, a pyrexia of unknown origin in an Asian is considered to be tuberculous in origin until proven otherwise. Tuberculosis is still rife in most parts of Africa, India, south-east Asia, and South America. In 1981 it was estimated that 10 million new cases occurred each year. The main source of infection with the human strain of *Mycobacterium* tuberculosis is airborne droplets from an 'open' case of pulmonary tuberculosis. Infection typically begins in the mid or lower zones of the lung, and the initial exposure results in pulmonary tuberculosis. The initial peripheral sub-pleural lesion is known as the Ghon focus, and the combination of the Ghon focus and involvement of the hilar lymph nodes is known as the primary complex. In most instances, tuberculin reactivity develops, and microbial growth in the lungs and extra-pulmonary sites is inhibited, often producing visible calcific deposits on X-ray, in which viable bacilli often persist. Viable bacilli may also persist elsewhere.

Both pulmonary and extrapulmonary tuberculosis can develop at any time in an infected person. Certain factors are known to reactivate tuberculosis, including poor nutritional status, steroids, immunosuppressants, reticuloendothelial malignancies, trauma, and possibly pregnancy. Virtually any part of the body can be affected. The clinical manifestations of the primary pulmonary infection vary with age. Symptoms are more liklely to be noted in the very young, who react with more extensive regional lymphadenitis, and are more prone to miliary-meningeal disease. Often the initial infection is asymptomatic, but the child may be unwell, with anorexia, cough, and pyrexia. The lymphadenitis may compress a bronchus, causing atelectasis, or may rupture into the bronchus, seeding organisms distally, and causing a symptomatic pneumonia.

The most common form of the disease, chronic pulmonary tuberculosis, typically begins in the sub-apical region, and may progress through caseation to cavitation and drainage into the bronchial tree. Aerosolization of the material draining from the cavities may result in bronchogenic spread, and further cavitation. Clinically the onset may be insidious or abrupt, with cough—initially dry, later productive of mucopurulent sputum, malaise, anorexia, haemoptysis, night sweats, and loss of weight. Examination may be normal. The chest X-ray may show infiltrates, cavities, fibrotic changes, and calcification. The sputum may be positive on direct Ziehl–Neelsen (ZN) staining, and is generally culture-positive. Occasionally the clinical examination reveals the signs of a pleural effusion, which is confirmed radiologically. Here aspiration reveals the organism in approximately half the cases, and pleural biopsy generally reveals granulomata.

Miliary tuberculosis is the result of haematogenous spread, and may occur before tuberculin-sensitivity develops. In children it results in an acute severe illness with high intermittent fevers, night sweats, and occasionally rigors, occasionally associated with peritonitis, meningitis, and pleural effusions. In adults the illness is usually more insidious, with symptoms for an average of four months before presentation. The symptoms are usually those of fever, malaise, and weight-loss. Headache should suggest the possibility of meningitis, which occurs in one-fifth of the patients with miliary tuberculosis. The chest X-ray almost always reveals a miliary infiltrate.

Tuberculous meningitis may present with headache or a change in mentation over a period of weeks. Cranial nerve palsies are not uncommon, but meningism is unusual. Tuberculomas may present as a space-occupying lesion, spinal involvement as nerve-root compression. Abdominal tuberculosis, although rare in the indigenous population in Britain, is not uncommon in immigrants from the Indian subcontinent. It may either present as peritonitis, with abdominal pain, malaise, distension, and fever, or it may affect the bowel. Tuberculous pericarditis presents either with the cardiovascular effects of the effusion, or with fever and other non-specific features. The diagnosis is usually made clinically and radiologically; pericardiocentesis is generally negative on ZN staining, and the fluid is culture-positive in less than half the cases.

Involvement of the spine typically affects the anterior portion of a vertebral body—often in the thoracic region; and the disc space between two involved vertebrae is usually destroyed and results in a gibbus. Tuberculosis of peripheral bones and joints is typically a combination of osteomyelitis and arthritis. The weight-bearing hip and knee joints are most commonly involved, but any joint may be affected, especially those with pre-existing arthritis.

The genito-urinary tract can be affected, either as renal tuberculosis, which typically presents with dysuria, haematuria, or loin pain, and few systemic features, or with involvement of the prostate, seminal vesicles, epididymis, and testis. Genital involvement in the male is suggested by the finding of a scrotal swelling, occasionally with a sinus. In females there may be involvement of the ovary and endometrium. Genital involvement in the female is suggested by menstrual irregularity and lower abdominal pain, and again there are generally few systemic symptoms. Tuberculous lymphadenitis similarly occurs in otherwise healthy individuals, and few have systemic complaints. Most patients with lymphadenitis present with cervical or supraclavicular nodes. The diagnosis is established by biopsy. Other sites are involved less commonly. These include the larynx, ear, eye, skin, and aorta.

Immigrants from the Indian subcontinent seem prone to reactivation, but the site of infection is not always clear. A common presentation in the Asian patient is a pyrexia of unknown origin, with night-sweats, malaise, and weight-loss, a normal chest X-ray, and negative results from a comprehensive range of investigations. In this situation a therapeutic trial with anti-tuberculous chemotherapy is warranted, and often results in a remission of fever and other symptoms.

Treatment of tuberculosis should be carried out by specialists in either infectious diseases or respiratory medicine. In 1976 the British Thoracic and Tuberculosis Association (now the British Thoracic Association—BTA) recommended daily treatment with rifampicin plus isoniazid for nine months, supplemented by ethambutol or streptomycin during the first two months. More recent studies have shown that the duration of therapy can be reduced from nine months to six months if pyrazinamide is added for the first two months. Thus in addition to its earlier recommendation, the BTA now recommends two months of treatment with rifampicin plus isoniazid plus pyrazinamide plus ethambutol or streptomycin, followed by four months of rifampicin plus isoniazid. The fourth drug may contribute little, and many specialists only give three drugs. Unwanted effects of treatment are common, and it is important that patients be informed of these before and during treatment, and that the warning be recorded in the notes. The most worrisome side-effects are optic neuritis from ethambutol, peripheral neuropathy from isoniazid, and hepatotoxicity, particularly from rifampicin, isoniazid, and pyrazinamide. Transient disturbances of liver function are not uncommon, and do not require discontinuation of therapy. Treatment with all drugs is halted if jaundice or other symptoms of hepatitis develop, and is restarted one at a time when liver function has returned to normal.

BCG vaccine contains an attenuated strain of the bacillus *Mycobacterium bovis*. A number of strains are prepared in different laboratories; but all of them originate from the original strain of Calmette and Guerin. In Britain, it is recommended that the following groups be vaccinated if found negative for tuberculin hypersensitivity:

(a) Contacts of cases known to be suffering from active respiratory tuberculosis. Children of immigrants in whose communities there is a high incidence of tuberculosis may for this purpose be regarded as contacts. Newly-born babies who are contacts need not be tested for sensitivity, but should be vaccinated without delay.
(b) Health Service Staff.
(c) Schoolchildren between their tenth and fourteenth birthdays.
(d) Students—including those in teacher-training colleges.

The dosage of BCG is 0.1 ml of vaccine administered intradermally (reduced to 0.05 ml for infants under three months of age) at the insertion of the deltoid muscle. The tip of the shoulder should be avoided. In girls, for cosmetic reasons, the upper and lateral surface of the thigh may be preferred. The efficacy of BCG vaccine remains controversial. Protection studies in British schoolchildren have shown over 70 per cent efficacy, but in other areas of the world some studies have shown little or no protection. BCG vaccine is relatively safe. Almost all children develop a raised papule at the injection site, which occasionally develops into a slow-healing abscess. Usually the papule gradually heals, leaving a pitted scar that identifies children who have had BCG. Disseminated BCG infection is very rare, occurring in less than one in a million vaccinated individuals. Contraindications to receipt of BCG include tuberculin sensitivity, immuno-compromised persons, steroids, and pregnancy. Vaccine should not be given into skin affected by eczema or any septic condition, and is not recommended in persons who are febrile.

(b) Malaria

Malaria is distributed throughout Latin America, with the possible exceptions of Chile, Argentina, and Uruguay; and is present throughout tropical Africa and the Near, Middle, and Far East. Only Australasia, Europe, and North America can be regarded as malaria-free and safe for the traveller. A relatively new problem is the emergence of chloroquine-resistant *P. falciparum* malaria, which is now distributed in most of Latin America, south-east Asia, the Indian subcontinent, East Africa, and Central Africa. Malaria is transmitted from man to man by *Anopheles* mosquitoes, but can be transmitted by blood transfusion, by the sharing of needles among drug addicts, and by vertical transmission.

The hallmarks of malaria are the paroxysms of fever, chills, and rigors. Patients in addition may complain of non-specific symptoms, including malaise, myalgia, and headaches; and the infection can readily be mistaken for a viral illness. Examination may reveal splenomegaly and a tender liver, and, depending upon the type and severity of infection, there may be anaemia, icterus, retinal haemorrhages, flow murmurs, signs of congestive heart-failure, and delirium and minor behavioural changes associated with the high fever. Cerebral malaria, which occurs as a complication of *P. falciparum* malaria, is associated with disturbance of consciousness, convulsions, focal neurological signs, acute organic brain syndromes, with intellectual impairment and behaviour changes, and movement disorders.

The febrile paroxysms are related to the rupture of red blood-cells, but the precise cause for the intermittent fever is not understood. Anaemia is a common complication, and extensive haemolysis may occur in association with the high parasitaemias of *P. falciparum* infection. Anaemia may also result from sequestration of red blood-cells in the spleen, and possibly by an autoimmune process. Dyserythropoiesis also occurs, but disseminated intravascular coagulation is not a feature. *P. falciparum*-infected erythrocytes undergo membrane changes that result in sluggish blood flow, hypoxia, and increased capillary permeability; and renal failure, heart failure, and cerebral features are the result of such pathological changes.

The diagnosis of malaria depends upon the identification of the malarial parasites in stained blood-smears. Greater numbers of parasites are found during paroxysms, but practitioners should not wait until the next febrile episode before obtaining blood. Careful examination of the peripheral blood film enables the identification of *P. falciparum*, *P. ovale*, *P. malariae*, and *P. vivax*. Mixed infections (for example, *P. falciparum* and *P. vivax*) occasionally occur, and this may only be recognized when the patient has unsuspected chloroquine-resistant *P. falciparum* and fails to respond to treatment.

The diagnosis of *P. falciparum* infection must be established with haste, since patients can deteriorate rapidly if left untreated. A diagnosis of malaria can only be excluded by obtaining negative blood-smears on several successive days. Parasite counts can be extremely useful in the management of *P. falciparum* malaria, and provide a baseline from which the response to therapy can be assessed. Moreover, *P. falciparum* is more likely if more than 5 per cent of the red blood-cells are parasitized.

P. falciparum malaria does not have a latent phase with liver forms, and the relapses characteristic of *P. vivax* and *P. malariae* are not found in infections with *P. falciparum*. The incubation period of *P. falciparum* malaria is usually several weeks and is almost inevitably acquired during travel to endemic areas. Rare exceptions include cases where infection occurred in or near to airports.

If *P. falciparum* infection can definitely be ruled out, therapy for malaria can be organized from the practice, since all malarial parasites except *P. falciparum* are sensitive to chloroquine. Conversely, if *P. falciparum* is suspected, or cannot be ruled out, or there is a possibility of a mixed infection, then the patient should be hospitalized and the response to therapy closely supervised.

Oral chloroquine is the drug of choice for the treatment of all malarial infections not due to *P. falciparum*. These infections can be treated in the practice, providing close contact is maintained with the patient. Chloroquine phosphate is normally given at a dose of 600 mg base, followed by 300 mg base after 6 hours, then a further 300 mg base for 2 days. Dosage adjustments are made in children. No dosage reductions are required in renal failure. Patients with non-*falciparum* malaria are given a course of primaquine after treatment with chloroquine to eliminate the exoerythrocytic forms in the liver. The usual dose is 15 mg for fourteen days. Dosage adjustments are made in children. Primaquine can induce haemolysis in patients with gluclose 6-phosphate dehydrogenase (G6PD) deficiency, and patients should be screened prior to primaquine administration. Pregnancy is a contraindication to the receipt of primaquine. Instead, pregnant women should receive chloroquine for the treatment of each relapse. The treatment of *P. falciparum* malaria or malaria recently acquired overseas should be undertaken in hospital, and is beyond the scope of this book.

Many Asian patients do not consider themselves to be at risk for malaria and other diseases when they travel to Africa or Asia. Thus it is important for practitioners to educate patients generally about the potential hazards of travel whenever the opportunity arises. Patients should be advised to avoid mosquito bites by keeping arms and legs covered when outdoors after sunset. They should also sleep in screened accommodation, or use mosquito nets and insect repellents and killer sprays.

In view of the increasing spread of *P. falciparum* malaria in south-east Asia, Africa, and Latin America, travellers are increasingly being given the combination of chloroquine and proguanil for antimalarial prophylaxis. Chloroquine is administered weekly and proguanil daily. Chloroquine should be administered one week before entering an endemic zone, and proguanil for several days before. Prophylaxis should be continued for at least four weeks after leaving. The most serious hazard of prolonged chloroquine therapy is irreversible retinal damage. Problems are said to arise if the total consumption exceeds 1.6 g/kg. On this basis, expatriates receiving 500 mg of chloroquine weekly can be given the drug for some years.

(c) Enteric fever

Enteric fever is the term used to describe the typhoid-paratyphoid group of fevers. These infections are caused by invasive members of the genus *Salmonella*, and are characterized by an acute bacteraemic illness, with typical features of fever, headache, abdominal discomfort, cough, splenomegaly, leukopenia, and a relative bradycardia. *S. typhi* is most frequently responsible for the enteric fever syndrome, but other *Salmonellae*, particularly *S. paratyphi* A and B and also some other *Salmonella* serotypes can cause a similar illness.

Enteric fever is most prevalent in the socio-economically deprived areas of the world. Several hundred cases are reported annually in Britain. The majority of typhoid cases are adults who have acquired their infection abroad, most commonly in the Indian subcontinent. A smaller number acquire their infection from a symptomless carrier at home, who originally imported the infection. *S. paratyphi* A infections are generally imported from the Indian subcontinent and *S. paratyphi* B infections are imported from the Mediterranean littoral, the Middle East, and the Indian subcontinent. Transmission usually occurs through ingestion of food or drink that has been contaminated by the excreta of a human case or carrier. Person-to-person spread is unusual.

After an incubation period of around ten to fourteen days, there is usually an insidious onset, with one or more symptoms of malaise, chills, headache, myalgia, abdominal discomfort, non-productive cough, and constipation. There may be a gradual elevation in temperature, which is classically described as 'stepwise'—rising in the evenings and falling to a lesser extent in the mornings. The fever may be remittent, but is usually sustained during the second week of illness, when a relative bradycardia may be evident. The presence of rose spots towards the end of the first week of illness, although not pathognomonic, is a useful diagnostic feature. They consist of smaller macules, usually on the lower chest and upper abdomen, are several millimetres in diameter, and are generally sparse—often there are only four or five lesions. Examination may further reveal modest splenomegaly, lower abdominal tenderness, and occasional chest crepitations.

During the second and third weeks, the patient becomes progressively enfeebled, disorientated, and delirious, with abdominal distension. Diarrhoea may occur at this time, but the patient is just as likely to remain constipated throughout the whole illness. It is during the third week that the greatest incidence of abdominal complications occurs. Subsequently the fever begins to settle, and has usually returned to normal by the end of the fourth week. The features of *S. paratyphi* and other causes of enteric fever are similar to the above, although the illness is generally milder, of shorter duration, and the rash may be more profuse.

The principal complications of typhoid include relapse, which seems to be uninfluenced by antibiotics and occurs in 5–2 per cent of cases, intestinal haemorrhage, intestinal perforation, pneumonia, myocarditis, pyelonephritis, neuropsychiatric manifestations, and abscess formation. These complications are now less common with the advent of specific antimicrobial therapy.

The diagnosis of enteric fever is made by isolating *S. typhi* and other *Salmonellae* from blood, marrow, stool, or urine. Stool cultures are positive in less than half the patients, and urine cultures even less frequently so. The marrow may be positive when blood cultures are negative. The white blood-cell count is helpful, since leukopenia or a normal white-cell count is found in the majority of cases. The liver-function tests may be mildly deranged, urinalysis may reveal proteinuria and pyuria, and there may be coagulation abnormalities compatible with mild disseminated intravascular coagulation. The role of the Widal test in diagnosis is extremely limited, first by cross-reactions with other *Salmonellae*, and secondly by background antibodies due to vaccination or exposure overseas, by the variable response to the H and O antigens, by occasional false-positive reactions, and by difficulties in diagnosing enteric fever caused by non-typhoid *Salmonellae*.

In the pre-antibiotic era, the mortality rate from typhoid fever was around 15 per cent, mostly from the gastrointestinal complications. It is important that any patient with fever and malaise who has recently returned from Africa, Asia, or central or southern America be admitted to hospital if the aetiology has not been rapidly established. If a diagnosis of enteric fever has been confirmed in the home setting then the patient should be admitted to hospital, preferably to a specialist unit, for medical supervision.

Chloramphenicol is the drug of choice, and in adults is commonly given at a dosage of 1 g every six hours, the total course lasting for fourteen days, though longer courses are necessary for septic foci. Generally the fever resolves within four to five days. Chloramphenicol resistance has been noted in Mexico, southeast Asia, and the Indian subcontinent, and in these cases treatment with ampicillin or cotrimoxazole has proved effective. However, ampicillin resistance has also been reported. Additional therapy includes fluid and electrolyte replacement.

Convalescent carriage of *S. typhi* and other *Salmonellae* is common, and clears spontaneously in the majority of cases. Food handlers should be prevented from returning to work. The management of chronic carriage poses difficulties, since prolonged courses of antibiotics often fail to eradicate the organisms. In this situation cholecystectomy may be beneficial when there is evidence of gallstones.

The prevention of typhoid and related infections is dependent upon scrupulous food hygiene and safe water. Travellers should refrain from drinking water that has not been boiled, and from eating foodstuffs that have not been adequately prepared, cooked, and stored. Typhoid vaccine provides around 70–80 per cent protection for up to three years. The basic course of immunization consists of two 0.5 ml doses separated by four to six weeks. A single does is sufficient to boost immunity, even if a period of more than three years has elapsed since the last vaccination.

(d) Hepatitis

Serological surveys have identified the existence of hepatitis B globally, and it is conservatively estimated that there are 200 million carriers of hepatitis B virus (HBV) worldwide. The distribution of chronic carriers provides a good measure of the rate of infection. On this basis, the world can be divided into areas of high infection-rate, such as sub-Saharan Africa, the Far East, and Oceania; moderate infection-rate, including the Middle East, Central Asia, South America, eastern Europe, and the Arctic; and low infection-rate, including North America, western Europe, and Australasia.

Although transmission of hepatitis B can occur within families by non-sexual means, by far the most common means of infection are through the sharing of contaminated needles by intravenous drug abusers, and by sexual transmission. Thus the incidence of acute hepatitis B infection in adult Asians in Britain seems to be no greater than in the indigenous white population.

Hepatitis B does not constitute a risk to the ordinary traveller, but health-care workers and students who are engaged in medical and dental practice in countries with a high infection rate are at increased risk compared to that in Britain, and should be adequately immunized before travelling overseas. A recombinant yeast-derived hepatitis B vaccine and a plasma-derived vaccine are both currently available. They are both given as a series of three injections at time zero, one month, and six months. The antibody response is rather slow, and the first two injections should be given some months before travel.

Hepatitis A is endemic in all parts of the world, but the incidence appears to be decreasing in the industrialized nations of northern Europe and North America. Hepatitis A is highly contagious, and is a recognized hazard of travel to areas of the world with poor hygienic conditions. There is no vaccine against hepatitis A, but infection can be prevented with immune serum globulin (ISG), which can be given pre- and post-exposure. In the case of type A hepatitis, all family members and close contacts should receive ISG as soon as possible after the exposure. Work and school contacts do not need to be treated, but ISG has been used effectively in homes for the mentally handicapped and in nursery schools. ISG does not always prevent infection, and excretion of hepatitis A virus and subclinical hepatitis may develop. Prophylaxis with ISG is also recommended for persons visiting highly endemic areas such as the Indian sub-continent. Protection is considered to last for approximately six months.

(e) Rabies

Rabies, an acute infectious encephalomyelitis caused by a rhabdovirus, is enzootic in all continents except Australasia and Antarctica. Most other disease-free areas are islands, or less commonly peninsular land masses, where quarantine regulations can be stringently enforced. The disease exists in two epidemiological forms: urban rabies, which is propagated chiefly in unimmunized dogs, and is prevalent in Mexico, South and Central America, Africa, and Asia; and sylvatic rabies, where the disease exists in a wide range of wild animal species.

The extent of the human rabies problem in the Third World is uncertain. The disease poses an immense public-health problem in many Third World countries, and the human toll in some regions is formidable. From estimates of hospital admissions it is suggested that at least 17 000 cases occur annually in India alone. This figure is probably an underestimate, since many cases never reach hospital, and, of those that do, the clinical course defies diagnosis in at least 20 per cent of cases. The risk of exposure in many countries is high. A survey of missionaries and foreign-aid workers has revealed an overall one in six chance of one of the family members requiring postexposure treatment, based on a stay of four to five years in the tropics (Bjorvatin and Gundersen 1980).

The incubation period of rabies is very variable, and is often prolonged. Approximately 80 per cent have an incubation period ranging from one week to three months, and at least 5 per cent have an incubation period in excess of one year. Human rabies is rare in Britain—on average a case is diagnosed every one to two years. Virtually all of the cases seen in recent years were infected in the Indian subcontinent.

The presenting features are generally non-specific, and even after hospitalization the initial course does not always suggest rabies. The onset is marked by one to seven days of prodromal symptoms comprising fever, malaise, anorexia, nausea, vomiting, diarrhoea, sore throat, cough, myalgia, and headache as the most common complaints. An early symptom of considerable diagnostic significance is an abnormal sensation involving the bitten area, most commonly pain or paraesthesia; but these are noted in less than half of the cases. Few signs occur early in the clinical course, so unless the doctor's attention is drawn to a recent exposure, or healed bite-wounds are noted, it is unlikely that the diagnosis will be considered.

The prodrome is followed by one of two basic patterns of disease—'furious' and 'dumb' rabies. 'Furious' rabies is characterized by agitation, hyperexcitability, hyperactivity, and purposeless movements, either occurring spontaneously or provoked by a variety of stimuli. Often there is frothing at the mouth, difficulty in swallowing, and intense spasms affecting the muscles of deglutition and respiration, which may follow attempts to drink, but may be precipitated by other stimuli, such as eating, swallowing accumulated saliva, etc. Approximately 50 per cent exhibit hydrophobia, the overwhelming fear of water that is precipitated by attempts to drink, and sometimes by the sight, sound, or mention of water. The patient is usually febrile, and may develop a variety of CNS abnormalities including convulsions, autonomic dysfunction, cranial nerve palsies, etc. Deterioration is marked by the evolution of a flaccid paralysis and onset of coma. Untreated cases survive for an average of three to seven days once symptoms develop.

'Dumb' rabies poses a greater diagnostic problem, since the spasms and hydrophobia so characteristic of rabies rarely occur. There are approximately four cases of furious rabies for every case of dumb disease. The paralysis of dumb rabies typically starts in the bitten limb, then spreads rapidly and symmetrically. Sphincter control is lost, and paralysis of the muscles of deglutition and articulation typically occur as a terminal event. Survival tends to be longer than four patients with furious rabies, the average period being from seven to twelve days.

Routine laboratory tests are unhelpful. Examination of the CSF reveals a picture of a viral meningoencephalitis, and the EEG and CAT scans are non-diagnostic. The diagnosis is confirmed by isolation of the virus from saliva, by immunofluorescence of skin biopsy specimens (which may reveal the presence of virus within the nerves supplying hair follicles), by immunofluorescence of corneal impressions, and by serology. The most rapid test is skin biopsy; but the test is not always positive. The most successful test overall is the detection of rabies antibodies; but the patient may die before antibody becomes detectable. Post-mortem diagnosis is made by the demonstration of virus within the brain by immunofluorescence, by electron microscopy, and by virus isolation; and by the demonstration of Negri bodies.

Rabies is inevitably fatal. Three human cases have recovered, but here survival was partly attributed to anti-rabies treatment prior to the onset of symptoms. Intensive care does prolong life, but unfortunately does not alter the prognosis. Medical and nursing attendants, family members, and other close contacts are at an incredibly small risk of contracting rabies; and there is little justification for the panic measures that accompany a diagnosis of rabies in Britain. Patients with suspected rabies should be admitted to an isolation unit, and standard isolation precautions are all that are required.

Rabies human diploid cell strain (HDCS) vaccine grown on human embryonic lung fibroblasts is licensed in Britain, and is available for pre- and postexposure use. Pre-exposure immunization is routinely given to certain professional groups (that is, workers in quarantine facilities, port workers, etc.), but should be considered for persons travelling overseas. It is not necessary for travel to Europe, North America, South Africa, the Mediterranean countries, the Near East, Australasia, Hong Kong, Malaysia, and Japan; but should definitely be considered for individuals travelling to the Indian subcontinent and Indo-China, and for prolonged travel in rural Africa. Rabies vaccine can be prescribed in the normal way, and can usually be obtained by the patient within 24 hours of presenting the prescription to a large national chain of chemists. Vaccine is administered on days 0, 28, and 56, or on days 0, 7, and 21. Two doses, either by the intramuscular or intradermal routes, usually evoke antibody responses. Reactions are minimal.

Bite or scratch wounds or mucous membranes contaminated by saliva must be washed with copious amounts of soapy water or water alone. Postexposure rabies treatment should be given without delay. Hyperimmune rabies immune globulin (HRIG) or antirabies serum should be administered, particularly when the bite is severe, that is, when it involves the head or neck, or the hand, or is deep, or is large enough to require stitching. Suturing should be avoided if at all possible. Postexposure treatment with HDCS or other potent tissue-culture vaccine if available is administered on days 0, 3, 7, 14, 28, and 90. Vaccine and HRIG is available through the Public Health Laboratory Service.

(f) Others

Detailed information on some of the rarer tropical diseases and infections (for example bilharzia) can be found in textbooks (see further reading at end of chapter).

Childhood infections

Mumps, measles, diphtheria, pertussis, tetanus, and varicella zoster virus (VZV) infections, and many other 'childhood' infections, occur to the same extent and severity in Asians born in the United Kingdom as in their white compatriots.

There is evidence however that Asians in Britain are at a higher risk from congenital rubella syndrome (Miller *et al.* 1987). This is partly attributed to a higher susceptibility to rubella in Asian than non-Asian women, as shown by antenatal serological data from selected public-health laboratories. However, it also seems that Asian women may be less likely to request diagnostic investigation for possible rubella in pregnancy than non-Asian women. In addition, Asians in Britain are at a higher risk from polio if they return to the Indian subcontinent, since the disease is not uncommon in some areas (PHLS 1986).

Surveys of immunization uptake amongst Asians have been limited. In Bradford (Baker *et al.* 1984) Indian and Pakistani children had higher uptakes than British and half-Negro children. A similar pattern is seen in Leicester and Glasgow (Bhopal and Samim 1988), but not amongst first-generation Asian immigrants in Nottingham, who are often unprotected (Morgan *et al.* 1987).

Detailed information on the incubation period, infectivity, and features of these infections can be found in textbooks (see further reading at end of chapter). Since most of these conditions can be prevented, this section will concentrate on immunizations and, in the case of pertussis, tetanus, and VZV, specific treatments.

(a) Mumps

Live-attenuated mumps vaccine is currently available in this country for people over the age of twelve months, and since autumn 1988 has been available as a combined mumps-measles-rubella (MMR) preparation. Trials of live-attenuated mumps vaccines indicate that they are highly cost-beneficial, with a protective efficacy of greater than 80 per cent for periods of up to eight years after vaccination. In the United States, there has been a greater than 95 per cent decline in the incidence of mumps after vaccine licensure, and a proportional decline in the number of mumps-related deaths and cases of mumps encephalitis.

(b) Measles

Live-attenuated measles vaccine is available to prevent the disease, and in Britain this is supplied as a single dose during the second year of life. In the USA, following rigorous implementation of the measles-virus vaccination programme, measles case reports have fallen by approximately 99 per cent, with a concomitant decline in mortality. A similar, but less impressive, pattern has been achieved in England and Wales, where vaccine acceptance in 1983 was 58 per cent. A combined mumps-measles-rubella (MMR) vaccine was introduced in autumn 1988, and should replace measles vaccine in the second year of life. With increasing vaccine usage the incidence of measles will hopefully diminish from the current level of around 5000 cases a year. Mumps-measles-rubella vaccine should be given irrespective of previous measles vaccine, or of a history of measles, mumps, or rubella infection.

(c) Rubella

Live-attenuated rubella vaccines have been licensed since the early 1970s. In the UK the policy has been to vaccinate schoolgirls between their tenth and fourteenth birthdays, and to vaccinate other susceptible women of childbearing age. This was later extended to include seronegative women during pregnancy, who were offered vaccine *post partum*. The UK Congenital Rubella Surveillance (CRS) Programme has shown little reduction in the incidence of congenital rubella syndrome; whereas in the US, where rubella is given as a combined mumps-measles-rubella vaccine, and a very high proportion of children are immunized, there has been a decline in both congenital rubella syndrome and post-natally acquired rubella. A combined MMR vaccine was introduced into the UK in autumn 1988. Rubella vaccination of girls aged ten to fourteen years will continue, with single antigen rubella vaccine and the target of 95 per cent uptake. When a high uptake of mumps-measles-rubella vaccine in young children has been achieved, and the elimination of rubella has been demonstrated, the decision may be taken to stop the vaccination of schoolgirls.

Rubella virus vaccine produces seroconversion in approximately 95 per cent of recipients, and more than 90 per cent protection against clinical rubella. Susceptible recipients of rubella vaccine may have viraemia, with complications of mild fever, rash, lymphadenopathy, arthralgia, and arthritis. These are uncommon, and are more likely to occur in adults than in children. Pregnancy is an absolute contraindication to vaccination, although it does not appear to induce damage. As with all other live-virus vaccines, rubella vaccine is contraindicated in any patient who is immunocompromised.

(d) Diphtheria

Diphtheria vaccine consists of a formalized preparation, and is given as a routine childhood immunization, beginning at three months and with an interval of six to eight weeks between the first and second dose and four to six months between the second and third doses. A reinforcing dose of diphtheria and tetanus toxoid vaccine combined is recommended for children at school entry, preferably after an interval of at least three years from the last dose of the basic course. individuals who may be exposed to diphtheria at work should be considered for an 'adult type, low-dose booster—say every ten years or so; but in the UK the routine boosting of other individuals is deemed unnecessary, in view of the disease being adequately controlled.

(e) Pertussis

Treatment is essentially supportive, and it is advisable that all infants and children with complications are admitted to hospital. Antibiotics are of no value during the paroxysmal stage, but do eliminate organisms from secretions, and render the patient non-infectious within several days. There is some evidence that erythromycin may abort or ameliorate the illness if given in the early catarrhal stage of the illness. Thus all contacts can be treated with erythromycin 35–50 mg/kg/24 hours in four divided doses for fourteen days. Atelectasis is treated by intensive physiotherapy, convulsions with anti-convulsants, pneumonia with antibiotics, for example, ampicillin; secretions are sucked from the pharynx, and oxygen is given during the paroxysms; and nursing in oxygen is recommended should cyanosis occur. Steroids appear to be of value in lessening the frequency and severity of the paroxysms, and should be considered in severe cases.

Pertussis vaccine used in Britain, the USA, and most other countries consists of a suspension of killed organisms. Pertussis vaccine is available in monovalent form, but is almost always given in combination with diphtheria and tetanus vaccines, either as plain vaccine, or, more commonly, adsorbed with aluminium hydroxide or phosphate. Efforts to produce a component vaccine with fewer side-effects are being made in many countries.

Pertussis vaccine is almost always given with diphtheria and tetanus toxoids. The standard single-dose volume is 0.5 ml, and adsorbed preparations should be administered by deep subcutaneous or intramuscular injection. In Britain, the Department of Health and Social Security Joint Committee on Vaccination and Immunization (DHSS JCVI) recommends a basic course of three doses of adsorbed vaccine, beginning at three months of age, with an interval of six to eight weeks between the first and second doses and four to six months between the second and third doses. However, if whooping cough is prevalent, it suggests an alternative course of triple vaccine with one month's interval between the first and second and second and third doses, commencing at the age of three months. Such a course should be followed at twelve to eighteen months of age by a dose of adsorbed diphtheria and tetanus toxoid vaccine, since the intervals of one month are not considered to be adequate for the diphtheria and tetanus antigens. Reinforcing doses are otherwise not recommended. Adsorbed (that is, adjuvanted) vaccine is preferred to the plain vaccine, since it is more immunogenic and causes fewer local reactions. There is no need to re-start the course or repeat earlier injections if the basic course is interrupted. Monovalent vaccine can be given when the pertussis component has been omitted from previous vaccinations.

Because the incidence and severity of pertussis decreases with age, and because of adverse reactions, pertussis immunization is not recommended after the sixth birthday in Britain. In exceptional cases, such as persons with chronic pulmonary disease exposed to children with pertussis, or health-care personnel exposed during outbreaks, a reduced booster dose may be contemplated. Routine pertussis vaccination of hospital personnel is not recommended.

In Britain, after undue publicity about adverse reactions, a fall in vaccination rates to 30 per cent in 1978 resulted in the occurrence of the two largest epidemics since the 1950s. During 1978–1980, comparison of the attack-rates among diphtheria, tetanus and pertussis (DTP) and diphtheria and tetanus (DT) recipients gave a vaccine efficacy of 84 per cent, which increased to 93 per cent when the analysis was restricted to bacteriologically confirmed cases. In addition, whooping cough in unvaccinated children is more severe, lasts longer, and is more likely to be associated with an abnormal chest radiograph and hospitalization than the disease in vaccine recipients.

Pertussis vaccine is one of the relatively few remaining whole bacterial vaccines, and contains many biologically active substances. It is therefore inherently toxic, causing a spectrum of adverse reactions after vaccination. In a recent study (Cody *et al.* 1981) comparing the nature and rates of reactions after adsorbed DTP and DT vaccines, local redness, swelling, and pain, and simple generalized reactions such as irritation and fever ($>38°$ C) were two to five times more common after DTP vaccine than after DT vaccine, occurring in roughly 30 per cent to 50 per cent of the vaccinees. Vomiting occurred after 6.2 per cent and 2.6 per cent of DTP and DT immunizations respectively, and crying lasting from one to twenty-one hours after 3.1 per cent and 0.7 per cent respectively. Convulsions and hypotonic hyporesponsive episodes within forty-eight hours of immunization each occurred after one in 1750 DTP injections, and unusual high-pitched crying after one in 926. No serious persisting neurological sequelae were noted among the 15 752 DTP recipients. Similar post-vaccination febrile convusion rates were found in studies in Australia, Germany, and the Netherlands (Ehrengut 1974; Hannik and Cohen 1979; Feery 1982). Although seemingly high, the incidence of febrile convulsions after vaccination is considerably lower than occurs during pertussis (0.5 per cent to 2.0 per cent of cases), and is possibily no higher than the background incidence of convulsions in children in this age-group.

The most severe reactions following pertussis immunization are permanent neurological damage and death. Many cases of coma, prolonged convulsions, and persistent neurological complications have been reported, but their incidence has been a matter of much speculation, with estimates of one in 5000–10 000 (Dick 1974) to one in 1.25 million immunizations (Griffiths 1978). To establish the association between pertussis vaccination and serious acute neurological illness, the National Childhood Encephalopathy Study studied more than a thousand children aged two months to three years presenting with acute neurological illness, and 1955 case controls (Miller *et al.* 1981). The study should, in theory, have included all serious neurological illnesses occurring in the entire child population during the study period who were admitted to hospital, and, by making assumptions about immunization rates, the risks attributable to vaccination were calculated. A significant association with serious neurological illness was shown for pertussis vaccine, but not for diphtheria and tetanus vaccine. The estimated attributable risk of serious neurological disorders after DTP vaccine in previously normal children irrespective of outcome was one in 110 000 doses of DTP, that is, one in 37 000 children, and for neurological sequelae one year later one in 310 000 injections, or approximately one in 100 000 children. In a further study 134 700 children received three doses of DTP vaccine, and a similar number completed courses of DT vaccine (Pollock and Morris 1983). No major difference between DTP and DT vaccine recipients was found when children who had been admitted to hospital were compared. The authors concluded that there was no convincing evidence that DTP caused major neurological damage.

In the UK, pertussis vaccine is absolutely contraindicated in children who have a history of any severe local or general reaction to a preceding dose. If the child is suffering from any acute illness immunization should be postponed until it has fully recovered.

The Joint Committee on Vaccination and Immunization considers that there are certain groups of children in whom whooping-cough vaccine is not absolutely contraindicated, but who require special consideration as to its advisability. These groups are: children whose parents or siblings have a history of idiopathic epilepsy; children with a documented history of cerebral damage in the neonatal period; and children with a personal history of convulsions. A personal or family history of allergy has in the past been considered a contraindication to vaccination, but is no longer considered to be so.

(f) Tetanus

The treatment of tetanus generally demands intensive nursing and supportive care, and description of this is beyond the scope of this chapter. The wound, should it be evident, may require surgical debridement. Large doses of penicillin are administered to eliminate the organism, and antitoxin is given to neutralize tetanospasmin.

The prevention of tetanus depends upon pre- and post-exposure vaccination, and passively administered antibody. Tetanus toxoid vaccine is prepared from purified toxin which is 'toxoided' with formalin. Since plain highly purified formalin toxoids are generally of poor immunogenicity, the World Health Organization recommend that only adjuvant DTP preparations be utilized in immunization programmes. For primary immunization of young children, adsorbed tetanus toxoid is usually given with adsorbed diphtheria toxoid (DT) or with adsorbed diphtheria toxoid and pertussis (DTP) vaccines. Non-adsorbed tetanus and DTP vaccines are also available, but they are not so potent as the adsorbed preparations, and are generally reserved for persons who reacted adversely to a previous dose of adsorbed vaccine and are considered to be inadequately protected. Plain vaccine is not recommended for primary immunization, and is probably insufficiently immunogenic in the presence of passively administered antibody.

The reader is referred to the section on diphtheria for information on the primary immunization schedule. The DHSS JCVI recommends a reinforcing dose of combined DT vaccine for children at school entry, preferably after an interval of at least three years from the last dose of the basic course, and a further booster at age fifteen to nineteen years on leaving school. Thereafter a reinforcing dose is recommended by the DHSS only in the event of an injury which it is considered might give rise to tetanus. Because of the risk of hypersensitivity, the DHSS recommended that tetanus vaccine should not be routinely given to any patient who has received a booster dose within the preceding five years, unless the wound is regarded as carrying an unusually high risk of tetanus; and even then vaccine is not necessary if a booster has been given during the preceding year. Tetanus immune globulin is indicated only in persons whose wounds carry a high risk for tetanus, and who have either never been vaccinated against tetanus or have only received a single dose.

A single dose of tetanus toxoid produces seroconversion in around 98 per cent of vaccinees. Three doses evoke protective antitoxin levels in 100 per cent of infants. Similar antibody responses are found in breast- and bottle-fed children, malnourished and well-nourished children, malaria-infected and non-infected children, and children or pregnant women in holoendemic areas taking or not taking chloroquine. Splenectomized patients respond normally to booster injections with tetanus toxoid, but patients with onchocerciasis, or being treated for tuberculosis, have a diminished response.

Complications are more common in adults, and numerous reports of adverse reactions to tetanus toxoid have appeared in recent years. None the less the overall incidence appears to be very low. Neurological reactions to tetanus toxoid are extremely rare, and have an estimated incidence of one per 833 000 vaccinees (Quast *et al.* 1979; Ehrengut 1986). Virtually all cases have a history of multiple tetanus toxoid injections.

Reinforcing doses at frequent intervals can precipitate hypersensitivity reactions, and should be avoided. Generally it is not recommended that tetanus toxoid be given to anyone who has experienced a serious reaction, including anaphylaxis, angioneurotic oedema, serum sickness, or a neurological complication. If an anaphylactic or other allergic reaction is suspected, intradermal testing with diluted tetanus toxoid may be useful before deciding to discontinue tetanus toxoid immunization.

(g) Polio

Polio vaccines are available as live and inactivated preparations. Live oral polio vaccine (OPV), containing attentuated strains of poliomyelitis virus types I, II, and III, is routinely used for immunization in Britain. A single dose may give protection, but a course of three doses produces solid immunity against all three types. Oral polio vaccine is given as a course of three separate doses with intervals of six to eight weeks between the first and second dose, and four to six months between the second and third doses, generally at the same time as DPT. In infants, three drops of vaccine are dropped directly into the mouth; in older children the vaccine is given on a sugar lump. Breast-feeding does not interfere with the antibody response. Reinforcing doses are given before school entry (at the same time as the reinforcing dose of diphtheria/tetanus vaccine), and at fifteen to nineteen years of age, before leaving school.

The risk of vaccine-associated poliomyelitis is extremely small for immunologically normal vaccinees (approximately one case per nine million doses distributed) and their contacts (one case per seven million doses distributed). The risk is acknowledged as increasing with age, and some authorities, for example, the US Public Health Service, prefer the use of inactivated polio vaccine for the primary immunization of adults. In this country the Joint Committee on Vaccination and Immunization recommend the use of OPV.

Inactivated polio vaccine contains polioviruses of all three types inactivated by formaldehyde, and is recommended for people in whom live virus vaccines are contraindicated, that is, the immunocompromised, their siblings, or other household contacts. Primary and reinforcing doses are given at the same time as for OPV.

Reinforcing doses of OPV and IPV for adults are not necessary unless they are travelling to countries where poliomyelitis is endemic or epidemic, or are health-care workers in possible contact with poliomyelitis cases. For those at continuing risk a single reinforcing dose should be administered every ten years.

(h) Varicella zoster virus

Uncomplicated varicella or zoster requires no treatment. Pruritis can be relieved by calamine lotion. Varicella in an immunocompromised patient can be a serious, even fatal, condition; and admission to hospital for intravenous acyclovir could be life-saving. There are few benefits to be gained from the use of acyclovir in the immunologically normal patient with zoster. Healing and acute pain are shortened by a few days, but unfortunately there is no effect on post-herpetic neuralgia. In the immunocompromised patient, however, treatment with acyclovir is advisable. Topical idoxuridine (IDU) is, by contrast, messy, since the affected area must be covered in gauze which is kept continuously soaked with IDU in dimethylsulphoxide for around four days. More importantly, IDU appears to be less effective than acyclovir.

Congenital infections and their prevention

Transmission of infection vertically is uncommon nowadays, and probably occurs with the same frequency in white children and children born to Asian parents. Vertical transmission of hepatitis B and malaria are two notable exceptions.

(a) Vertical transmission of hepatitis B

The patterns of infection in endemic areas of Asia and Africa are different from those seen in Europe and North America, where the vast majority of cases occur in teenagers and young adults. In the economically-deprived countries, serological surveys indicate that most infected persons have already been infected by their early teens. Perinatal transmission has been documented frequently enough to suggest that this is possibly the most important mechanism for maintenance of hepatitis B virus in the Third World. Unlike infection acquired later, perinatally-acquired hepatitis B is characterized by chronicity, which may ultimately lead to cirrhosis and hepatocellular carcinoma.

Infants at greatest risk for perinatally-acquired infection and chronicity are those born to mothers who are hepatitis Be antigen (HBeAg) positive. Approximately 80–85 per cent become chronic carriers. By contrast, children born to mothers who have antibodies to the e antigen that is, are anti-HBe positive—or have no HBe or anti-HBe, are far less likely to become infected, although occasional cases do occur. The precise modes of infection are unknown, but HBV can be detected in vaginal secretions, breast milk, and cord blood, as well as being present in maternal blood, and transmission may occur through abrasions or ingestion, or across mucous membranes. In approximately five per cent of cases infection is deemed to have occurred *in utero*.

HBV infection in infants can only be prevented by identifying high-risk infants. Women with symptomatic hepatitis B infection in the third trimester are readily identifiable. In contrast, chronic carriers are usually asymptomatic, and can only be identified by screening. Routine screening of all pregnant women in Britain is not cost-effective. However, women of Asian descent, particularly those from the Far East, are a high-risk group wherever they live, and screening is considered prudent. These women should be tested for HBsAg during pregnancy. Infants born to mothers who are both HBsAg- and HBeAg-positive during the third trimester are at the greatest risk; the likelihood of transmission is considerably reduced if the mother is HBsAg-positive and anti-HBe positive.

Postexposure treatment of infants at risk should be organized jointly between the departments of Obstetrics, Paediatrics, and Microbiology. Hepatitis B immune globulin (HBIG) alone reduces the incidence of hepatitis B infection by approximately 70 per cent, and a similar level of protection is obtained with hepatitis B vaccine. Optimal protection of around 90–95 per cent is obtained through the combined use of HBIG and HBV. Infants of HBV-infected mothers do not need isolating from their mothers. Breast-feeding is a possible route of transmission of HBV, and in developed countries, such as Britain, where the risk of gastroenteritis from inadequately sterilized bottles and equipment is low compared to the situation in the Third World, breast-feeding should probably be avoided.

(b) Vertical transmission of malaria

The placenta is normally an effective barrier to *Plasmodium* species, but vertical transmission can occur with all species of malarial parasite. Vertical transmission of malaria is unusual in Britain, but should be borne in mind in infants whose mothers had *vivax* malaria treated during pregnancy with chloroquine alone.

Conclusion

Asians in Britain develop the same infectious diseases as the indigenous population, but are more at risk of important infections such as malaria or typhoid. The general practitioner should be more alert to those infections which are more prevalent amongst Asians, and be especially vigilant when seeing patients who have recently returned from travelling abroad. He is also ideally placed to practise preventive medicine, and educate his patients about the benefits of vaccination and the risks of foreign travel.

References

Baker, M. R. Bandaranyake, R., and Schweiger, M. S. (1984). Difference in rate of uptake of immunisation among ethnic groups. *British Medical Journal*, **288**, 1075–8.

Bhopal, R. S. and Samim, A. R. (1988). Immunisation uptake of Glasgow Asian children: paradoxical benefit of communication barriers? *Community Medicine*, **10**, 215–20.

Bjorvatin, G. and Gundersen, S. G. (1980). Rabies exposure among Norwegian missionaries working abroad. *Scandinavian Journal of Infectious Diseases*, **12**, 257–64.

Cody, C. L., Baraff, L. J., Cherry, J. D., Marcy, S. M., and Manclark, C. R. (1981). Nature and rates of adverse reactions associated with DTP and DT immunizations in infants and children. *Paediatrics*, **86**, 650–60.

Dick, G. (1974). Reactions to routine immunization in childhood. *Proceedings of the Royal Society of Medicine*, **67**, 371–2.

Ehrengut, W. (1974). Uber konvulsive reaktionen nach pertussis schutzimpfung. *Deutsche Medizinische Wochenschrift*, **99**, 2273–9.

Ehrengut, W. (1986). Central nervous system sequelae of vaccinations. *Lancet*, **i**, 1275–6.

Feery, B. J. (1982). Incidence and type of reactions to triple antigen (DTP) and DT vaccines. *Medical Journal of Australia*, **2**, 511–15.

Griffiths, A. H. (1978). Reactions after pertussis vaccine: a manufacturer's experiences and difficulties since 1964. *British Medical Journal*, **1**, 809–15.

Hannik, C. A. and Cohen, H. (1979). Pertussis vaccine experience in the Netherlands. In *International symposium on pertussis*, DHEW (NIH) Washington: US Government Printing Office. 279–82.

Miller, D. L., Ross, E. M., Alderslade, R., Bellman, M. H., and Rawson, N. S. B. (1981). Pertussis immunisation and serious acute neurologic illness in children. *British Medical Journal*, **282**, 1595–9.

Miller, E., Nicoll, A., Rousseau, S. A., Sequeira, P. J. L., Hambling, M. H., Smithells, R. W., and Holzel, H. (1987). Congenital rubella in babies of South Africa women in England and Wales: an excess and its causes. *British Medical Journal*, **294**, 737–9.

Morgan, S., Aslam, M., Dave, R., Nicholl, A., and Stanford, R. (1987). Knowledge of infectious diseases and immunisations among Asian and white parents. *Health Education Journal*, **46**, 177–9.

PHLS (Public Health Laboratory Service) (1986). *Communicable Disease Report. Suspected poliomyelitis ex Pakistan*, **86/41**, 1.

Pollock, T. M. and Morris, J. (1983). A seven-year survey of disorders attributed to vaccination in North West Thames Region. *Lancet*, **i**, 753–7.

Quast, U., Hennessen, W., and Widmark, R. (1979). Mono and polyneuritis after tetanus vaccination (1970–77). *Developments in Biological Standardisation*, **43**, 25–32.

Further reading

Department of Health and Social Security. (1988). *Immunisation against infectious diseases*. HMSO, London.

Mandell, G. L., Douglas, R. G. and Bennett, J. E. (1985). *The principles and practice of infectious diseases*, 2nd edn. Wiley Medical, Chichester.

Manson-Bahr, P. E. C. and Bell, D. R. (ed.) (1987). *Manson's Tropical Diseases*, 19th edn. Baillière Tindall, London.

Two Department of Health booklets are recommended to GPs for use by patients intending to travel overseas: 'Before you go', (SA40, February 1988) and 'While you're away', (SA41, February 1988). Free copies are obtained by telephoning 0800 555 777, at any time, free of charge. Bulk copies may be ordered from DHSS Leaflets Unit, PO Box 21, Stanmore, HA7 1AY.

Further information

Vaccination requirements change from time to time, and information on the current requirements for any particular country may be obtained from the:

DoH
Alexander Fleming House
London SE1 6BY   Telephone 01-407-5522

Scottish Home and Health Department
St Andrew's House
Edinburgh EH1 3DE   Telephone 031-556-8501

Welsh Office
Cathays Park
Cardiff CF1 3NQ   Telephone Cardiff 825111

Department of Health and Social Services
Dundonald House
Upper Newtownards Road
Belfast BT4 3FS   Telephone 0232 63939
or from the embassy or legation of the appropriate country.

Current advice on malaria prophylaxis is available from:
The Malaria Reference Laboratory
The Ross Institute
Keppel Street
London WC1   Telephone 01-636-3924

Continually updated advice on computer is available, for those with the appropriate equipment and modem, through the Communicable Diseases (Scotland) Unit (041-946-7120); or a computer print-out of a suggested schedule for a given itinerary is available from Masta, PO Box 14, Gosport, Hants, PO12 3SJ.

16   Skin diseases

Derek Barker

Introduction

Although the management of skin diseases in a multi-ethnic community presents special challenges to both general practitioner and consultant dermatologist, the ideal should always be that each patient, whatever his or her ethnic origin, feels confident that their doctor has understood their account of the presenting problem. In addition to making an accurate diagnosis the doctor must appreciate the cultural background of the patient and the significance of the skin complaint, adapting explanation and treatment accordingly. In real life this ideal situation is probably seldom realized, although increased understanding of these factors should enable the doctor to improve the service offered.

This chapter first deals generally with the differences in the ways that skin disease affects the white and Asian communities, and moves on to discuss how Asian patients with particular skin complaints can be managed. A problem-orientated rather than disease-specific approach has been adopted in describing clinical management, and minimal emphasis has been given to describing those disorders where diagnosis and clinical management are unaffected by the patient's ethnic origin. Inevitably this has meant that several common and important skin diseases, such as acne and psoriasis, are given relatively little attention. The chapter ends with a list of further reading.

The Asian patient: key issues

The prevalence of individual skin diseases in the two communities within the UK has not received close study, and we are very dependent on anecdotal evidence and individual experience. Although comparative epidemiological data are essentially lacking, the clinical impression is that, with the exception of certain imported tropical infections, the skin diseases which affect the white and Asian communities in the UK are not markedly different. There are, however, profound linguistic and cultural distinctions between the two groups, and indeed within the Asian population itself, which affect the diagnosis and management of skin disease. Clearly many Asian patients maintain contacts with family members living in their country of origin. The geographical flow of individuals in both directions accounts for 'imported' skin diseases, such as leprosy and leishmaniasis, seen amongst Asians. On the other hand few parts of the world are beyond the reach of a modern travel agent, and holiday-makers from the white community may return home with malaria or cutaneous larva migrans.

Some diseases which affect both communities do show a variable prevalence; photosensitivity is commoner in the white community, and melasma or lichenified eczema in the Asian. The presence or absence of erythema, normally a useful pointer to dermatological diagnosis, is obscured by highly melanized skin, and is a feature which cannot be relied upon in assessing an Asian patient. Psychological responses to skin conditions vary between ethnic groups, and this may be difficult to assess when there are language and cultural differences between patient and doctor. Indeed, it is important to appreciate the differences within the Asian population, and also between the generations; for example the reactions of second-generation, UK-born, teenagers to a skin problem may be very different to those of their traditional and religiously orthodox parents.

(a) Cultural and psychological variations

In very traditional Asian families skin disease can represent a much greater social stigma than in the white community. This may reflect long-held fears concerning contagious diseases. The presence of even a relatively minor skin disease, or indeed any disfigurement, in a teenage Asian girl may affect her marriageability, and the dowry due from her family under the arranged marriage system. This situation is particularly poignant if the disease is only partially controllable, as is the case with psoriasis or eczema. It is essential for a doctor faced with this predicament to give a clear explanation about the infectivity or non-infectivity of the problem, and also to make clear the possibilities of inheritance by future generations. In addition, describing possible causes (and non-causes) along with the likely natural history and prognosis can be helpful.

It is, however, an over-simplification to assume, as many people do, that such problems are inevitable in, or particularly associated with, Asian patients. It is a constant, and probably justified, complaint of patients from all ethnic groups that their doctors do not really understand what it is like to have a chronic or disfiguring skin disease. The anxieties which Asian patients communicate are familiar: are they the only person with the problem? Will there ever be a cure? Why is the treatment so slow to work?

The reaction of different individuals to a single disease is well illustrated by considering vitiligo. In this condition there is destruction, probably auto-immune in origin, of melanocytes in the basal layer of the epidermis. As a result symmetrical depigmented patches develop, with the face, limbs, and trunk being frequently affected. Occasionally vitiligo remits spontaneously; but the natural history is usually one of slow progression. Apart from the appearance, and the inevitable sensitivity to sunlight, the affected areas of skin are entirely normal. On the untanned skin of white-skinned people, patches of vitiligo are scarcely visible. The disorder is however of very profound significance in dark-skinned Asians. It represents a very obvious cosmetic disability, and patients often receive the diagnosis with considerable alarm. In some individuals the psychological impact may be heightened by confusing it with the hypopigmented patches of leprosy.

Some Muslim patients believe that vitiligo is acquired by eating white foods. Many may have already been advised by relatives to severely modify their diets to eliminate foodstuffs such as milk, yoghurt, and egg white. In addition they may have already adopted traditional remedies, such as holy water or sand from Mecca. Older Hindu beliefs may portray vitiligo as a punishment for sins committed in a previous life, although such views are no longer widely held. Nevertheless, it is difficult to exaggerate the hurt and humiliation that vitiligo can cause, to the extent that there are reports of some affected individuals who found it almost impossible to go outdoors or maintain any social contacts.

Appropriate examination of patients with skin problems often necessitates partial or extensive undressing. Awareness of sensitivities concerning exposure of the body, particularly amongst more orthodox and conservative Asian women, can avoid considerable distress.

It used to be said that Asians were more likely to consult traditional healers (Muslims—*hakims*; Hindus—*vaids*), although the growth of alternative medicine in the United Kingdom generally means that this now also occurs in the white community. There is no research evidence on which to evaluate these different approaches to medical care, but it is perhaps fair to observe that alternative practitioners are often perceived by their patients as providing more individual treatment than is the custom in Western medicine. Such treatment is the legitimate wish of all patients with skin diseases, white, Afro-Caribbean, or Asian. Religious observance substantially affects the day-to-day lives of many Asian patients, and the practitioner must be aware of this and be sensitive to his patients' views. For example, contact with alcohol or pig products is forbidden to Muslims, and therefore to offer a devout Muslim a topical application containing alcohol or a leg-ulcer dressing made from porcine dermis would be very upsetting. An orthodox male Sikh asked to cut his hair in order to facilitate treatment of a scalp disorder would be deeply distressed. Similarly, a female Sikh patient with hypertrichosis may not be able to bring herself to cut or shave the hair in any way; although some, less strict Sikh women would not find this difficult. Although exemption from the strict dietary rules of Ramadan is given to the sick, many orthodox Muslims will have problems taking regular oral medication during this period, for religious reasons. This may not be something that the patient will raise with the doctor, but can be an important factor in failure to respond to therapy.

Qureshi (1986) has dealt with another avoidable cultural problem. 'The English do not like the smell of curry on the clothing. Muslims abhor the smell of alcohol on the breath, and Sikhs hate smoking. Such patients will go to great lengths to avoid waiting in the same room, resulting in cultural misunderstanding.' Adding all these difficulties to the obvious ones of language we can see the obstacles there may be to a mutually acceptable consultation. Ways of combating such problems are described in Chapter 5.

(b) Imported disease

Leishmaniasis, in the form of 'oriental sore', is common in the Middle East and Pakistan. The causative agent is *Leishmania tropica*, transmitted by the bite of the sand-fly. Affected patients develop scaly, fibrotic, or ulcerated plaques on exposed skin. Self-healing with residual scarring is usual, although patients with incomplete resistance may develop the chronic leishmaniasis recidivans. In Bradford, many patients seen with leishmaniasis have recently spent a prolonged period in Pakistan; but in fact the disease is widespread throughout the Middle and Far East. Skin biopsy is diagnostic. The majority of patients need no active treatment; but where it is required, a good response is usually seen with intra-muscular sodium stibogluconate. Surgical excision, cryotherapy, and rifampicin have all been used to treat leishmaniasis, and are less toxic, if less effective, treatments.

Leprosy, especially new untreated cases, is much less common, but is occasionally detected amongst recent Asian arrivals to the United Kingdom. The numbers involved, however, are small: only 19 cases were notified for England and Wales during 1985 (OPCS 1987). Patients with a high degree of resistance to *Mycobacterium leprae* develop the tuberculoid form of the disease, which consists of a small number of hypopigmented anaesthetic patches, often associated with peripheral nerve enlargement; where this occurs the diagnosis is usually easily made. Individuals with poor resistance can develop the lepromatous form of the disease.

This is associated with multiple cutaneous modules, papules, and plaques, or simply skin-thickening, which is especially noticeable on the face. The skin lesions in lepromatous leprosy teem with mycobacteria. The proper approach for general practitioners encountering this condition is to refer suspected cases to hospital Skin Departments for biopsy. It is never too early to start reassuring victims of this disease that treatment with modern drugs such as dapsone, rifampicin, and clofazimine is highly effective, although management of leprosy-reaction neuropathy and some of the late complications can be quite testing. No case of leprosy has been transmitted within the United Kingdom this century. Despite this reassurance contacts in this country may sometimes manifest anxiety verging on hysteria.

Tuberculosis, both pulmonary and extra-pulmonary, is commoner in Asians than in the indigenous white population. The same is not true, however, of the classic cutaneous form of the disease lupus vulgaris. Lupus vulgaris is common in India and Pakistan; but perhaps the striking appearance of an indurated plaque associated with a variable degree of scarring leads to early recognition and treatment. Asian patients have been seen locally with 'cold', subcutaneous, tuberculous abscesses and tuberculous skin ulcers. Treatment with rifampicin and INAH is highly effective.

Two tropical diseases, 'creeping eruption' and 'Madura foot', merit brief consideration. Creeping eruption or cutaneous larva migrans resembles an itchy, erythematous thread under the skin, and is caused by the larval stage of an animal hookworm (for example, *Ankylostoma* spp.). These most unwelcome visitors are normally acquired by walking barefoot on infected soil or beaches.

Injury to the foot, with subsequent subcutaneous fungal infection, is responsible for the development of mycetoma, or Madura foot. The affected foot enlarges, and subcutaneous nodules with multiple discharging sinuses develop. Various combinations of systemic anti-fungal agents may be helpful; but involvement of the underlying bone may necessitate amputation.

(c) Obscured diagnosis

The examination of patients with skin diseases yields information in two ways: firstly, through scrutiny of the morphology of individual lesions; and, secondly, by observing the way in which the total population of lesions are distributed over the body.

Ethnic origin does not influence the distribution of lesions in any way, but can considerably affect their individual appearance. In white-skinned patients, it is possible to appreciate quite minor degrees of erythema, and even such subtle distinctions as the purplish colour of lichen planus, or the pulsating erythema of tetracycline-induced fixed-drug eruptions. Pigmentation makes these variations much less easy to recognize, and this can present a problem in intensely melanized individuals. To take two examples. Psoriasis in Asians usually appears silvery and scaly, rather than red and scaly; but the plaques are still sharply demarcated from uninvolved skin, and are still commonly found on the elbows, knees, and sacrum. Secondly, lichen planus may be so deeply pigmented that the classical purplish colour is indistinguishable. The papules are still pruritic and polygonal, however, with involvement of the buccal mucosa just as likely.

Any inflammatory skin disease may induce post-inflammatory depigmentation; but naturally this is much more obvious in dark Asian skin than in white. Simple napkin eruptions in Asian infants may exhibit marked post-inflammatory depigmentation. This change can sometimes be so striking as to draw attention away from the actual diagnosis.

(d) Altered prevalence of skin diseases

Clinical experience suggests that some skin diseases, while afflicting all ethnic groups, seem to select out one community in particular. Since white skin is so poorly protected against ultra-violet light-exposure it is hardly surprising that the great majority of patients presenting with photosensitivity or solar keratoses are in fact white. Chilblains and acrocyanosis of the feet are cold-related circulatory disorders. They are relatively common in Asian women, probably because the sandals which they wear are quite inadequate protection during

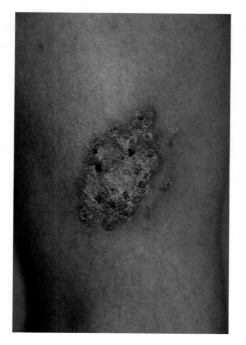

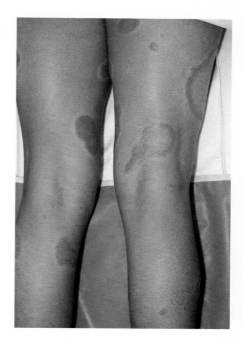

Fig. 16.1 Cutaneous leishmaniasis.

Fig. 16.2 Leprosy.

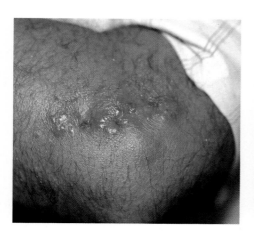

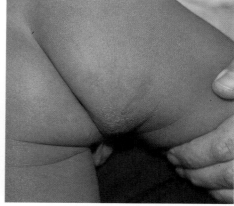

Fig. 16.3 Tuberculous bursitis with involvement of overlying skin.

Fig. 16.4 Cutaneous larva migrans.

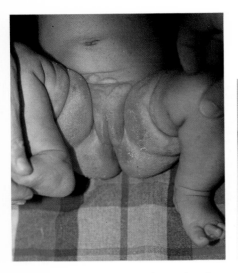

Fig. 16.5 Napkin eruption, showing depigmentation.

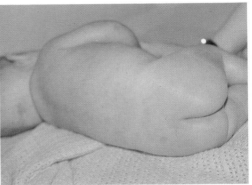

Fig. 16.6 Extensive 'Mongolian spot' in an Asian baby.

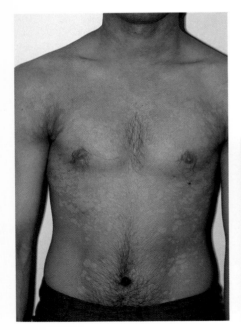

Fig. 16.7 Pityriasis versicolor: a superficial yeast infection.

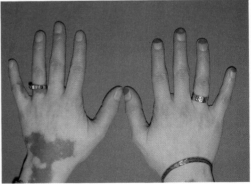

Fig. 16.8 Vitiligo involving the hands.

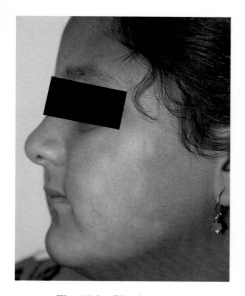

Fig. 16.9 Pityriasis alba.

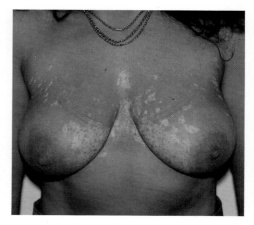

Fig. 16.10 Hypopigmentation *before* camouflage.

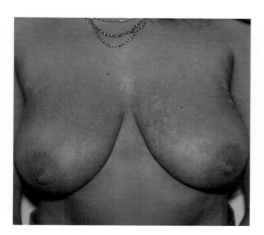

Fig. 16.11 Hypopigmentation *after* camouflage.

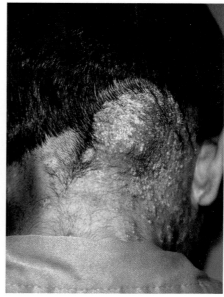

Fig. 16.12 Scalp ringworm (tinea capitis).

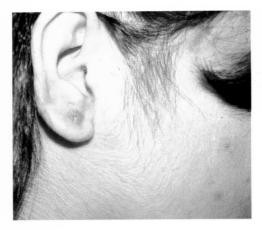

Fig. 16.13 Ear-ring keloid and facial hypertrichosis.

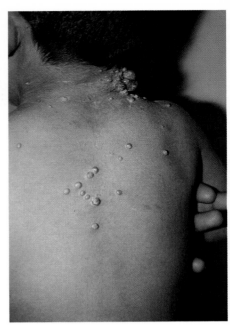

Fig. 16.14 Molluscum contagiosum.

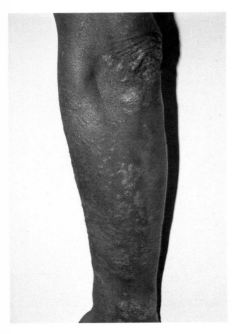

Fig. 16.15 Psoriasis in an Asian man (with acknowledgements to Dr L. G. Millard).

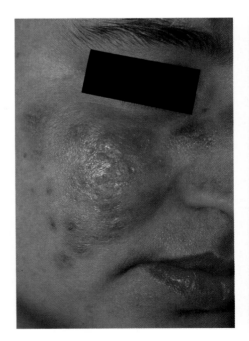

Fig. 16.16 Discoid lupus erythematosus.

a British winter (or for that matter many British summers). Shoes and boots, as well as being expensive, may be regarded as 'masculine', and are unlikely to be worn. Moreover, shoes, socks, or even tights are incongruous with the *kameez* (tunic) and *shalwar* (loose trousers) worn by many Muslim women. Reluctance to change dress is a matter of cultural expression rather than religious observance. Drug therapy of chilblains or acrocyanosis is not really helpful.

(e) Communication

Communication is probably the major hurdle to overcome. In a small survey of twenty-five Asian patients attending the Skin Department in Bradford it was found that ten could not speak and understand English, and fifteen found nurses' instructions hard to follow. At present we have no Asian-language-speaking professional within our department, although twenty of the survey patients would have welcomed this. Fifteen patients found the development of a skin disease, and the necessity of a hospital visit, 'emotionally upsetting'. On the other hand seven patients had been educated in the United Kingdom, and were quite capable of managing and understanding their condition.

Lack of a common language is frustrating for both doctor and patient. Asian patients may go to considerable lengths to bring interpreters from within the family, but this is not always a satisfactory solution, since those accompanying the patient will miss work or school as a result, and may not, in any case, be able to understand and explain medical terminology. The opportunity for a patient to talk to someone who understands in their own language is obviously highly desirable, but this opportunity is seldom provided.

Management of individual skin problems

(a) Disorders of pigmentation

A pigmented sacral macule, or 'Mongolian' spot, is seen in infants of all ethnic groups, but is common in Asians. It resolves spontaneously, and requires no treatment. Very rarely, large Mongolian spots require to be differentiated from bruises. This is simple, since the pigment involved, melanin, does not evolve into the yellowish colour which characterizes haemosiderin in the skin.

Pigmentation of the face, particularly the cheeks and forehead, is fairly common in young Asian women, but can occur in both sexes and at all ages. It is important to be clear about terminology. Chloasma is a term best reserved for pigmentation in the female associated with pregnancy or the use of oral contraceptives. Melasma is the term applied to patchy facial pigmentation in either sex and from any cause. Both melasma and periorbital pigmentation in Asians are so common as to be virtually normal variants. All patients with disfiguring facial pigmentation should be offered cosmetic camouflage advice.

The pigmented areas are frequently still responsive to ultra-violet light-exposure, and should therefore be 'protected' with sunscreens (for example, ROC 15 Total Sunblock, or Spectraban 15).

Patients may enquire about skin-lightening preparations. These are based on hydroquinone, and are widely available in retail chemists serving populations with a high percentage of Asians or Afro-Caribbean customers. When this problem was investigated recently by Boyle and Kennedy (1986) they identified no less than forty-one over-the-counter skin-lightening preparations containing this material. Hydroquinone inhibits tryosinase, which prevents the conversion of the amino acid tyrosine to dihydrophenylalanine, a precursor of melanin. Dermatologists use combinations of hydroquinone and retinoic acid for treating melasma. Self-treatment with hydroquinone carries the risk of producing irritant dermatitis, contact allergic dermatitis, and unwanted hypopigmentation. Patients employing this type of medication should be followed up with very great care. Monobenzylether of hydroquinone is more potent still, and even more likely to cause unwanted hypopigmentation. It is prohibited in cosmetic preparations in the United Kingdom.

There are many causes of depigmentation. Vitiligo is progressive and difficult to treat; consequently every effort should be made to find an alternative cause for the problem. As already mentioned, many inflammatory skin diseases may leave residual hypopigmentation.

Pityriasis (tinea) versicolor is a common and frequently symptomless infection of the stratum corneum by the yeast *Pityrosporum orbiculare*. The rash usually affects the trunk and upper arms. The lesions are approximately annular, tan-coloured macules which may be confluent or perifollicular. Fine scaling is visible if the lesions are abraded. Infection commonly leads to macular hypopigmentation of the skin, which becomes visible in white patients after sun-bathing, and in Asian patients at any time. The depigmentation may persist for months. *Pityrosporum orbiculare* cannot be cultured using ordinary techniques, but spores and hyphae are easily visible on microscopic examination of skin scrapings. Any broad-spectrum anti-fungal will control this infection, although relapses are frequent. A cosmetically acceptable regime is clotrimazole cream applied nightly to all affected areas for ten to fourteen days. Ketoconazole 200 mg orally is also effective if given for a similar period; but the hepato-toxic side-effects of this drug restrict its use to the few severely affected patients who fail to improve with correctly employed topical treatment.

It is surprising that vitiligo is so often confused with the depigmentation produced by pityriasis versicolor, since the resemblance is only superficial. The lesions of vitiligo are widespread and symmetrical. The depigmentation produced is total. The lesions of pityriasis versicolor are confined to the trunk and upper arms; they are hypopigmented but not depigmented. The pigment—loss produced by the yeast is the result of a fatty acid (azaleic acid) synthesized by the organism. Interestingly, this agent is currently undergoing preliminary trials as a therapeutic depigmenting agent in melasma.

As already mentioned, true vitiligo is a major cosmetic problem, particularly in patients whose skin-colour is black or brown. Once more cosmetic camouflage is the only approach guaranteed to be both safe and helpful. Vitiliginous areas often slowly repigment if treated regularly for months with potent fluorinated topical steroid preparations (Kandil 1974; Kumari 1984). This may be at the cost of inducing some skin atrophy, and the regime should be used with great caution. Treatment with a systemic photosensitizer, such as a psoralen, followed by exposure to ultra-violet light (PUVA) or natural sunshine, has slowly produced perifollicular repigmentation of vitiliginous areas. This is a field for experts, and the regime is by no means universally applicable. It is possible that Asian patients with vitiligo respond better to topical steroids and PUVA than whites, although many patients within both groups fail to improve substantially with any treatment. If all else fails, and the vitiligo is very extensive, the best cosmetic result may be produced by bleaching the few remaining areas of uninvolved skin with 20 per cent monobenzylether of hydroquinone is a cream base.

Pityriasis alba is a common cause of annular, slightly scaly patches on the face, particularly in childhood. Involvement of the upper arms and shoulders is not uncommon, and occasionally the disease can be generalized. Pityriasis alba affects all ethnic groups, but in Asian children is the cause of prominent patchy hypopigmented lesions. The condition is probably a chronic low-grade eczema. Parents should be reassured that eventual spontaneous resolution is usual. Treatment with emollients or hydrocortisone ointment may be helpful.

Chemical-induced depigmentation is a rare but well recognized complaint. It is usually an occupational problem encountered in the rubber and automobile industry, following exposure to para-tertiary-butyl phenol. Contact leucoderma has been described in Hindu women who employed self-sticking coloured plastic discs on the '*bindi*' site on the central forehead, rather than the traditional vermilion powder (Bajaj *et al.*, 1983). The problem has been blamed on the adhesive, and an associated depigmentation may develop at other sites—for example, areas of skin in contact with plastic watch-straps, or the straps of synthetic footwear (Pandhi and Kumar 1985).

(b) Alopecia and scalp disorders

In addition to being 'a woman's crowning glory', the hair, and its colour, style, and length, are matters of considerable cultural significance. Muslim parents will shave the hair of an infant as soon as possible after birth. The hair is also shaved after pilgrimage to Mecca (*haj*). Conversely, uncut hair of the scalp and body (*kesh*) is one of the five signs that a strict Sikh will observe.

Many skin disorders involving the scalp and hair are the cause of considerable distress. Exact diagnosis may be difficult, even for a dermatologist. Alopecia areata is the common cause of patchy, non-scarring hair-loss in children of all ethnic groups; the disease is by no means rare in adults. It is an auto-immune disease, which can affect any hairy area, although it is usually only noticeable, or worth treating, when it involves the scalp. The condition commonly remits spontaneously; but second or third attacks, particularly if associated with atopy or nail-pitting, carry a poor prognosis. Potent topical steroids are widely prescribed, although their value is still uncertain. Over the last few years topical minoxidil, and the induction of contact dermatitis, have been used to treat this condition. As yet none of these methods can be said to have achieved an established place in effecting long-term, cosmetically valuable, regrowth. If psychologically acceptable to the patient the provision of wigs is a very satis-factory cosmetic solution for those severely affected.

Diffuse hair loss is a fairly frequent complaint. One type is produced by slow continuous pulling on the hair. It is usually seen in the frontal or parietal areas of the scalp, where numerous broken hairs will be visible. Traction alopecia was seen in the white community when 'pony tail' hair-styles for girls were common. The problem has been described in Sikh boys (Singh 1975), who twist their hair into a tight twisted plait on top of the head, and Libyan women (Malhotra and Kanwar 1980), who hold their hair in place with a tight scarf or *maharama*. When the traction is removed it may take many months for any significant regrowth of hair to occur.

In childhood patchy alopecia with scarring is likely to be due to a fungal infection. Hitherto in urban areas the cat ringworm (*Microsporum canis*) was likely to be responsible. Since 1979 in Bradford, children from the Pakistani community have presented with a more inflammatory scalp ringworm, resulting from infection with the fungus *Trichophyton violaceum*. This phenomenon has also been noted among London's Bangladeshi community (Barth 1984). This species of fungus has apparently been 'exported' to the United Kingdom, and is now becoming more common. Eleven of the twelve affected individuals identi-fied in Bradford have been Asian, although the fungus has just been isolated from the first white patient. The fungus has been isolated from the nails as well as the scalp. From a dermatological point of view this innovation does make the diagnosis of scalp ringworm more complicated. Hairs invaded by *M. canis* fluoresce a turquoise-blue colour under Wood's light. Those invaded by *T. violaceum* do not. In both conditions Griseofulvin should be prescribed on a weight-related basis for six to eight weeks.

Androgenic alopecia is the commonest cause of non-scarring diffuse hair loss in adults of all ethnic groups. The process can affect either sex, but the male-pattern alopecia is the most familiar variety. In women the disease progresses more slowly, and seldom progresses to complete baldness.

Not all diseases of the scalp are the cause of significant hair-loss. Fine scaling of the scalp is known as pityriasis capitis or dandruff. Other manifestations of seborrhoeic eczema may be present. Regular use of a detergent shampoo will be helpful. Some patients will benefit from shampoos containing selenium sulphide, tar solution, or zinc pyrithione. If the scaling is thick, two per cent salicylic acid in a water-soluble base is helpful. More active eczemas of the scalp will require treatment with a topical steroid gel or lotion. Atopic eczema commonly affects the scalp in childhood, and is frequently infected. Scalp psoriasis is common in all ethnic groups, but will usually respond to treatment with pomades containing salicylic acid, tar, or dithranol. Long hair or complex hairstyles may make the treatment of Asian women difficult.

(c) Hirsutism and hypertrichosis

Hypertrichosis is the development of unwanted or excessive hair in either sex and at any site. Hirsutism is the development by a female of body hair in a male secondary sexual pattern. Mild degrees of hirsutism or facial hypertrichosis are not uncommon in young adult women, and Asians do seem particularly subject to this problem. In fact, hirsutism seems more acceptable in traditional Muslim women, and less acceptable in 'westernized' individuals. Naturally black hair is more visible than fair hair, and this may serve to excacerbate the difficulty.

Rarely, hirsutism may be one manifestation of virilization, along with deepening of the voice, decrease of breast size, temporal hair recession, and acne. In practice, the vast majority of patients do not have polycystic ovaries or androgen-secreting tumours, although any hirsute patients with a history of amenorrhoea or oligomenorrhoea should be referred to a gynaecologist. Some drugs, such as minoxidil, can also produce hypertrichosis. The great majority of patients are said to have idiopathic or constitutional hirsutism, which presumably is the result of a minor abnormality of androgen metabolism or production.

In many cultures, hair, and particularly beard hair, is a symbol of masculinity. The development of hirsutism may be the source of great humiliation and anxiety. It is unfortunate that the images of women portrayed in the media are hairless apart from the scalp and eyebrows. The first step in managing such patients is the reassurance that they are normal. Cosmetic treatment is essential, and patients should be told that no form of hair-removal will make the hair grow more rapidly or thickly. Shaving is cheap, easy, safe, and can be performed by the patient herself. However, although women may be able to shave their legs and axillae, there can be great psychological difficulties in shaving the face. On the whole, waxing is a reasonably satisfactory means of dealing with the limbs. Electrolysis is the only permanent method of hair-removal, but it is time-consuming, expensive, and can cause scarring if unskilfully performed. Because of the time involved it is applicable to visible sites only.

Ethnic origin may affect the acceptability, or otherwise, of hair-removal techniques. Sikh women may find any type impossible to use. Muslim patients do not find hair-removal difficult, and may already shave their axillary and pubic hair for religious and hygienic reasons. There are cultural differences of this type even among European women: those from the west will usually shave axillary hair but leave pubic hair unshaven, while in eastern Europe the opposite is true. A number of systemic agents have been employed to reduce the rate of growth of body or facial hair. Low doses of systemic steroids will suppress endogenous androgen production. Cyproterone acetate and the diuretic spironolactone both have anti-androgen effects, which may diminish the rate and thickness of hair-growth. The drugs need to be given on a permanent basis, and are not effective enough to obviate the necessity for physical removal of hair. Their long-term use is difficult to justify in young women.

(d) Generalized pruritus

Generalized pruritus is a common and very demoralizing problem. There are many dermatological and medical causes of this symptom. Despite extensive investigation, some patients will remain whose itching is totally unexplained. These individuals are said to have idiopathic pruritus if they are young, senile pruritus if they are old, and psychogenic pruritus if they are ungrateful. Unexplained generalized itching seems to be a particularly common and troublesome problem within the Asian community. The first step when confronted with a patient is to establish whether there is a simple cutaneous cause for the itching. In an individual with no previous history scabies must be the first diagnosis to be considered. Atopic eczema, urticaria, lichen planus, and dermatitis herpetiformis are all notoriously itchy skin-complaints. Even if there is no obvious rash there still may be a simple cause for the problem. Xeroderma in the elderly, contact with fibreglass or biological washing-powders, or the wearing of wool by atopics, can all be associated with marked pruritus.

Chronic renal failure is frequently associated with generalized itching, although few patients actually present in this way. Infectious hepatitis or any form of obstructive jaundice commonly causes pruritus, possibly because of retained bile-salts. Intrahepatic cholestasis is thought to be the mechanism responsible for the pruritus that may occur in the last trimester of pregnancy. Weight-loss, night sweats, or lymphadenopathy will suggest the diagnosis of a lymphoma. Generalized pruritus can also occur with iron-deficiency anaemia, polycythaemia, diabetes mellitus, hypothyroidism, and hyperthyroidism. These disorders are easy to exclude by simple investigations. The majority of cutaneous causes of pruritus have a specific remedy available. Additional symptomatic treatment with an antihistamine may also be beneficial. It is important to note that the anti-pruritic effect of antihistamines in diseases such as atopic eczema and lichen planus is related to their central sedative action. Newer antihistamines with a purely peripheral action, such as terfenadine, are valuable in urticaria, but are less effective in reducing other types of pruritus, as they do not possess this property.

The incidence of organically-caused itching does not appear to differ between the white and Asian communities; but inevitably a substantial number of patients will remain for whom a cause for this itching cannot be found. It seems that some dermatologists have formed the impression that Asian patients are particularly well-represented in this latter group. When this problem was investigated in my own clinic the conclusion was reached that many of these patients were atopics, with typical atopic itching but minimal eczema. Certainly, as judged by comparison of serum IgE levels, groups of Asian patients with itching alone and those with frank atopic eczema were indistinguishable (Greenwood and Barker 1985).

Such patients, and elderly individuals with xeroderma, may improve with emollients and topical steroids. Rarely, a speculative course of systemic steroids may be warranted where symptoms are unendurable; although even this approach is not assured of success.

(e) Artefacts and adornments

Not all skin-disease has an organic basis. Simulated disease is not uncommon, but can be difficult to recognize. Dermatitis artefacta (DA) affects accessible sites. The lesions are often geometrical in shape, and may show superficial necrosis or ulceration. They are difficult to explain in terms of common skin disorders, and, inexplicably, fail to heal. A few patients are frankly psychotic; but the vast majority have no obvious psychopathology. Gentle probing may reveal background anxieties or problems. In many individuals it is difficult to see what benefit results from the simulation, and DA seldom, if ever, represents simple malingering for a clearly definable purpose.

Direct confrontation is rarely a profitable approach in these patients. With children, it may be beneficial to explore the home circumstances; some adults will accept that their problem is 'stress'-related. Dermatitis artefacta will heal naturally if the area can be occluded, but relapses are all too frequent.

Ear-piercing, and even multiple ear-piercing, is a socially acceptable artefact in the white and Asian communities. Nose-piercing in the UK is traditional in the Asian female community, and is also currently practised in the white community. Asian females may use a nose ring, or a nose stud. It is more a matter of fashion and tradition than religion. Skin-piercing commonly results in infection and keloid formation, and may be the cause of the high incidence of nickel-sensitivity in women. Unmarried Asian females usually wear costume jewellery. Gold bracelets and ear-rings are usually worn by married women, and are presents from their husband's family. Ankle-chains were traditionally worn by Hindu women; but these have now spread to the white and Muslim communities.

In many Asian countries women stain their nails, palms, and soles with the vegetable dye henna. This will certainly be done for very special occasions such as marriage, and many Muslims will also do so to celebrate the festivals of *Eid*. Elderly Muslim men may use the dye simply as a cosmetic to stain greying hair and beards. Some years ago it was reported from the Sudan that this pigment was augmented by the synthetic dyestuff paraphenylenediamine (PPD) (El-Ansary *et al.* 1983). This substance, a known potent, if infrequent, skin sensitizer, is used in the west as the basis of permanent hair-dyes. The combination of henna and PPD is toxic if ingested, and has been used as a suicidal agent.

Other Asian cosmetics may be harmful. *Surma* is a fine powder, rather like mascara, but which is applied to the conjunctival surfaces of the eye rather than the eyelids. Originally it contained antimony sulphide, but latterly lead sulphide has been substituted. Ali and colleagues (1978) found that *surma* was quite widely used by children, and could be associated with raised blood-lead levels—'cosmetic' plumbism.

(f) Lumps and bumps

Keloids represent excessive and inappropriate fibroblastic response to cutaneous injury. Their development is precipitated by injury, although this may be very slight. Distinction is usually drawn between hypertrophic scars, in which the firm, thickened, and red tissue still conforms to the dimensions of the original injury, and true keloids, where the masses of abnormal tissue are often rounded, painful, and greatly exceed the dimensions of the original wound. It is not clear why some individuals are particularly prone to keloid formation. It is commonest in Afro-Caribbean and Asian patients, but can affect any ethnic group. Sites such as the chest and upper arm are frequently involved. It is better not to perform minor surgery in sites of predilection if this can possibly be avoided. Hypertrophic scars or small keloids may respond to intralesional injections of triamcinolone, although steroids administered in this way may produce hypopigmentation, and patients must be warned about this possibility. Large amounts of keloid tissue can be surgically excised, and the margins of the keloid sutured together. Initially results are very good; but unfortunately relapse is common.

Trauma may damage the skin in other ways. Lichenified hyperkeratotic nodules have been noted on the forehead of Shi'ite Muslims (Vollum and Azadeh 1979). These follow the use, for many years, of a 'prayer stone', which touches this area during the devotions that are performed five times daily. Age and associated actinic exposure were also thought to be aetiological factors. Prayer nodules have also been reported developing on the dorsum of the foot, because of the posture adopted (English *et al.* 1984).

Milia are small white or yellowish cysts containing keratin. They are usually most noticeable on the face, and are most common in infants and adolescent girls. More rarely milia develop secondary to a blistering disorder, such as epidermolysis bullosa or porphyria cutanea tarda. Milia are clearly epidermal, and may develop from sebaceous or sweat-gland remnants. Facial milia in infants do not require treatment. In adolescents, the overlying epidermis can be incised, and the contents of the cyst expressed with a fine sterile needle. This process is easy, but tedious, and the more sensible patients can easily treat themselves. Although there is no information about the prevalence of milia, they certainly are commonly seen in teenage Asian girls in clinical practice. The familiar umbilicated papules of molluscum contagiosum contain myriads of poxvirus particles. The disease is usually seen in children and young adults, where perigenital lesions are common. Despite the name, the disorder does not appear to be easily transmitted. Traumatic damage or inflammation of the papules usually leads to their resolution, and this fact has been exploited in treatment strategies such as squeezing with fine forceps or freezing with liquid nitrogen. In fact neither of these treatments are practical in apprehensive small children. Since there is almost always spontaneous resolution in twelve to eighteen months a painless placebo is preferable in this group. Tetracycline cream is widely used. Children of all ethnic groups may catch this disorder, but I have only seen the largest lesions, 'giant' molluscum contagiosum, develop in Asian children.

(g) Infections

Bacterial Impetigo is a superficial infection of the skin by *Staphylococcus aureus*, either alone or in association with the haemolytic streptococcus. Fragile blisters and pustules develop, which evolve into the classical golden-yellow crusted lesions. The same organisms can cause secondary infection, or impetiginization, of scabies, head-lice infestation, or atopic eczema. These infections can affect all ethnic groups in the United Kingdom, and usually respond to systemic antibiotic treatment with erythromycin or penicillin combined with flucloxacillin. The same bacteria are associated with the disease ecthyma. This disorder most frequently involves the legs. Blisters develop, which rupture to leave firm adhrent crusts. When the crusts are removed shallow ulcers remain, which eventually heal with scarring. Ecthyma is now quite uncommon; but the few cases which occur in my practice are invariably young Asians with ecthyma of the shins, whose problem began during a stay in the Indian subcontinent. There is no obvious explanation for this phenomenon; but of interest is the occurrence, in India, of another pustular skin disease which affects this site ('Pustular dermatitis atrophicans of the legs'). It seems to represent a superficial and deep pustular folliculitis; but no definite predisposing factor is recognized.

Viral Warts, herpes simplex, and herpes zoster are common in the white and Asian community. Ethnic origin does not seem to affect the presentation of these infections in any way; but Asian patients are more likely to develop post-inflammatory depigmentation following herpes zoster (shingles). Molluscum contagiosum has been discussed in the previous section.

Fungal and other infections Apart from the importation of *T. violaceum*, dermatophyte infections affecting the Asian communities in the UK closely resemble those seen in whites. Both groups are commonly affected, and the conditions are probably underdiagnosed. Infestation with *Sarcoptes scabeii*, or scabies, is common in the white and Asian communities, but Afro-Caribbean individuals may be less susceptible. The development of severe and intractable itching associated with scaling and burrows on the finger-webs, wrists, penis, and other sites should be, but often is not, immediately diagnostic. Scabies responds within seven to ten days of anointing the whole body with gamma-benzene hexachloride cream or lotion. All members of the family should be treated, whether clinically affected or not. The regime can be repeated once, after a week, but should not be performed more frequently. Complex treatment regimes like this will fail unless completely understood by the patient. If those concerned are not fluent in English then an interpreter is essential.

Psoriasis and eczema   Psoriasis is a common, non-infectious, skin disorder affecting perhaps one to two per cent of the adult population in the UK. The disease affects patients of both sexes and of any age, but with a peak incidence in the twenty to thirty-five age-group. Well-defined erythematous plaques develop, covered in silvery scales. The lesions are usually symmetrical, with elbows, knees, and scalp sites of predilection. In Asian patients the lesions of psoriasis will often be dark, rather than erythematous, but the distribution and silvery scaling should make the diagnosis obvious. The treating of male Asian pateints with a coal-tar or dithranol regime is not associated with any particular problems; but female patients may find the disease much more of a social stigma, and the amount of the body exposed during courses of treatment unacceptable. Photo-chemotherapy (PUVA) is a widely used technique for treating severely affected patients, but is not very easy to apply to the dark-skinned individual because melanin is an effective barrier to ultraviolet light transmission. The use of metho-trexate or etretinate can be highly effective, but these are more toxic agents, unsuitable for use in the setting of general practice.

Eczema is not a single disease, but rather an inflammatory skin reaction pattern induced by a number of internal and external factors acting alone and in com-bination. Two types of eczema are worthy of closer scrutiny.

Atopic eczema produces an itchy rash, often beginning at three to six months of age, on the face and napkin areas. It later localizes to the hands, feet, buttocks, and flexures. It may occur in association with asthma, hay-fever, or urticaria, and commonly runs in families. Overall atopic eczema tends to improve with age. It is difficult to know whether or not atopic eczema is actually commoner in the Asian community, but in my practice many of the more severely affected paediatric patients are Asian. The disease seems to be commoner in the United Kingdom than in India or Pakistan, although it certainly occurs worldwide. Asian atopic patients almost always report an improvement in their eczema if they return to India or Pakistan for a visit.

The skin may be generally dry; but active eczema is scaly, erythematous, and excoriated. Chronic eczematous patches may show lichenification. Secondary infection (usually with *Staphylococcus aureus*) results in weeping and crusting, with increased itch and soreness.

The serum IgE level will usually be raised, and most atopics will have multiple positive prick tests to common ingestants and inhalants. It must be clearly explained that regular treatment is essential, and that eczema is helped but not 'cured' by therapy. The maximum possible benefits should be obtained from the regular use of emollients (for example, Aqueous Cream, Unguentum Merck, or E45 Cream). Bath oils such as Balneum and Oilatum should be employed as soap-substitutes.

The daily application of a topical steroid can be very helpful. Only hydrocortisone preparations are safe enough to be used regularly in the paediatric age group. One per cent hydrocortisone cream or ointment is cheap and safe, with Vioform-HC cream being useful if secondary infection is present. Dry skin will benefit from ten per cent urea cream, with or without hydrocortisone. Coaltar paste is helpful for dry, thick, lichenified eczema. Sedative antihistamines used at night can be helpful if nocturnal itching is a major problem. The management of atopic eczema in childhood involves one of the most complex treatment regimes that parents are called upon to perform themselves. Adequate, and often repeated, explanation is necessary. The assistance of an interpreter is invaluable if there are language difficulties.

The other form of eczema that appears to be particularly troublesome in the Asian patients, although it affects all groups, is lichen simplex. The persistent thickened or lichenified plaques that develop on the limbs, or neck, are also known as neurodermatitis. Topical steroid therapy alone is not very effective in this disorder. Plaques of lichen simplex are best managed by occlusive bandaging with tar-impregnated dressings. Superficial X-ray therapy may be used by dermatologists with access to this form of treatment. Relapse is unfortunately common, whatever form of treatment is employed.

Conclusion

Within the United Kingdom, with the rare exceptions of the imported diseases, there appear to be no major differences in the skin disorders that affect the white and Asian communities. Asian patients, particularly those from a very traditional background, are however more likely to be alarmed by the development of a skin disease. Obvious language difficulties may make a history more difficult for a non-Asian doctor to take, and he or she may miss the cultural significance of some aspects of the history even if help with translation is provided.

When it comes to physical examination, female Asian patients may find it impossible to accept scrutiny by male doctors. The colouration of individual lesions may present difficulties for physicians accustomed only to the apperance of rashes occurring on white skin. The distribution of lesions over the body should however still be a reliable guide.

Once a diagnosis is made the Asian patient may find it more difficult to accept the limited degree to which many skin disorders respond to therapy. There are occasionally ingredients of topical preparations that are religiously objectionable. For these, and other reasons, Asian patients may wish to consult traditional healers.

References

Ali, R. A., Smales, O. R. C. and Aslam, M. (1978). Surma and lead poisoning. *British Medical Journal*, **2**, 915–16.

Bajaj, A. K., Govil, D. N. and Bajaj, S. (1983). Bindi depigmentation. *Archives of Dermatology*, **119**, 629.

Barth, J. H. (1984). Tinea capitis—*Trichophyton violaceum* in East London (letter). *Clinical and Experimental Dermatology*, **9**, 625.

Boyle, J. and Kennedy, C. T. C. (1986). Hydroquinone concentrations in skin lightening creams. *British Journal of Dermatology*, **114**, 501–4.

El-Ansary, E. H., Ahmed, M. E. K., and Clague, H. W. (1983). Systemic toxicity of Para-phenylenediamine. *Lancet*, **i**, 1341.

English, J. S. C., Fenton, D. A. and Wilkinson, J. D. (1984). Prayer nodules. *Clinical and Experimental Dermatology*, **9**, 97–8.

Greenwood, R. and Barker, D. J. (1985). Pruritus and atopy in Asians. *Clinical and Experimental Dermatology*, **10**, 179–80.

Kandil, E. (1974). Treatment of vitiligo with 0.1 % betamethasone 17-valerate in isopropyl alcohol—a double-blind trial. *British Journal of Dermatology*, **91**, 457–60.

Kumari, J. (1984). Vitiligo treated with topical clobetasol propionate. *Archives of Dermatology*, **120**, 631–5.

Malhotra, Y. K. and Kanwar, A. J. (1980). Tractional alopecia among Libyan women. *Archives of Dermatology*, **116**, 987.

OPCS (Office of Population Censuses and Surveys) (1987). Communicable Disease Surveillance Centre. *Communicable disease statistics 1985*, Series MB2 **No. 12**. HMSO, London.

Pandhi, R. K. and Kumar, A. S. (1985). Contact leukoderma due to 'bindi' and footwear. *Dermatologica*, **170**, 260–2.

Qureshi, B. (1986). Skin problems encountered in multi-ethnic groups. *Dermatology in Practice*, **4**, 11–16.

Singh, G. (1975). Traction alopecia in Sikh boys. *British Journal of Dermatology*, **92**, 232–3.

Vollum, D. I. and Azadeh, B. (1979). Prayer nodules. *Clinical and Experimental Dermatology*, **4**, 39–47.

Further reading

So far as I am aware no textbook exists which specifically deals with the skin problems of the Asian community within the UK. Essential reading for those with an interest in this subject is:

Bhutani, L. K. (1984). *Colour atlas of dermatology*, (2nd edn). Interprint, New Delhi.

This book describes, and beautifully illustrates, the patterns of infective and non-infective skin diseases in an Indian setting

Acknowledgments

I should like to thank, for their advice, several colleagues at Bradford Royal Infirmary: Dr W. M. Edgar (Consultant Microbiologist), Ms Yasmin Ahmed (Social Work Department), and Sister B. Smith (Sister in charge, Dermatology

Department). I am also most grateful to Ms Ruby Khan, of Bradford Community Relations Council, for permission to use material from her survey of our Department. Mrs Shahnaz Bahadur and Mrs Gurpaul Sandhu kindly read the manuscript. I am of course responsible for any errors or infelicities that remain.

17 Psychological and psychiatric disorders

Philip Rack

Introduction

There are many different Asian communities in the UK, and the practitioner who has Asian patients from a particular community must familiarize himself or herself with the needs and problems of that community, and that can only be done locally. Moreover, within each community people act as individuals, guided no doubt by culture and custom, but not necessarily constrained by them. Generalizations, including those made in this chapter, should be interpreted with care.

In all communities, while there is strength, both private and communal, there is also unhappiness; and this is true of the Asian communities in the UK. There are Asian women whose days are spent in loneliness and social isolation, cut off from family and neighbourhood networks. Many older Asian women speak little or no English. Some are confined to the home, by their husbands or their own timidity, and are seldom seen; others may become surgery-haunters—perhaps because a visit to the doctor is one of their few opportunities for a culturally-sanctioned outing. There are Asian men in their fifties who are prematurely aged because, having lost their jobs, they have lost the objective for which they came to the UK, and with it, their self-respect. There are parents and parents-in-law who expect respectful obedience from the next generation but do not get it. Some Asian teenagers are confused about questions of career, lifestyle, or arranged marriage; most of them love their parents, and are made unhappy by their own feelings of rebelliousness. A few of them suffer actual physical maltreatment, and some run away from home. There are thoughtful intelligent parents who recognize the intergenerational schisms in the family, but can find no way to resolve them, and are distressed by that.

Issues of these kinds must be understood by psychiatrists and general practitioners dealing with functional disorders. Unhappiness is not the same as mental illness, and in most cases it is endured or overcome without help from doctors; but those kinds of stress can lead to mental or physical symptoms, and even to overt breakdown. It is often difficult for an Asian person to discuss personal and emotional problems with a doctor, (especially a male, white doctor); so causes may be denied while symptoms continue to proliferate. In that situation the practitioner has to make diagnostic judgements on the basis of hints, evasions, and observations of family dynamics. That is never easy, but becomes a little less difficult the more we can learn about the general background of the patient, the family and the community.

Background

Although a systematic description of the origins of the Asian population in the UK is given in Chapter 1, a brief account is also provided here, because it is relevant to considering the background to the psychological problems of this migrant population.

Most Asians in the UK who are more than about thirty years old arrived as immigrants in the 1960s. They came by invitation, for those were the years of economic expansion, and there was a need for unskilled labour. In those days thousands of migrant workers were being recruited in southern Europe (for example, Turkey, Yugoslavia, Greece) to work as Gastarbeiters in the factories of the industrial north (Germany, Holland, Scandinavia). Britain, because of its colonial history, had access to other areas of recruitment, which included the Caribbean islands to the west, and India, Pakistan, and Bangladesh to the east.

Most of the original migrant workers in Europe were young men, and either were single or left their families behind. Their aim was to find work and return home rich after a year or two; they had no intention of permanent settlement. Many of them came from areas which were economically backward by the standards of their own countries, and they did not have much formal education; but they had initiative and courage. They were prepared to take whatever work was available, sacrificing personal happiness for a year or two for the sake of the family and dependants back home, to whom regular remittances were sent. (For a more detailed account see Power and Hardman (1978). The Asian immigrants to the UK were not called 'migrant workers', or perceived as such by the British; but they had the same aims and characteristics as the European Gastarbeiters (Dahya 1973; Anwar 1979; Rack 1982*b*, 1985). They saw themselves (originally) as transient, even though as Commonwealth citizens they had (until 1963) the legal right of permanent residence in the 'mother country' (unlike Gastarbeiters elsewhere in Europe). They also had the right to send for their wives and children to join them. Some did so, and the rising numbers of unfamiliar-looking people with different habits provoked a backlash in certain sections of the British population, leading to a series of increasingly-restrictive immigration laws. Seeing the door closing, more Asians sent for their relatives while they could, thereby adding to British fears of being 'swamped', and fuelling the British xenophobia which was later to erupt into overt racism.

The pioneering Gastarbeiter (whether Turk in Germany or Pakistani in the UK) usually chose to keep to his own community, mixing as little as possible with his British neighbours, and learning no more of the local language than was necessary for survival. But if he was joined by his family, and his children started going to school, this separatist stance was no longer tenable. His children learned English even if he did not; they watched television and were affected (a devout Muslim might say 'infected') by British culture. Even now in many families the parents still cherish the thought of going 'home' eventually, but to their children 'home' is the UK. This contradiction within the family, and often within the mental processes of an individual, lies at the root of many of the psychological and psychiatric problems of that generation of Asian patients; they are no longer transient migrants, but have not fully accepted the self-image of settler, and are experiencing the psychological consequences of that ambivalence and marginality. (Rack 1982*b*; 1986). On top of all that, additional stresses are inflicted by the dominant 'white' majority culture. An outside observer might have supposed that Britain's colonial history would have produced an atmosphere of tolerant liberalism, a cosmopolitan culture in which newcomers would be easily absorbed. But that has not been the case: it seems that the British people do not easily adopt a multicultural perspective; they tend to be ethnocentric. History shows that every group of immigrants which has arrived in the UK in the last hundred years, including those who came as refugees, has been subjected to abuse and persecution (Nicolson 1974); and the abuse is greatest against those whose difference is marked by their skin colour.

Racial violence attracts the attention of the media when incidents occur in some deprived inner-city area; riots are news. But the violence which members of ethnic minorities themselves experience in their daily lives gets little publicity. Sometimes this violence takes the form of physical assault and harassment—faeces or petrol-soaked rags pushed through letter-boxes; usually it is expressed more subtly, in terms of disparaging jokes, dismissive assumptions, and negative stereotypes—all of which are seen by the victims as manifestations of tacit contempt. There is widespread discrimination in, for example, employment and promotion. Public institutions and authorities (such as the Health Service) have been extremely slow to change any of their systems and procedures to accommodate new multicultural needs.

Asians are not evenly distributed throughout the country; they came to certain cities because their labour was needed in old-fashioned (labour-intensive) industries, and in times of economic recession it is those industries, and those cities, which tend to have the worst economic and social problems. In a climate of high unemployment, low public expenditure, and widening gulfs between the 'haves' and the 'have-nots', racial prejudice has come to the surface as never before. It is not immigrants, or ethnic minorities, or black people who are the cause of social and economic problems; but they make convenient scapegoats.

It is quite difficult for comfortable middle-class white practitioners to appreciate the extent and severity of racism as it affects black people at the present time; but for those who bother to look, the evidence is incontrovertible. It must be kept in mind, especially in relation to psychological and psychiatric disorders (Wilson 1978, 1981; Burke 1984, 1986; Fernando 1986, 1988).

Mental illness rates

Psychiatric morbidity statistics must be considered in the context of what is known generally about migration and mental health. Epidemiologists have studied this for over a century, (ever since asylum superintendents in America in the 1850s started to report large numbers of immigrant admissions e.g. Ranney 1850), and the usual finding has been that immigrants are significantly more vulnerable to mental disorders than non-migrants (Pollock 1913; Odegaard 1932, 1936; Malzberg 1969). There are exceptions, however: some studies show morbidity-rates for immigrants which are actually lower than those of the host population (Murphy 1973, 1977, 1982; Rack 1982a).

The results of some recent research studies in Britain are summarized in Table 17.1. It will be seen that in some surveys the Asian rates of mental hospital admission are somewhat higher, but in other cases they appear to be lower, than those of the local indigenious population; and, in those studies which make a distinction between Indians and Pakistanis, the findings in different places are contradictory.

Table 17.1 *Mental hospital admission rates summary table*

Country of origin	England and Wales, 1971 (Cochrane 1977)		Bradford 1968–70 (Hitch 1975)		Manchester 1973–75 (Carpenter and Brockington 1980)		South East Thames 1976 (Dean *et al.* 1981)	
	All admissions		First admissions only					
	M	F	M	F	M	F	M	F
INDIA	85	79	88	59			149	123
					236	325		
PAKISTAN	68	68	134	191			59	55

(Figures are percentages of British-born admissions, calculated in each case from rates given by the authors.)

General conclusions cannot be drawn, presumably because of local differences which may be related as much to patterns of service-provision as to racial or demographic differences; on balance, when the age and sex variables of each group are taken into account, we may tentatively suggest that Asian admission rates do not differ very significantly from national base rates. This stands in contrast to the statistics for Afro-Caribbean groups, which are generally much higher. Given the stresses to which all non-white groups are subjected, this is a surprising finding.

That evidence alone does not prove that Asian communities are particularly mentally stable or 'tough'. Admission figures do not reflect morbidity, they reflect the take-up of services; and there are many reasons why Asians are slow to seek psychiatric help. They include language and communication—obviously crucial in this field; there is also a tendency to express mental distress in somatic terms (see below); and in all Asian cultures a great stigma is attached to 'insanity'. However, some Birmingham research does support the idea that Asians there are less stressed than might be expected. The researchers took a translated version of the Langner 22-item Questionnaire, revalidated it on Asian samples, and used it in a series of community surveys. Surprisingly, the results revealed less mental and emotional disorder among the Indian and Pakistani samples than among the indigenous sample (Cochrane and Stopes-Roe 1977, 1981). This work has not been repeated, and awaits confirmation elsewhere.

Diagnostic pitfalls

Depression and anxiety

Many Asian patients show a tendency to express their depression or anxiety in purely physical terms, and this somatization of distress is well-recognized by psychiatrists working in India and Pakistan, so it is not simply a matter of language (Rao 1966). Because of somatization many cases of depression, anxiety, and other emotional disorders are treated by GPs, possibly without recognition by either doctor or patient that the complaints are psychosomatic. Pain is a very common presenting symptom, and can lead to a dismissive diagnosis of 'hypochondriasis'—which by itself is never a complete diagnosis. The pain is often in the head or abdomen, but may occur in any limbs, or throughout the whole body, when it has been called 'body-ache'. Its characteristics are changeable and vague, and often do not correspond to any organic syndrome. Some patients complain of gas in the stomach, chest, or head, which is probably a way of expressing the sensation of physical tension. Anergia and loss of interest may be expressed as generalized bodily weakness. (For a more detailed description and discussion see Rack 1982*b*.) Depressive illness should always be considered in such cases. Organic causes must obviously be excluded, and ones which might be overlooked include anaemia due to iron deficiency or to infestation; osteomalacia (vitamin D deficiency), which can present with fugutive joint-pains and nothing else; and tuberculosis, which, in its various forms, is somewhat more prevalent in Asian communities.

When anxiety or depression is suspected, and direct questions are asked about mood, patients may still decline to admit the existence of any emotional symptoms or any psychosocial causes. None the less, if the patient seems depressed and no other cause can be found for the complaints, a trial of antidepressant medication is often worthwhile. If endogenous depression is the correct diagnosis the prognosis is good, provided that the medication is taken as prescribed and for a sufficient time. (That is a requirement which must be clearly explained and reinforced.) If the depression or anxiety are reactive to external factors the patient may be unwilling to confide the true problems at the first visit, but may gain confidence to do so later; or another member of the family may provide the missing information.

Sexual dysfunction is a fairly common complaint of Asian men, and may take the form of erectile impotence, premature ejaculation, or the *dhat* syndrome. '*Dhat*' (also known as *jiryan*) consists of the conviction that sperm is leaking from the body in the urine, and its loss is causing progressive bodily weakness. *Dhat/jiryan* seems to be specific to the Indian subcontinent (Carstairs 1956). It is often associated with impotence. All forms of sexual dysfunction are difficult to treat. Many Asians patients expect to be cured by aphrodisiac or hormone injections, and are even more reluctant than Europeans to accept psychodynamic explanations. Joint therapy with both sexual partners is seldom possible or acceptable. The best hope is that the dysfunction is a manifestation of a generalized anxiety-state or depressive illness, in which case treatment can be given for the underlying condition. Even so, full sexual function may not return immediately, probably because of secondary anxiety. Further discussion on sexual dysfunction is contained in Chapter 10.

It used to be thought that depressive illness was less prevalent in Asian than in European cultures, but recent work suggests that this is not so. It has probably been underdiagnosed in the past because of the tendency to somatic presentation.

Schizophrenia

Schizophrenia exists with approximately equal frequency in most countries which have been surveyed (WHO 1972), including India and Pakistan; and it occurs among Asian immigrants in the UK. In contrast to affective disorders, the problem here is not underdiagnosis but overdiagnosis, because symptoms which in a European would be indicative of schizophrenia do not necessarily have the same significance in an Asian patient. One of the cardinal symptoms of schizophrenia is paranoia—the belief that one is being persecuted. Some complex and systematized delusions can be recognized at once—they could not possibly be true; but in other cases, less extreme or at an earlier stage, there may be only a general expression of grievance and victimization, or even just a suspicious and evasive manner of responding to questions. Is this paranoia? From what we know already about inequality and discrimination it is apparent that many Asians do actually experience victimization or persecution in their everday lives—so in that case a cautious approach and suspicious attitude to strangers (including doctors) may not be at all pathological. Time, and repeated visits, may be required before trust is established. When it is, the doctor may have some difficulty in believing the stories which are told about the police, Department of Health or Social Security officials, immigration officers or other authority-figures, or about the bitterness of some intrafamily disputes; but it is important to keep an open mind, and not jump to conclusions about 'paranoid' behaviour.

Particular care should be taken with people who have been refugees. This includes most of the Vietnamese, Tamils, and East African Asians. A great number of such people—more than was previously recognized—have been victims of torture or other forms of deliberate violence. They do not necessarily wish to reveal this history, but may 'clam-up', and become evasive or panic-stricken when faced with anything resembling an interrogation. The psychological effects of extreme trauma can show themselves years later, even in old age (Bram 1983; Davidson 1983; Jagucki 1983).

Another diagnostic problem (which applies in many cross-cultural situations) is that beliefs which seem to the doctor to be erroneous and bizarre, and therefore delusional, may be quite normal. An example is belief in magic. In Pakistan, India, and Bangladesh, the individual's subjective world is peopled by djinns and other dangerous spirits, and all kinds of adversity may be attriubted to their malignant influence. Similar beliefs exist in most other parts of the world; in fact 'western' scientific scepticism represents a minority culture in numerical terms. Pain and illness can be produced, it is thought, by an evil-minded person employing witchcraft or sorcery. An Asian patient might express the idea that his or her symptoms are due to the malevolence of (for example) a hostile sister-in-law, even thought she is not in the household, and perhaps not even in the country. Such beliefs are not evidence of paranoid psychosis, and they are not confined to the uneducated or illiterate; they may be held by highly sophisticated and intelligent people; but the more 'Westernized' will probably be hesitant or sheepish in mentioning them to a doctor, fearing ridicule. Asian patients may often be observed wearing *tavees*, which are charms or amulets obtained from a spiritual healer. In the case of Muslims, the *tavees* usually contain some verses from the Quran, and they are intended to protect the wearer against the evil eye and the machinations of enemies.

A cardinal rule of psychiatry is that a belief should not be classified as a delusion simply because it is erroneous; it must also be outside the range of normal beliefs for the culture to which the subject belongs. Thus for one person to claim to receive messages direct from God is pathological, while for another it is not. Judgement is based not on the oddity of the claim as it appears to an outsider, but its congruence or incongruence with the patient's own culture, and its compatibility with his or her personality and other longstanding beliefs. It would be unreasonable to expect every doctor to have an anthropologist's knowledge of all the belief-systems which he or she might encounter in a multi-cultural society such as Britain; so it is a question of taking advice each time the issue arises. Usually the best people to advise will be the patients own relatives or friends, who will say whether or not the patient is 'mad' in their judgement. Occasionally one has to beware of distortions due to personal antipathies or ulterior motives, and that can be a problem. In such a situation a practitioner who has a circle of friends spanning various cultures may be able to seek informal advice elsewhere, with due regard to confidentiality. (A practitioner working in a multicultural community who has no such multicultural friendships might like to ask himself or herself why not.)

Sometimes it may be the patient's relatives who offer unexpected explanations of illness; for example a man might suggest that his wife is possessed by the devil or an evil spirit. That is an acceptable explanation of abnormal behaviour, and is not limited to schizophrenia, but applies equally well, if not more so, to hysteria. There is nothing to be gained by entering into an argument; the cultural explanation is, in its own way, as valid as the scientific one, and it has a valuable de-mystifying benefit. We do harm by demolishing a set of explanations if the ones we offer instead will not be understood or accepted. In order to retain the family's co-operation one should not object to the use of faith-healing or alternative medicine at the same time as 'western' medicine. Religious healers (*pirs*) and practitioners of *Unani-Tib* and Ayurvedic medicine (*hakims* and *vaids*) are available and popular among the Asian communities in the UK (Aslam 1979); and they deal with a great deal of minor psychiatric disorder. In fact every practitioner should act on the assumption that an Asian patient whom he or she is treating is also receiving concurrent treatment from an alternative healer—and has at least as much confidence in the other one. But the very fact that the patient is consulting a western doctor indicates some confidence in western medicine, and this can be built upon. Problems arise if the *hakim*—or anyone else—advises the patient not to take the medicine which the doctor has prescribed; a great deal of patience may be required to resolve such conflicts.

Another diagnostic problem in relation to schizophrenia is the acute reactive, stress-induced, or psychogenic psychosis. Among indigenous British subjects, stress can produce many different reactions, including anxiety, depression, hysterical symptoms, and phobias—in fact the whole range of neurotic syndromes. It can also produce psychosomatic disorders. Rarely, however, does stress produce psychotic symptoms—delusions, hallucinations, thought-disorder, confusion, and loss of contact with reality. Those symptoms are usually interpreted as pointers toward a diagnosis of schizophrenia; and any recent stresses in the patient's life tend to be relegated to the role of trigger-factors or precipitants, not primary causes.

That generalization is not entirely satisfactory even for indigenous British patients, and it is certainly not applicable across all cultures. In other parts of the world, even in some European countries, psychiatrists diagnose reactive psychosis frequently, and distinguish it from schizophrenia. The reason why reactive psychosis is rare (or rarely diagnosed) in the UK is unclear. Among Asian patients schizophreniform symptoms, including some of Schneider's 'first-rank' symptoms of schizophrenia, can and do occur in response to stress, in subjects who have no evidence of schizophrenia in their family history or pre-morbid personality. The onset of the disorder is usually acute and often dramatic, and at first it may be impossible to say whether or not this is the beginning of a genuine schizophrenic illness. Urgent treatment is required, probably including hospitalization and neuroleptic medication; but a history of serious life-stresses immediately preceding the onset, and a rapid initial response to treatment, should suggest a reactive condition. The management of such patients should include attention to social and environmental factors; and they ought not to be labelled 'schizophrenic' too readily, as that label has long-term implications, and in reactive psychosis the subsequent history is not necessarily that of schizophrenia.

Hysteria and hysterical behaviour

Hysteria is the most culturally variable of all psychiatric conditions. This is because hysterical symptoms are intended (unconsciously) to attract attention. They are therefore a kind of communication, and communication has to employ the local idiom if it is to get a response. In the UK today we rarely see the kind of dramatic conversion symptoms described in classical textbooks—para-plegias, fits, aphonias, and the like. Instead we have a positive epidemic of teenage overdoses, and a burgeoning fashion for anorexia and bulimia. Asian teenagers who have grown up in the UK are learning to use the locally-accepted methods of signalling distress (such as overdose); but more dramatic forms of attention-seeking are also seen, such as pseudo-epileptic fits, hallucinations, and possession states. Recent research from Birmingham (Merrill 1988) has shown that over the past five years, self-poisoning among young white women has decreased by 33 per cent; but among young Asian women there has been a 33 per cent increase; young Asian women may be more than twice as likely to self-poison as their white counterparts. The main contributory factors seem to be culture-conflict between older and younger family members, and racism (Merrill and Owens 1986). Insanity carries a great stigma in many Asian families, so to behave in an 'insane' way is a sure means of arousing anxiety and gaining attention, and is used as such. Women and girls are somewhat more likely than men to use hysterical mechanisms, probably because they have less power in a male-dominated culture, and fewer ways of claiming attention for their feelings; and people who cannot communicate verbally because of language barriers are naturally likely to communicate by acting-out.

Obsessions and phobias

Contrary to some previous beliefs, obsessional compulsive and phobic states do occur in Asians; their relative prevalence-rates are not known. Symptoms may include compulsive checking and handwashing; obsessional intrusive thoughts which are frequently painfully unacceptable to the sufferer, for example immoral or obscene throughts; agoraphobia; social phobias; and specific phobias. Diagnosis can be difficult with patients who have incomplete command of English, as they may have great difficulty in describing the exact nature of the disability; but once the possibility of the condition is recognized appropriate questions will usually elicit the symptoms.

Confusion can arise occasionally in relation to religious observances. A devout Muslim should engage in prayer several times daily at set times, and prayer should be preceded by washing. There are also dietary prohibitions, and during Ramadan one should fast from dawn to sunset (which is not easy in northern latitudes in summer). As in other religions, some believers take these instructions more literally and conscientiously than others; and a few are so meticulous that their practice borders on obsession, or becomes an overt obsessional neurosis. Treatment is very difficult, but might be aided by obtaining the support of an Imam.

Language problems and the use of interpreters

A majority of 'Asians' in the UK were actually born here, or arrived in childhood, and have few or no problems with language; but that does not apply to the older generation, especially older women, as is shown in the data presented in Chapters 5 and 14. When such patients visit a doctor they are often accompanied by a relative or friend who speaks better English. This arrangement has to be accepted; often the companion not only interprets, but provides emotional support for the patient in a frightening situation. He or she is sometimes also an additional source of useful information. There are problems, however. An interpreter who is emotionally involved with the patient is likely to intrude his or her own opinions and interpretations (consciously or not) into the translation—and this is particularly damaging when psychosocial factors or interpersonal problems are part of the picture. Husbands are sometimes inclined to speak for their wives instead of translating for them. Children should not be used as interpreters; this practice is common, not least because a parent will often bring one of his or her children along for the purpose; but it should be resisted except in an emergency. Not only is it distasteful to ask a child to transmit intimate medical or emotional details, but the person who acts as interpreter is, for the time being, in a position of great power *vis-à-vis* the non-English-speaker. When we bear in mind the hierarchical structure of many Asian families and the importance of filial respect, and realize that this tradition is frequently under strain in families in the UK, we can begin to imagine the effect on family dynamics of putting a son or daughter in such a position. If the interpreter is a neighbour, and not a family member, considerations of confidentiality may apply.

It is generally better to obtain the services of an independent interpreter, preferably one with professional training. This is becoming standard practice in some psychiatric hospitals, and it is not impossible to arrange in general practice. A local office of Social Services may be helpful; many of them have lists of interpreters available for the main locally-required languages. An even better arrangement is to have a colleague who speaks the patient's language. This might be a doctor, nurse, health visitor, or social or community worker; and such a person is more than a translator, if he or she understands the nature and significance of what is said. (For further discussion see Rack 1982*b*; 1987; Bavington and Majid 1986; and Chapter 5).

Treatment

As always, the key to successful treatment is correct diagnosis. Once this is achieved, treatment may follow the same lines as for any other patient. It is important to explain the illness to the patient, and if possible to a relative. The explanation should include diagnosis, treatment plan, and prognosis. Care should be taken to ensure that explanations and instructions are understood. Some patients who are apprehensive, or overpolite, or have an imperfect command of English, may answer 'Yes' to everything, without taking it all in.

Asian patients may ask questions which are different from those asked by English patients. They often wish to know about causes. It is not sufficient to state: 'You have an obsessional neurosis', or 'Your son has schizophrenia'. They want to know why—and this means not only; 'Why do you say that?', but also 'Why did it happen?', and also 'Why me?' (or 'Why him?'). A practitioner who has no explanation to offer loses credibility. Another question is about what the patient and the family can do themselves to hasten a cure. What about diet—sleep—rest—daily timetable of activity—sexual life? Would a change of environment be helpful—a trip to Indian perhaps? An Ayurvedic practitioner would include advice about all these in his treatment regimen; and a doctor who merely prescribes pills and nothing else is quite unimpressive in comparison. Pills are in any case less impressive than injections; and any medication which does not have a perceptible effect on the first day is likely to be abandoned. This is a particular problem with tricyclic antidepressants, which have a seven to ten day latency of onset; so persuasive explanations and careful supervision may be needed to ensure compliance. On the other hand, the idea that a well person requires regular injections in order to remain well (as with depot maintenance of chronic schizophrenia) seems to be accepted by many Asian families as well as, if not better than, by English ones.

Pharmacotherapy

All the usual psychotropic drugs may be used; but there is some evidence that lower doses may be required to achieve therapeutic effects, and avoid side-effects. The reasons for this are not known, nor do we know to which drugs it applies; through anecdotal evidence is strongest for the tricyclic group. In research experiments using clomipramine it was found that the same single dose produced higher plasma levels in Asian subjects than in matched English controls, which suggests that there is a genuine metabolic difference in absorption or detoxification of this compound. (Allen *et al.* 1977; Lewis *et al.* 1980). Similar results were found with fluphenazine (Lewis and Rack, unpublished). More research is desirable, and, until it is done, the best rule seems to be to start with somewhat lower doses than usual, and work up slowly. Monoamine oxidase drugs should be given only if the prescriber is satisfied that the accompanying dietary restrictions are perfectly understood and will be followed; and often that is not the case. Aslam and Stockley (1979) reported evidence of incompatibility between some 'western' drugs and substances used by *hakims* or in Asian cooking; and this possibility should be considered if unusual side-effects are reported.

Psychotherapy

Of all medical procedures psychotherapy is the most dependent on communication; so if there is a significant language problem individual psychotherapy is impossible. The only solution is to find someone else who understands the patient's language—and not only the vocabularly, but the nuances of expression—who can carry out psychotherapy, under supervision if necessary. Such a person might be a colleague, or possibly a member of the patient's family.

The view has been expressed that interpretive or analytic psychotherapy on a 'European' model is not appropriate in cultures which are less individualistic and more family-orientated, and where the self is conceptualized differently. It has been suggested that traditional Asians are not sufficiently psychologically-minded, and lack the power of introspection and self-analysis. These generalizations contain some truth; but like all stereotypes, they must not be applied too readily. Some experienced therapists claim that individual psychotherapy is effective provided that techniques are modified where necessary (Bavington and Majid 1986). A more directive approach may be appropriate; as noted above, Asian patients may appreciate counselling, as well as medication.

Group therapy is also possible, and has been found to be a very effective technique in some situations. (Bavington and Majid 1986; Das, unpublished). Family therapy is certainly possible. In fact it is the norm, and not only in cases where family dynamics are causative. Asian families expect to be involved in the treatment of one of their members; they will continue to have great influence on the patient while he is under treatment, and this influence can be made use of by bringing some of the most significant members into the therapy situation, and working with them. A practitioner who works in this way has the additional advantage of learning about the norms and expectations of the family, and will be less likely, then and in the future, to make culturally inappropriate interpretations or recommendations.

Conclusion

There is a complex interplay between culture, migration, racism, and mental health. In addition the presentation of psychological and psychiatric disorders is strongly influenced by factors such as culture, religion, and language. Knowledge and understanding of the background, characteristics, and needs of the local community will enable the practitioner to provide appropriate and sensitive care to his Asian patients.

References

Allen, J. J., Rack, P. H., and Vadaddi, K. S. (1977). Differences in the effects of clomipramine on English and Asian volunteers; preliminary report of a pilot study. *Postgraduate Medical Journal*, **53**, Suppl. 4, 79.

Anwar, M. (1979). *The myth of return*. London, Heinemann.

Aslam, K. (1979). *The practice of Asian medicine in the United Kingdom*. Thesis for Ph.D., University of Nottingham.

Aslam, K. and Stockley, I. H. (1979). Interaction between curry ingredient (Karela) and drug (Chlorpropamide). *Lancet*, **i**, 607.

Bavington, J. and Majid, A. (1986). Psychiatric services for ethnic minority groups. In *Transcultural Psychiatry*, (ed. J. Cox), pp. 87–106. Croom Helm, London.

Bram, G. (1983). Breakdown in elderly Polish refugees. In *The psychosocial problems of refugees*, (ed. R. Baker), pp. 39–41. British Refugee Council, London.

Burke, A. W. (ed.) (1984). Transcultural psychiatry, racism and mental illness. *International Journal of Social Psychiatry*, 30th anniversary double issue, **30**, 1–2.

Burke, A. W. (1986). Racism, prejudice and mental illness. In *Transcultural Psychiatry*, (ed. J. Cox), pp. 139–57. Croom Helm, London.

Carpenter, L. and Brockington, I. F. (1980). A study of mental illness in Asians, West Indians and Africans living in Manchester. *British Journal of Psychiatry*, **137**, 201–5.

Carstairs, G. M. (1956). Hinjra and Jiryan. *British Journal of Medical Psychology*, **29**, 128–38.

Cochrane, R. (1977). Mental illness in immigrants to England and Wales. *Social Psychiatry*, **12**, 25–35.

Cochrane, R. and Stopes-Roe, M. (1977). Psychological and social adjustment of Asian immigrants to Britain; a community survey. *Social Psychiatry*, **12**, 195–6.

Cochrane, R. and Stopes-Roe, M. (1981). Psychological symptom levels in Indian immigrants to Britain; a comparison with native English. *Psychological Medicine*, **11**, 319–27.

Dahya, Badr (1973). Pakistanis in Britain; transients or settlers? *Race*, **XIV**(3), 241–77.

Davidson, S. (1983). The psychosocial aspects of holocaust trauma in the life cycle of survivor refugees and their families. In *The psychosocial problems of refugees*, (ed. R. Baker), pp. 21–31. British Refugee Council, London.

Dean, G., *et al.* (1981). First admissions of native-born and immigrants to psychiatric hospitals in South-east England, 1976. *British Journal of Psychiatry*, **139**, 506–12.

Fernando, S. (1986). Depression in ethnic minorities. In *Transcultural psychiatry* (ed. J. Cox), pp. 107–38. Croom Helm, London.

Fernando, S. (1988). *Race and culture in psychiatry*. Croom Helm, London.

Hitch, P. J. (1975). *Migration and mental illness in a northern city.* University of Bradford Ph.D. Thesis.

Jagucki, W. (1983). The Polish experience: 40 years on. In *The psychosocial problems of refugees* (ed. R. Baker), pp. 32–8. British Refugee Council, London.

Lewis, P., Vadaddi, K. S., Rack, P. H. and Allen, J. J. (1980). Ethnic differences in drug response. *Postgraduate Medical Journal*, **56** (Suppl. 1), 46–9.

Malzberg, B. (1969). Are immigrants psychologically disturbed? In *Changing perspectives in mental illness* (ed. S. C. Ploy and R. E. Edgerton). Holt, Rinehart, and Winston, New York.

Merrill, J. (1988). Self-poisoning by Asians. *Update*, **37**, 931–4.

Merrill, J. and Owens, J. (1986). Ethnic differences in self-poisoning: a comparison of Asians and white groups. *British Journal of Psychiatry*, **148**, 708–12.

Murphy, H. B. M. (1973). The low rate of mental hospitalisation shown by immigrants to Canada. In *Uprooting and after*, (ed. C. A. Zwingmann, and M. Pfister-Ammende), Springer-Verlag, New York.

Murphy, H. B. M. (1977). Migration, culture and mental health. *Psychological Medicine*, **7**, 677–84.

Murphy, H. B. M. (1982). *Comparative psychiatry*. Springer-Verlag, New York.

Nicolson, C. (1974). *Strangers to England: immigration to England 1100–1952*. Wayland, London.

Ødegaard, O. (1932). Emigration and insanity. *Acta Psychiatrica Scandinavica*, Copenhagen, **Suppl. 4**.

Ødegaard, O. (1936). Emigration and mental health. *Mental Hygiene*, **20**, 546–53. Reprinted (1973) in: *Uprooting and after* (ed. C. Zwingmann and M. Pfisterammende). Springer-Verlag, New York.

Pollock, H. M. (1913). A statistical study of the foreign-born insane in New York state hospitals. *State Hospitals Bulletin*, (Special No.). **5**, 10–27.

Power, J., in Collaboration with Hardman, A. (1976, revised 1978). *Western Europe's migrant workers* (MRG report no. 28). Minority Rights Group, London.

Rack, P. H. (1982*a*). Migration and mental illness: a review of recent research in Britain. *Transcultural Psychiatry Research Review*, **XIX**(3), 151–72.

Rack, P. H. (1982*b*). *Race, culture and mental disorder*. Tavistock, London.

Rack, P. H. (1985). Migration and mental health: a matrix of variables. In *Psychiatry, the state of the art* (Proceedings of the 7th World Congress of Psychiatry at Vienna, 11–16 June 1983). *Vol. 8: History of Psychiatry, national schools, education and transcultural psychiatry*. Plenum, New York.

Rack, P. H. (1986). Migration and mental illness. In *Transcultural Psychiatry* (ed. J. Cox), pp. 59–75. Croom Helm, London.

Rack, P. H. (1987). Patients from other cultures. In *A handbook for trainee psychiatrists* (ed. K. J. B. Rix), pp. 197–206. Baillière Tindall, London.

Ranney, M. H. (1850). On insane foreigners. *American Journal of Insanity*, **7**, 53.

Rao, A. V. (1966). Depression: a psychiatric analysis of thirty cases. Indian Journal of Psychiatry, **8**(2), 143–54.

WHO (World Health Organization) (1972). *The international pilot study of schizophrenia*. WHO, Geneva.

Wilson, A. (1978). *Finding a voice: Asian women in Britain*. Virago, London.

Wilson, A. (1981). *Black people and the Health Service*. Brent Community Health Council, London.

18 Terminal care and bereavement

Dewi Rees

Introduction

Those caring for dying patients and their families need to understand the cultural and religious idiom of their patients. Within a stable society, with accepted customs and patterns of thought and language, this is relatively easy. In a multifaith and culturally mixed society it is more complex. Among Asians attitudes to death and bereavement vary with different religions, caste, and socio-economic backgrounds. But one attitude remains constant; this is the concept of the 'good death', epitomized by a voluntary and peaceful acceptance of death, for which spiritual preparation is important.

Death and dying

A distinction needs to be made between death and dying. Most people are apprehensive about dying, though less frequently of death, hoping that their distress may be eased or even prevented. Attitudes to death differ, but may be listed as an expectation that death is:

1. extinction; or
2. a gateway into a new life.

Between these two polarities other attitudes occur, commonly:

1. uncertainty regarding the nature of death;
2. feeling cheated by the premature onset of death, so that important aspects of one's life remain unfulfilled; or
3. a death-wish.

Of the two main polarities, Asians reject the finality of death; rather, they see it symbolically as a birth into a new life. Many will accept it as an aid to spiritual progress. For the Muslim or Christian Asian, this new state may be in paradise, purgatory, or hell. The Buddhist, Sikh, or Hindu will think in terms of reincarnation; seeing death as an aspects of *karma*, the universal moral law, and their approach to it as something which may enable them to wipe out past misdeeds and begin the next life with a clean slate.

Definition

Death transcends all cultures and ethnic boundaries, yet surprisingly few people have a clear understanding of when a person is terminally ill. A definition helps to clarify the uncertainties, and the definition I find helpful is this:

A person is terminally ill when, following correct diagnosis and appropriate treatment, the disease remains progressive, death is inevitable in the short term, and the practical need is for care not cure. And by *care* we mean good symptom-control, with support for the patient and his family.

Family support is seen here as an important aspect of preventive medicine, helping to reduce the increased morbidity and mortality known to be associated with bereavement. But sometimes family support can be destructive. This is apparent in the reverence Indian society shows to the *suttee*—the 'true wife'—who cradles her husband's head on her lap as his funeral pyre is lit, and thus joins him in death. The practice of suttee was abolished in 1829 by the Governor General, Lord William Bentinck, and the Indian penal-code still forbids it. But the practice continues sporadically, the most recent case occurring in September, 1987, in the Rajasthan village of Deorala.

Emphasis on *correct diagnosis* may seem pedantic in a situation where empathy and a caring attitude may seem more important than exact technological assessment. But misdiagnoses do occur; and people are not infrequently considered to be dying from cancer, who do not have cancer, and would recover if properly treated. Care in diagnosis is most important among Asians. They are more likely that the indigenous population to have diseases rarely encountered by British doctors, and this makes them especially likely to be the victims of fatal diagnostic errors.

The distress of dying

The distress of the dying patient has many causes, and these extend beyond the physical to the psyche. They include intellectual questionings, which may be introspective (why is this happening to me?) or outward-looking (what will happen to my children, when I am dead?). There may be emotional conflicts, housing problems, and family quarrels to be resolved. Financial problems are common, especially among low-income groups. Within all this there is a need for the patient to retain the spiritual orientation that gives meaning to his dying. For the immigrant Asian, these problems have to be resolved in an alien culture, with its own spiritual and moral poverty, that has been described as more difficult to bear than the material poverty of India. Pain, that common complaint of the dying person, can itself be multi-focal and have many causes. The factors involved in the perception of pain are shown in the following statement:

Of these the most important factor is the patient's psychological state. This is in dynamic relationship with people and the environment, so that changes in personal relationships and the environment can have important effects on

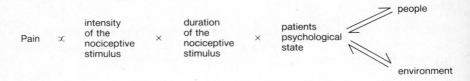

$$\text{Pain} \quad \propto \quad \begin{array}{c}\text{intensity}\\\text{of the}\\\text{nociceptive}\\\text{stimulus}\end{array} \quad \times \quad \begin{array}{c}\text{duration}\\\text{of the}\\\text{nociceptive}\\\text{stimulus}\end{array} \quad \times \quad \begin{array}{c}\text{patients}\\\text{psychological}\\\text{state}\end{array} \quad \begin{array}{c}\text{people}\\\\\text{environment}\end{array}$$

the pain experienced by a patient. Pain-thresholds are likely to be low if a patient feels unsupported and isolated in an alien environment. This seems to happen often with immigrant women who have not integrated into their new environment, and remain isolated in language and cultural identity. Among Muslim women, in particular, there can be a poor integration with the host community; and this has been suggested as a possible cause for the high incidence of early death from breast cancer reported among immigrant Muslim women.

The same general principle applies to other causes of distress, as is shown in the following statement:

$$\begin{array}{c}\text{The distress}\\\text{of dying}\end{array} \quad \propto \quad \begin{array}{c}\text{type}\\\text{of}\\\text{symptoms}\end{array} \quad \times \quad \begin{array}{c}\text{number}\\\text{of}\\\text{symptoms}\end{array} \quad \times \quad \text{duration} \quad \times \quad \text{intensity} \quad \times \quad \begin{array}{c}\text{people}\\\text{patient's}\\\text{psychological}\\\text{state}\\\text{environment}\end{array}$$

Some of the most important causes of distress for the dying patient and his family are listed in Table 18.1. It will be seen that the emotional distresses include most of the Stages of Dying listed by Kübler-Ross (1970), viz. denial, anger, bargaining, depression, and acceptance.

Communication

Good communication is essential for the proper assessment of a patient's needs. Diagnosis precedes therapy, and treatment based on an inadequate case-history will not be effective. Important symptoms will be missed if not stated, and socio-economic problems that could be resolved, overlooked.

Next to pain, poor communication is the most important cause of distress to the dying patient. Poor communication is often the result of haste; of being focused on the next patient or visit, instead of the present problem. Good communication starts with sitting down and slowing down, to create a time-space where the patient's areas of concern can be expressed and dealt with. Open-ended

Table 18.1 *Sources of potential distress for the dying person and his family*

physical	emotional	mental
pain	denial	poor communication
weakness	anger	dementia
loss of taste	depression	stupor/coma
dyspnoea	fear	
dysphagia		
anorexia		
vomiting		
incontinence		
sweats		

questions may enable these areas to be explored more fully, the aim being to enable the patient to have access to the basic information he desires for his decision taking. Such queries as 'have you all the information you require?', 'is there anything else we need to talk about?', 'what have the hospital doctors told you about your illness?' can reveal important uncertainties that need to be discussed.

For people dying in a foreign land and an alien culture, the situation is more difficult. With a high proportion of immigrant Asians unable to converse in English and illiterate in their own language, the problems become more complex. This deficiency in linguistic skills is most prevalent in women and elderly Asians. Among Muslims, the tradition that the family head acts as spokesman for the patient makes the situation even more complex, especially if neither is fluent in English. The presence of an interpreter then becomes a basic requirement for an adequate patient–doctor dialogue. Often a younger member of the family will undertake this role, but occasionally an outsider is needed. The domiciliary assessment of a terminally ill Asian woman is likely to be conducted in the presence of her husband as family head, with a teenage daughter as interpreter; and other members of the family may also be present. The scenario may seem crowded, but it is within the cultural pattern; and the patient is less socially isolated than she would be in an in-patient unit.

Management

The management of physical distress is well described in textbooks on terminal care. This care does not vary greatly with ethnicity, though Muslim patients should not be given medications containing alcohol or pork. In terminal care betadine is frequently used as a dressing for fungating growths. This is an alcohol solution, and should not be used for Muslim patients. The same restriction applies to surgical spirit, which contains 70 per cent alcohol. Pork insulins and beef insulins are taboo for Muslim and Hindu patients respectively, although decisions on the appropriateness of an insulin will usually have been taken before the patient becomes terminally ill. Dietary taboos must be observed, though most religions allow some relaxation of dietary laws for the terminally ill. Thus the Muslim patient may be allowed to take life-maintaining fluids and medicines during Ramadan. Immigrant Asians are commonly low-income groups, and often need financial help. Care should be taken to ensure that they receive all the appropriate benefits for the sick that are available from the state and charitable sources. In this area, a consultation with a social worker is often helpful.

Deaths in the Asian population

The size and demography of the Asian population in Britain is described in Chapter 6. It is relevant here to restate the extent of mortality. In 1984, of the 566 881 deaths registered in England and Wales, 4279 were of persons born in the Indian subcontinent.

The mortality rate among immigrants from the Indian subcontinent is less than among the indigenous population, but is steadily rising; the increase being roughly two-fold between 1971 (0.45 per cent of all deaths) and 1984 (0.75 per cent of all deaths) (OPCS 1985).

These figures may underestimate the true mortality among Asian immigrants, because some return to their country of birth to die when terminally ill (Jain *et al.* 1985).

Use of medical and social services

Proper use of medical and social services is essential for good terminal care. Possible failures by primary-care teams to meet the needs of Asian patients are more likely to be inherent in the difficulties of British general practice than peculiar to Asian patients. These broad assertions are generally true for terminal care. Asian patients show no apparent reluctance to use hospice services, domiciliary or in-patient, or to accept the wide range of palliative care and pain-relief available (Rees 1986). But terminal care has a broader spectrum than physical palliative care. Social and community care are equally important. There is some evidence that Asians receive less community services (home helps, meals on wheels, chiropody, social workers) than the indigenous population.

Place of death

In India and Pakistan dying patients are likely to be taken home from hospital by their relatives. This reflects the predominant desire within the family for a death to occur at home, where the patient can be comforted by his family, and the appropriate sacred readings, prayers, and rites undertaken.

Traditionally, it is important for devout Hindus to die on the floor with the head to the north. Various reasons are given for this, the most common being the need to be close to Mother Earth. Also some believe that the body should be free from physical constraints or boundaries, and in alignment with the North–South magnetic currents of the Earth. At the moment of death, sacred *tulsi* leaf and *Gangajal* (Ganges water) should be placed in the person's mouth, and, if this has not already been done, the body should be placed on the floor, and a *diva* lit to illuminate the way for the soul. For the Muslim patient it is different. At the moment of death, the Muslim should be facing Mecca, either sitting or lying with his face turned towards the sacred city. Position at death is not important to the Sikh or Buddhist.

Presence of a religious leader

When a Muslim or Sikh is dying the presence of a religious leader is not necessary. It is essential when the patient is a Buddhist, and the priest should be of the same Buddhist sect, if this is possible. A Hindu family may ask a priest to visit, if one is available. The visit of a guru or holy man to a dying Hindu is considered particularly helpful and auspicious.

Alternative healers

People who know they have incurable illness will sometimes seek help from unorthodox medical practitioners of the kind described in Chapter 7. This may involve the use of homoeopathic or naturopathic drugs, treatment by healers, colour therapy, and visits to holy shrines or to unusual cancer-cure centres.

One would expect similar patterns to be present among Asians, especially since Indian cultures have their own traditional medical practices. Although little has been written on this aspect of terminal care, Asians in the United Kingdom do not appear to use unorthodox practitioners more than the indigenous population. About 6 per cent of elderly Asians consult an alternative healer each year, whereas over 90 per cent will visit their general practitioner (Blakemore 1982). Terminal patients who emigrated from the Indian subcontinent sometimes return home to seek a cure, though in my experience without success. If alternative healers are used, it is sensible to accept their involvement. Their intention is usually good, though with a terminal illness, the success rate is not likely to be high. In Pakistan, faith-healers are seen by many people as the main source of health care. Attempts by doctors to discredit them have usually met with hostility from the people. The Psychiatry Department of Rawalpindi Medical College has adopted a system of integrating faith-healers into the primary mental-health-care team. The response has been excellent, many faith-healers being keen to be part of the team (Mason 1987). Problems do arise with faith-healers when the expectation of cure is raised too high. This occurred with a seventeen year old Sikh patient of mine, but was resolved by the healer when she informed the family that her promise to cure could not be achieved. Thereafter, she provided good support for the family, though their grief was intense when the youth died.

Place of death

It has been said of the English that 70 per cent of terminally ill patients prefer to die at home, but that 70 per cent of their relatives prefer the death to occur in hospital. This slightly ironic statement could not be said of Asians. Among them, patients and relatives still prefer death to occur at home, where the traditional customs can be maintained and family rites can be observed. In India dying patients are often removed from hospital by their relatives. In Pakistan, a colleague found few deaths occurred in the mission hospital where he worked, mainly because relatives would take the dying patient home, even though the distance might be great. Hospital was a place in which to be cured, not to die.

But people are pragmatic, and if socio-economic conditions make home-care impracticable Asians will request hospital or hospice admissions. Hospice admission was in fact requested by the husband of the first Hindu patient I attended. She was a thirty-seven year old woman, the mother of three young children; and, in common with many Asian immigrants, she could not speak English. She was bed-fast with non-Hodgkins lymphoma, and needed considerable nursing care. The family could not provide the husband with adequate support, and realizing that he could not care for his wife and children while continuing to work, he asked for admission. The patient was admitted to a hospice, and died eight weeks later. None of the customary rites were observed or requested at her death; but later the family expressed gratitude for 'the great and marvellous treatment provided'.

In contrast, the family of a fifty-one year old Muslim, with terminal hypernephroma, asked the hospital to discharge him home, where they could care for him. For the three weeks before he died, he was rarely alone, his companions being mainly men, though his wife was sometimes present. Nursing support was provided by the district nurse and hospice domiciliary care team. With the agreement of the family, continence was maintained with a self-retaining catheter, and pain-relief ensured with parenteral buprenorphine. When needed, the eldest son acted as interpreter and spokesman, but referred decision-making to an uncle. The patient died peacefully in the early hours of the morning, surrounded by male members of the family, all at the time asleep. Later his body was flown to Pakistan for burial.

Going home (to die)

Not all terminally ill Asians wish to die in this country. Some choose to return to the land of their birth. The number who do so is not known, but 8 per cent of those seen by me returned to their homeland when they realized the seriousness of their illness. Others would have done so if they had known the poor prognosis while still fit to travel. Some return to die. Others do so in the hope that in their native land a cure may be attained. Some, having gone home, return again to this country for final care.

The decision to 'return home' is usually taken only after the diagnosis and prognosis have been fully discussed and accepted. It can be costly; also important family and financial decisions may have to be taken quickly. Capital assets may need to be sold and money raised to pay for air travel. This occurred with a fifty-five year old Muslim with terminal lung cancer. He was hoping to be cured, but was informed of his poor prognosis to ensure he made realistic arrangements for his wife and children, who were recent arrivals in England and did not speak the language. Also his wife had been ill for many years, and was not capable of caring for the children. After sadly accepting the prognosis, he decided to return to Bangladesh. With advice from the social worker and elders of his mosque, he accepted loans from business friends to pay for air travel. Arrangements were made for his house (mortgaged) to be sold, and for the High Commissioner to oversee his finances in England. Within three weeks of accepting the prognosis, he had returned to Bangladesh with his family.

Among the terminally ill patients leaving this country, some will be taking opiates and other Schedule 2 drugs. If they need to take these drugs out of the UK then an appropriate licence should be obtained from the Home Office Drugs Board. Also, to ensure that no problems occur with the immigration authorities, prior consultation with the appropriate embassy or consulate is advisable.

Airlines expect to be informed when seat-reservations are made for seriously ill passengers who intend to use their flights. A Medical Certificate of Fitness for Air Travel is required from the passenger's doctor. The willingness of the airline to accept a terminally ill passenger depends on the information provided to their medical officer on this certificate. Airlines try very hard to accommodate terminally ill patients when there are strong compassionate reasons, but will not accept those who are moribund, and likely to die in flight. In general they will accept terminally ill patients, provided:

1. The flight will not make the patient worse.
2. They will not annoy or inconvenience other passengers.
3. They are not likely to cause an unscheduled diversion or delay.

The main in-flight hazards are caused by:

1. A fall in oxygen pressure, which may exacerbate hypoxia in patients with:
   (a) decompensated cardiac problems;
   (b) severe anaemia;
   (c) extensive lung disease; or
   (d) circulatory problems.
2. An expansion of gases within the body cavity of 30 per cent at 6000 feet. This is clinically important if the patient:

(a) has had recent abdominal surgery; or

(b) has a pneumothorax (British Airways Medical Services, no date).

Last words

The last throughts and words of the Asian patient are considered important for his future well-being. The devout Hindu will wish to die with the name of God on his lips and in his heart. If he cannot chant '*Ram, Ram*' himself, his relatives will do so for him, or will repeat '*Om*' or the *Gayatri Mantra*, or read chapter fifteen of the *Bhagvat Gita* or some other holy book.

The devout Sikh will be comforted by readings from the *Guru Granth Sahab*. Members of a Muslim family will recite readings from the Holy Quran in the presence of a dying relative, and will repeat with him the *Kalima*, the Muslim declaration of faith, 'there is no God but God, and Muhammad is His prophet'. These are among the first words that many Muslims hear, and the last he should utter.

Touching the body

If there is doubt about the propriety of touching the corpse, the family should be consulted first. Sikhs do not usually mind non-Sikhs touching the body, and Hindus are unlikely to object. Muslims are likely to be more particular. The body of a Muslim is considered to belong to God, and preferably should not be touched by non-Muslims. If a non-Muslim needs to touch the body, then disposable gloves should be worn.

Organ transplants

Amongst Hindus and Sikhs, there is no religious prohibition against organ transplants. Strict Muslims are likely to be against organ transplantation, though some may consider it acceptable.

Post-mortems

Amongst Hindus and Sikhs, there is no religious prohibition against post-mortem examinations. In Islam, post-mortem examinations are forbidden unless absolutely necessary for medico-legal reasons.

Burial and cremation

The prophet Muhammad said 'visit the graves, for surely visiting the graves lessens worldly loves and reminds you of the hereafter'. Burial is mandatory for Muslims. This should be done as soon after death as possible. In Eastern countries the body, enclosed in a simple shroud, which differs for men and women, is placed directly into the soil. The earth above the grave is then slightly raised, but otherwise the grave is unmarked. When a Muslim is buried in the United Kingdom, local by-laws are followed, and the corpse is placed in a coffin before burial. Recently, however, some local authorities have provided special areas in cemeteries which allow traditional Muslim burials. The Sikh attitude to the disposal of the body was expressed by the Guru Nanak, who said 'whether you burn the dead body in the sandalwood or throw it into the filth is immaterial'. Cremation is customary among Sikhs, the eldest son being expected to light the pyre or, in a crematorium, consign the coffin into the furnace. The ashes of the Sikh dead are scattered only on running water. In the Punjab the River Sutlej at Anandpur is often used. In the United Kingdom problems occur because of Government restrictions. Permission is required from the Ministry of Agriculture and Fisheries for the dispersal of cremated ashes on any stretch of water in England and Wales. The restrictions are tight, and the only water allowed for the dispersal of ashes is the tidal water of the River Severn, below Gloucester.

The disposal customs of the Hindus are similar to those of the Sikhs. Cremation is customary, though bodies of young children who have not fulfilled their time on earth are buried. Cremation is arranged as soon after death as possible, and in India often occurs within a few hours of death. Sometimes ashes are taken back to India to be scattered at a sacred or significant site, often the River Ganges or Brahmaputra. A friend who returned to Indian with the ashes of her husband scattered them at four separate sites, making it a pilgrimage for herself and her children.

The Sikh

After death the corpse is washed and dressed in normal clothes. The devout Sikh is buried with the five Ks, the visual symbols of Sikhism.

Friends and relatives visit the family, and accompany the body to the crematorium as a sacred duty. Before cremation, the body may be viewed by visitors, who may also express their grief with tears and lamentations. The clothed corpse, wrapped in a shroud and placed in a coffin, is taken to the *gurdwara* (temple) where prayers are said. At the cremation further prayers are spoken and a verse from the evening hymn, the *Kirlan Sohila*, is chanted as the body is consumed by the fire. Following the cremation the mourners, after washing their hands and faces, reassemble in the *gurdwara*, where a verse is recited from scripture, reminding the people that the gurus preached against wailing and crying at funerals. On returning home, a widow is bathed by her immediate family, and then taken outside for a walk, so as not to become obsessed with the dead. On the first day of death, friends bring food to the family. Subsequently and in the name of the deceased, the family provides all the food for visitors during the prescribed ten to thirteen days of mourning that follow. On the occasion I was enabled to visit a bereaved Sikh family, I found the deceased's bedroom had been cleared and turned into a prayer-room. Almost everything had been removed, including the pictures of the ten gurus—only the carpet had been retained. A covered dais (*manji*) surmounted by a canopy (*palki*p had been established in the room. Cushions were arranged on the *manji*, and on these were placed the *Guru Granth Sahab* (the holy book of the Sikhs), thus converting the prayer-room into a *gurdwara*. Those entering did so shoeless; with heads covered they knelt before the *Guru Granth Sahab* and placed money at the base of the *manji*, as a contribution to the communal food and to the poor. Then they took their places on the floor with the other sitters. The room had been prepared for an *akhand pat*: this is a complete reading of the *Guru Granth Sahab* during the ten to thirteen days of mourning. Not all Sikhs understand the *Gurmukhi* (Sikh alphabet), in which their holy book is written; but all friends will attempt to be present for at least part of the *akhand pat*. Sikhs, having no priests, use initiated elders to lead prayers and read from the Holy Scriptures in the *gurdwara*. Sometimes, as on this occasion, the reader (*granthi*) is able to read the *Gurmukhi* script, but does not understand it. On the final day of the *akhand pat* the family reassembles for the last reading. This is followed by a distribution of *Prashaad* (Sikh holy food), a hot semolina-based sweet blessed with the prayer of Guru Gobind Singh. If the family head has died a turban is now placed on the head of the eldest son, to indicate that he assumes the role of family head. Finally, the family provide all the mourners with a community meal (*langar*). The *Guru Granth Sahab, manji* and *palki* are removed from the prayer room; but a light may be kept in the room for some weeks, as a further act of remembrance of the deceased.

Muslims

The body of a Muslim belongs to God, and should not be touched by a non-Muslim. Although this precept must be observed, in practice one finds that Muslims may prefer the body to be laid out by nurses when a patient dies in a hospital or hospice. Determining the wishes of the family is essential before any action is taken. Also, disposable gloves should be worn if a non-Muslim needs to touch the corpse.

When a man dies, the body is washed by his father, son, or brother. In their absence, the duty may be performed by any male Muslim. When a woman dies, the body is washed by her mother, daughter, or sister. The eyes are closed and a piece of religiously pure material tied around the head and chin to close the mouth. Similar material is used to tie the feet and cover the body. The face is turned towards the *Kaaba* (most sacred place of Muslims in Mecca). During these offices prayers are said. The shroud must be of poor cloth, and will differ for men and women. Burial must take place as soon after death as possible, friends and relatives having been informed of the death. Flowers are not normally sent to a Muslim funeral, and there is no recognized colour for mourning. Women do not accompany men in the funeral procession to the grave-side, where prayers will be said and there will be readings from the Holy Quran. The earth above the grave will be slightly raised, but otherwise the grave will be unmarked.

By tradition, the family stay indoors for three days after the funeral. Relatives and friends will visit to provide companionship, prepare food, and do whatever tasks are necessary. Because the dead are expected to meet God, and hopefully find eternal peace, prolonged grieving is discouraged and considered wrong. But traditional patterns of mourning are expected to be followed. When a man dies, his widow is expected to remain in her own home for 130 days, and during this time she must not wear jewellery, bright clothes, or cosmetics. If the widow is pregnant, this restricted period lasts only until the child is born. If the widow is the sole bread-winner, she is allowed to go to work during the day, but must return to her house at night.

Hindus

After death, the corpse is washed and dressed in normal clothes. The body is placed in a coffin and taken to the crematorium, where cremation is performed as soon as possible, without, of necessity, waiting for family members to be present. Among Hindus the cremation and mourning customs vary with caste and locality. As with other religions, the auspicious rituals are concerned with the soul and not the corpse. Beliefs about the ultimate fate of the soul are dependent, within the laws of *karma*, upon immediate cremation and performance of the correct rituals, preferably by an appropriate priest. Outside India family mourning practices are not always known, and a suitable priest may not be available. Consequently, some of the important ceremonies are now being performed by proxy in India, without the immediate mourners being present.

In most cases, 'pollution' lasts ten to sixteen days, during which various prohibitions are observed, such as not shaving, not sleeping on the floor, not eating sweet food, and not offering food to guests. During this period, the ghost or *bhut pret* is thought to be wandering around. It may wish to cling to family members, and for this reason it is necessary to provide food, in the form of pinda and water, to enable it to form a new body. At the *sappinidkarma* ceremony that follows, the *bhut pret* is enabled to merge with the *pitrs*, or ancestors, and attain release to the place of the fathers.

At the ceremony I attended, following the death of a young wife, we were greeted at the door by a young man with the words 'you are welcome', and then, after removing our shoes in an anteroom, were admitted to the house. We joined some fifteen people sitting on the floor against the walls of the living room. The atmosphere was quiet, bright, and cheerful. Children walked freely without restriction. The fireplace had been made into a small shrine, with a garlanded photograph of the deceased, flanked by burning sticks of incense and surrounded by small grains of rice. Two men sat in the centre of the room behind a large metal bowl containing water. Symbolically, this was the river Ganges, where the ritual was being enacted. Beside the priest sat the widower's eldest brother, who, as family head, acted for the family. The drama of the rite was a trilogy between the priest, the family head, and the shrine, which represented the spirit or shadow of the deceased. The priest maintained a rhythmic chant, with changes of tone and pauses, which the brother answered with appropriate responses. At times, the priest cast water from the bowl and rice into the shrine. There was no reading from books. The ceremony proceeded rapidly in an Indian dialect, and one could not assess whether there was a strict adherence to a fixed liturgy or if spontaneous variations were introduced. Nevertheless, it was a moving experience.

After the rites of purification are completed, the priest lights the sacred fire and prays for the peace of the departed soul. Family mourning now ceases, except for the spouse and sons, who observe mourning for twelve months. Finally, the ritual is repeated every year on the deceased's anniversary.

Final journey

Some Asians return home to die. The corpses or ashes of others are sent back for burial or dispersal. This final return is indicative of the deep attachment people retain for the land of their birth, a *'hiriaeth'* (longing for) that Asians share with emigrants of other races. Corpses transported to the Indian subcontinent for burial are mostly Muslim, destined for Bangladesh or, more frequently, Pakistan. Their transportation is controlled by the regulations applicable for each sovereign state. The first requirement in the UK is that a certificate is issued by the coroner, authorizing removal of the body out of the country.

India requires:

1. the body to have been embalmed, hermetically sealed, and soldered in a zinc coffin, which is then enclosed in a wooden casket; and
2. the death, embalmment, and coroner's certificates to accompany the body.

Pakistan requires:

1. a certificate from the embarking authority confirming that the coffin has been inspected, is hermetically sealed, and is packed suitably for transport;
2. a certificate from the Community Physician stating that there is no infectious or contagious disease in the area; and
3. the passport and death certificate of the deceased.

The transportation of a corpse to another country is expensive. The cost by air freight depends on the weight and distance to be transported. For transportation by air to Karachi, there is a standing charge plus a *pro rata* rate per kilo. To the cost of air freight must be added undertaker's fees, the cost of the coffin, and, if undertaken, the cost of embalmment. If a relative accompanies the coffin, which is usual, there is increased cost, especially if the relative loses time from work.

There is no restriction on the transportation of ashes by air. The ashes of a cremated adult weigh approximately 15–17 kilos. Airlines will usually charge three times the normal cargo rate for their transportation.

Conclusion

The two most crucial events in life are birth and death. They are the least understood also, in terms of their meaning and ultimate significance. Every culture and race has sought to interpret these events, and embody their under-standing in philosophies and doctrines. Even in Western psychiatry the pattern is recurring, with Professor Carl Jung stating that, after the age of forty-five, the main concern of man's psyche is a preparation for death. With few exceptions, all races have given meaning to death in terms of a spiritual rebirth, seeing death as a gateway into a new life. This applies for the most ancient of religions— Hinduism—and the more recent, Islam (AD 622) and Sikhism (about AD 1500). Buddhism, which is based on the concept that life is a wheel of misfortune, provides in the *Bardo Thodol* (1957) (The Tibetan Book of the Dead) exact instructions for the dying person, that will enable the liberated soul to escape the misfortune of reincarnation. It is within these complexities of cultural ex-perience and interpretation that the British general practitioner has to work in his care of the dying Asian patient. He does so with his own legacy of the meaning of death severely weakened by the events of the past century. Most of western man's mourning customs—society's method of supporting the ber-eaved—have disappeared, and, for many, Christianity has been replaced by a philosophy of nihilism. Out of this lack, new forms of support for the bereaved are being developed, and a more positive approach to the mystery of death will evolve. But for the Asian, the same current of change will occur, and his children will be tested in their adherence to traditional attitudes to death and dying. In dealing with dying Asian patients, general practitioners will need to be aware of these future changes, and the added distress they will cause to the patient and his family.

Postscript on relevant literature

Among the first books dealing with the needs of Asian patients was the series written by Henley (1982, 1983*a*, 1983*b*). This was followed by publications by the Hospital Chaplaincies Council (1983) and Neuberger (1987). These books were written principally for health workers, hospital chaplains, and nurses.

They are simple, factual reports dealing with various aspects of care, but include important statements on the needs of dying patients. Written many centuries before these was the classic Mahayana Buddhist text, the *Bardo Thodol*, the Tibetan Book of the Dead.

There is now a growing and substantial literature on terminal care, but none deals specifically with the needs of Asian patients. The available textbooks have been written by Western authors—often hospice physicians with a primary interest in cancer care. Of these, I found the works of Twycross and Lack (1983, 1986) the most useful, though the writing of Kübler-Ross (1970) is more widely known. The standard work on bereavement is also by an English author, C. M. Parkes (1986).

Finally, the British Airways Medical Service provides a pamphlet free of charge to doctors on the transportation of seriously ill patients, including the terminally ill.

Acknowledgments

I was greatly helped by private communications from Shirley Firth on Hindu and Sikh Approaches to Death, and by Mr A. B. Taylor on the transportation of corpses and ashes.

References

Bardo Thodol, The Tibetan Book of the Dead (3rd Edn). (1957). Ed. Evan-Wentz. Oxford University Press, New York.

Blakemore, K. (1982). Health and illness among the elderly of minority ethnic groups living in Birmingham; some new findings. *Health Trends*, **14**, 69–72.

British Airways Medical Services (no date). *Your patient and air travel: a guide for doctors*. British Airways Medical Service, Queen's Building, (N121), Heathrow Airport (London), Hounslow, Middlesex.

Henley, A. (1982). *Asians in Britain: caring for Muslims and their families: religious aspects of care*. National Extension College, Cambridge.

Henley, A. (1983*a*). *Asian in Britain: caring for Sikhs and their families: religious aspects of care*. National Extension College, Cambridge.

Henley, A. (1983*b*). *Asian in Britain: caring for Hindus and their families: religious aspects of care*. National Extension College, Cambridge.

Hospital Chaplaincies Council (1983). *Our ministry and other faiths*. CIO Publishing, London.

Jain, D., Narayan, N., Narayan, K., Pike, L. A., Clarkson, M. E., Cox, I. G. and Chatterjee, J. (1985). Attitudes of Asian patients in Birmingham to general practitioner services. *Journal of the Royal College of General Practitioners*, **35**, 416–18.

Kübler-Ross, E. (1970). *On death and dying*. Tavistock Publications, London.

Mason, P. (1987). Faith healers in the mental health team. *The Lancet*, **ii**, 1029.

Neuberger, J. (1987). *Caring for dying people of different faiths*. Asten Cornish Publishers, London.

OPCS (Office of Population Censuses and Surveys) (1985). Deaths by birthplace of deceased 1984. *OPCS Minitor.* **DH1 85/2**. OPCS, London.

Parkes, C. M. (1986). *Bereavement. Studies of grief in adult life*, 2nd edn. Penguin, Harmondsworth.

Rees, W. D. (1986). Immigrants and the hospice. *Health Trends*, **18**, 89–91.

Twycross, R. G. and Lack, S. A. (1983). *Symptom control in far advanced cancer: pain relief.* Pitman Medical, London.

Twycross, R. G. and Lack, S. A. (1986). *Control of alimentary symptoms in far advanced cancer.* Churchill Livingstone, New York.

Index

abortion 153–4
acetylation, of drugs 142
acrocyanosis 276
adaptation to UK, difficulties 216–17
addresses and information
  alternative/complementary medicine 116
  Asian women's groups 191
  infectious diseases 270–1
  perinatal mortality 236
  pregnancy and congenital abnormalities 190
  self-help, voluntary, and support
      groups 168–9
  useful information services 39, 170–1
  vegans and vegetarians 129
  women's health 168–9, 171
adolescence 217, 284
  rickets 232, 234
advocacy schemes and advocates 67–8, 210
Afro-Caribbeans 50, 135, 162, 293
age
  Asian doctors 43
  fluency in English 63
  -structure of Asian population 76, 78, 87
airlines, terminally ill and 310
alcohol 119–120
  in medications, restrictions on 120, 274,
      307
alcohol-related disease 141–2
allergy, foods causing 122
allopathy 106
alopecia 279–81
  androgenic 280
  traction 280
alopecia areata 279–80
alphabets 8
alpha-feto-protein 178, 184, 205
alternative/complementary medicine 33, 93–
      116
  bizarre symptoms with 233–4, 301
  contraception 151–2
  elderly Asians, use of 247
  historical perspectives 93–4
  medical problems related to 142–3
  psychological and psychiatric disorders 297
  reasons for choice of 94–5
  skin disease 274
  terminally ill 309–10
  therapies available 95; see also individual
      therapies
amniocentesis 178, 205

amoebiasis 228–9
amoebic hepatitis 229
anaemia 121, 125–6, 139–40
  diagnosis in children 215
  haemolytic 140–1, 224
  hepatosplenomegaly with 233
  iron-deficiency, see iron-deficiency anaemia
  in pregnancy 179
  in vegetarians 121, 125–6, 139, 179, 219,
      231
anencephaly 203
antenatal clinic 176–7, 202
  timing of initial care 176–8
antenatal complications 179–81
antenatal period 218–20
'anticipatory learning' 97
antihistamines 282, 287
anxiety 112, 216, 294–5
aortic arch syndrome 145
appointment systems 37, 60
aromatherapy 95–6
artefacts and adornments, causing skin
      disease 279, 283–4
artificial feeding, infants 158, 211, 222
Asian population 3–7, 72–6, 194–5, 291
  births and perinatal deaths 76–83, 184–185
      see also perinatal mortality
  census data 72–3
  disease patterns 83–7
  distribution 5, 76–7
  elderly 14, 239
  fertility rates 79–80
  origins 4–7
  size and structure 74–6, 87
  by year of entry into UK 76, 79
  see also culture; migration
ASRA (Asian Sheltered Residential
      Accommodation) 246
asthma 99, 138
astrotherapy 97
atopic eczema 280–2, 286–7
autosomal recessive disorders 195, 223
Ayurvedic medicine 98–9, 116, 247, 300

baby milks 158, 222
  composition 213
  religious restrictions 121, 125, 212
Bangladeshi 4–5, 223
  age-structure 76, 78

population data   74–6
  year of entry into UK   76, 79
BCG vaccine   222, 253
beliefs, delusion and   296
Bengalis   5, 7, 63
  birthweights of   182
bereavement   212–14, 304–19
  perinatal death   188
  see also death and dying
beta-thalassaemia, *see* thalassaemia
betel nut   137
bhatura   118
births   76–82, 87
  registration   76–7
  of son   153
birthweights   182, 220
  perinatal mortality and   82–3, 220
blood pressure, measurement   132, 134
'body-ache'   294
bone diseases   124–5
bottle-feeding   158, 211, 222
breast cancer   137, 156–7
breast-feeding   125, 158, 187, 220, 222
  hepatitis B transmission   269
breast-screening   137–8
Buddhism   317–18
burials   214, 312–13, 315

Caesarean section   183–4, 186
calciferol   146, 180, 232
calcium absorption, impairment   124–5
cancer   136–8, 155–7
  incidence, Asians vs. non-Asians   85–6, 88,
    136–7, 155
cardiotocography (CTG)   181, 183
care, delivery of   35–8
career paths
  Asian doctors   43–5
  Asian nurses   52–3
carers, women as   159–62, 174
Caribbean, migration from   7
caste system   9
catering, for Asian patients   123–4
census data   72–3
cerebral malaria   234, 254
cervical cancer   136, 155–6
cervical cytology   136, 150, 155–6, 164
chain migration   5
chapati   118, 123–5
chaperons   36, 38
chest pain   131, 133
chilblains   276
child abuse   217–18
child rearing   157–9
children
  acquired diseases   225–30
  adaptation to UK, difficulties   217

atopic eczema   281, 286–7
clinical examination   215–16
clinical problems   216–18
consultations   214–16
cultural attitudes to illnesses in   211–14
diagnostic problems   233–4
diseases of uncertain aetiology   232–3
emotional and psychological disorders   216,
  290
growth patterns   210
hereditary disorders, *see* hereditary
    disorders
importance of   211
infectious diseases   225–30, 261–8
nutritional disorders   124–5, 211, 231–2
skin diseases   283–5
chloasma   277
chloramphenicol   257
chloroquine   255
chorionic villus sampling (CVS)   176, 178,
  184, 201
chromosomal abnormalities   178, 193, 220,
  225
cigarette smoking   122, 132–3
circumcision   222
clairvoyants   100
clinical examination, children   215
colostrum   158, 220
Commission for Racial Equality   47, 51, 170
communication   57–71, 172
  cause of distress for dying patient   306–7
  in consultations   64–5, 172, 214
  cross-cultural   57–9
  difficulties   57–8, 61, 172, 277
    after perinatal death   188, 214
  elderly Asians   241–3
  fluency and literacy   62–3, 150, 172, 241–3,
    307
  in general practice   35
  in genetic counselling   200, 206–7
  greetings and social conventions   62
  hysteria and hysterical behaviour   298
  modes of   60–1
  in pregnancy   172, 176
  in psychotherapy, importance   301
  skin diseases and   277
  as source of dissatisfaction   57, 94
  verbal and non-verbal   61
  ways to improve   63–9, 172–3
  see also culture; interpreters; language
compliance, poor, reasons for   99, 120, 133,
    135, 138
confidentiality   65, 299
congenital abnormalities   192, 220, 225
  risk of   197–9
  screening   175, 178–9, 184
congenital infections   268–9
congenital rubella syndrome   261–2

consanguineous marriage 194–200, 208, 220, 223–4
  attitudes to 207
  influence on pattern of disease 196, 208, 223, 225
constipation 101
consultations 214–16
contraception 150–3, 187
  methods 105, 151–2
contraceptive pill 105, 151
coronary angiography 131–2
coronary heart disease 131–3
  risk factors 132–3, 142
cosmetics, harmful 142, 215–16, 283–4
counselling 97, 160
  before, and in pregnancy 175
  bereaved parents 188, 214
  genetic disorders, *see* genetic counselling
cows' milk 125, 144, 222
'creeping eruption' 276
cremation 212–13, 312–13, 315
Crohn's disease 144
cultural bereavement 23–6
cultural factors in health and illness 17–27, 58–9
cultural stereotypes, avoidance 3, 22, 59, 237
culture 15, 59
  Asian, teaching to medical students 211
  Asian nursing recruits and 52–3
  attitudes,
    to handicaps 160
    to illness 211–14, 240, 247
    to sex 154, 295
  beliefs,
    as form of 'victim-blaming' 23, 25
    mental illness diagnosis and 296–7
  caring for elderly and 161, 237
  clash 19–20, 22, 26
  concepts of 17–19, 23
  conflict between generations 217, 298
  contraceptive methods and 151, 153
  diet and, *see* diet
  differences, barrier to successful
    communication 58–9, 94, 274
  of doctor 19, 22
  doctor's attitudes to, patient relationship 19, 22, 58–9, 94
  generalizations and lack of homogeneity 22, 25, 59, 194, 240–1
  of 'host' community, considerations 21–2
  inequalities of health and 21
  language appropriateness 61
  misuse of concept 20–5
  overemphasis on, in behaviour and symptomatology 23, 58
  as process of change (not static) 15, 22–3
  skin diseases and 273–5

socio-economic factors influencing 21–3
sub-cultures 19–23
women's role and behaviour 14–15, 150, 163
cutaneous larva migrans 276
cyanosis 215

dairy products, clarified 133
dandruff 280
death and dying 212–14, 304–13
  attitudes to 212, 304
  causes of 85–6
  distress of, causes 305–7
  final journey 316–17
  going home for 310–11
  last words 312
  place of 308–10
  registration, and mortality rates 85, 156, 308
  touching the body 213–14, 312, 314
  see also terminal care
depigmentation disorders 276, 278–9
  chemical-induced 279
depression 58, 294–5
deputizing services, Asians in 45, 48
dermatitis artefacta (DA) 283
dhat syndrome 154, 295
diabetes mellitus 130, 133–5
  in pregnancy 175, 181
  prolonged hypoglycaemia in 127, 143
diarrhoea, infective 227–9
diet 117–29
  in alternative medicine 102, 105
  cultural aspects 122–4
  in diabetes mellitus 135
  diseases linked 124–6
  medical emergencies and 126–7
  in pregnancy 174–5, 219–20
  restrictions, religious 118–22, 212, 307–8
  staple, regional differences 117
dietary history 128
diphtheria 263
diphtheria and tetanus (DT) vaccine 264, 266
diphtheria, tetanus, and pertussis (DTP)
    vaccine 263–6
discrimination 21, 24, 54, 292, 295
  Asian doctors 43, 45, 47–9, 54
  Asian medical students 46–7
  Asian nurses 50, 53–4
  elderly Asians 237
  UK trained Asian doctors 46
disease
  dietary factors 124–6
  ethnic patterns 83–7, 130
  hereditary, *see* hereditary disorders
  illness vs., concepts of relationship 20, 94

doctors, Asian, in NHS   40–9, 130, 173
  adaptation in practice, for Asian patients   47
  age and geographical distribution   43
  attitudes towards, discrimination   43, 45–6,
    55
  categories of   41–2
  characteristics   42–3
  from overseas but UK graduates   46–7, 55
  future policies and recommendations   47–8,
    55
  hospital   40, 43, 55
    career paths   43
  languages spoken   42
  at lower hospital grades, 'pool' of   41, 43
  numbers in Great Britain   40, 48
  postgraduate training   41, 43
  training, discrimination in   46–7, 55
  see also general practitioner (GP), Asian
doctor-patient relationship   19, 35, 172
  sources of communication errors   19, 57–9,
    94
dream guidance   99–100
'drug' interactions   104, 106, 247, 301
drug metabolism, fast and slow
        acetylators   142
duodenal ulcers   127, 143

ear-piercing   283
East Africa, Asians from   5–7, 245
eclampsia   180
ecthyma   285
eczema   286–7
  atopic   280–2, 286–7
education
  doctors   46, 211
  nurse   53–4
  see also health education
elderly Asians   237–49
  assessment of needs   238–41
  care of   160–2, 237
  cultural attitudes to illness and health
        care   240, 247
  discriminations and disadvantages   237–8,
    244
  ethnic diversity   240–1, 246
  facility in English   240–3
  health problems   238, 240
  household patterns, sizes and structures   161,
    243–5
  knowledge and use of welfare services   32,
    161, 240–1, 245–7
  life-experiences, diversity   238, 241, 248
  as minority member of minority group   238
  service design and provision   162, 238, 241,
    248
  size of population   14, 239
  status, in households   244

  stereotyping and assumptions on   237
  time spent outside home   244–5
emotional disorders
  in children   216
  in parents, effects on child   216–17
English language
  fluency and literacy   62–3, 150, 172, 241–3,
    307
  simplification   63–4
English for Pregnancy classes   69, 172
enteric fever   229, 256–7
epilepsy   145
  'hot water'   145
erythema   273, 276
erythromycin   263
ethnic diversity   4–5, 74–6, 150, 193
  of elderly Asians   240–1, 246
  see also Asian population
exorcisms   101
eye-contact   61

faith-healing   100–1, 297, 309
family
  extended   14, 161, 174, 187, 237
    history of genetic disorders   197
  history   214–15
  names   11–14
  pedigree   197–8
  precedence over individual   101, 301
  support   305
  systems and child rearing   159
  therapy   301
family-planning   151
fasting   11, 119–20
female doctors   60, 173
female modesty   47, 60, 173, 274
  in general practice   33, 36
fertility trends   79–80
fetal abnormalities, *see* congenital abnormalities
fetal death   183, 185
fetal distress   183
fluency, English   62–3, 172, 241–3, 307
folic acid deficiency   126, 139, 179
folklore remedies   102–3
follow-up visits   211
food-poisoning   126
food(s)
  avoidance (*perhaiz*)   122–3
  festive   119–20, 122
  forbidden   119, 121–2
  in hospitals   123–4, 307–8
  'hot' and 'cold'   122, 158
  staple   118
  see also diet
food-therapy (health foods)   101–2
forceps delivery   183
fungal infections of skin   285–6

garlic 102, 127
gastric ulcer 143
gastroenteritis 227–8
gastrointestinal disease 127, 143
gastrointestinal infections 227–9
  important features 228
GC1F allele 210–11
General Fertility Rate (GFR) 79–80
general practice
  Asians' experiences of and attitudes to 32, 34–5
  delivery of care to Asians 35–8
  discrimination against Asian doctors in 45, 48, 55
  future improvements 37–8
  human resources management 35–6, 38
  organization and facilities 36–8
    accommodation 36
    appointment system 37, 60
    medical records 36–7
  reasons for Asians in 43
  social class importance 34, 84
  sources of guidance for 38, 39
general practitioner (GP)
  alternative medicine role 32–3, 94, 106
  Asian 32–4, 173, 245
    adaptations, Asian patient treatment 47
    career paths 43–5
    in inner-city areas 43, 45, 48, 55
    number of 40
    problems experienced by 45
  attitude to holistic medicine 247
  experiences and difficulties with Asian patients 33–4, 38
  private, use of 33
  use of, by Asians 31–3, 84
    elderly 32, 245–6
  see also doctors, Asian, in NHS
genetic aspects, consanguineous marriage 195–6
genetic counselling 175, 200–2
  attitudes to 206–7
  consanguineous marriage, risks 196, 200, 223
genetic relationship, establishing 197
genetics clinic 200, 206, 208
giant-cell arteritis 145
giardiasis 228–9
gift food-poisoning 126
glucose 6-phosphate dehydrogenase (G6PD) deficiency 140–1, 224, 255
goal disparity, between doctors and patients 58–9
green pharmacy 103–4
greetings 62
group therapy 301
growth patterns, Asian children 210
Gujaratis 4, 7, 12

gulkand 105

haematological disorders 139–40, 200–3, 224
haemoglobin levels 140, 179
haemoglobinopathies 140–1, 200–3, 224
haemolytic anaemia 140–1, 224
hair-removal techniques 274, 281–2
hakims 104–6
  number 94, 247
  use of 32–3, 130, 142, 247
halal 119
handicaps, mental and physical 159–60
healing 93
  faith 100–1, 297, 309
health beliefs, factors influencing 18, 21
health education 162–3, 173
  cervical cytology 155, 164
  materials 163, 167–8
  in pregnancy 173, 176
  successful, key elements 162–3
health foods 101–2
health professionals, attitudes to 60
health services
  for elderly Asians 238, 245–8
  introduction of new roles, problem minimization 68
  provision 31–9
    future prospects 37, 47–9, 69–70
  use of 31–3, 38, 84, 294
    for terminal care 308
  see also general practice; National Health Service (NHS)
health visitors, Asian 53
heavy metals 99, 105, 142
height, of Asian mothers 182
helminthic infections 140, 179
  in children 230–1
henna 283
hepatic infections 229
hepatitis 258
  amoebic 229
hepatitis A infection (infective heptatitis) 229, 258, 282
hepatitits B serum globulin (HBIG) 268–9
hepatitits B virus (HBV) 218–19, 229, 258
  screening for 268
  vaccine 219, 258, 269
  vertical transmission 268–9
hepatitis Non-A non-B(NANB) 219, 229
hepatosplenomegaly 233
herbal medicine 103–4, 116
hereditary disorders 175, 184, 192–209, 223–5
  classification 193–4
  general population screening 202–3
  problems associated with study 192–3
  recurrence risk 200, 202, 204, 223–4

risk calculation   197–200, 223
  spectrum of   193–4
herpes zoster   285
Hikmat   104–6
Hindi language   7
Hindus and Hinduism   5, 8–9, 62
  astrotherapy   97
  birthweights of   182
  contraceptive methods   151–2
  death and bereavement   213, 313, 315–16
  dietary restrictions   120–1
  names   11–12
  place of death   308–9
  yoga   114
hirsutism   281
history, family and child's   214–15
homoeopathy   93, 106–7, 116
homozygosity, risk of   197–200, 223
honey   102, 157
hookworm   226, 230, 276
hospices   310
hospital, catering in   123–4
*Hospital medical staffing; achieving a balance;
    plan for action* (DHSS 1987)   43
hospital services, for elderly Asians,
    difficulties   247
household, multigenerational   161, 240, 243
household patterns, sizes and structures   243–5
human placental lactogen (HPL)   181
human resources management, in general
    practice   35–6, 38
hydroquinone   278
hygiene   123, 274
hyperemesis gravidarum   174
hyperimmune rabies immune globulin
    (HRIG)   260–1
hyperlipidaemia   133, 135
hypertension, coronary heart disease risk
    factor   132–3
hypertensive disease, in pregnancy   180
hypertensive reactions, monoamine oxidase
    inhibitors (MAOIs)   127
hypertrichosis   281–2
hypertrophic scars   284
hypochondriasis   58, 294
hypoglycaemia, prolonged, in diabetic
    patients   127, 143
hypoglycaemic agents, *Karela* interaction   127,
    143
hysteria and hysterical behaviour   298

ill-health, cultural factors influencing   20–5
illness   20
  cultural attitudes   20, 211–14, 240, 247
  religious attitudes   100
  as subjective response of patient   20

Immigrant Mortality Study   85
immigration, *see* Asian population; migration
immune serum globulin (ISG), hepatitis   258,
    268–9
immunization   150, 218, 222, 234
  childhood infections   261–8
  see also individual vaccines
impetigo   285
impotence   96, 154, 295
Indian childhood cirrhosis (ICC)   232–3
Indians
  age-structure   76, 78
  population data   74–6
  year of entry into UK   76, 79
infancy   222
infant feeding   125, 158; *see also* baby milks;
    breast-feeding
infections   225–30, 250–71
  in Asian children   226
  further information and addresses   270–1
  of greater prevalence in Asians   225–30,
    250–61
  skin   285–7
inflammatory bowel disease   143–4
information services, addresses, *see* addresses
    and information
inherited diseases, *see* hereditary disorders
inner-city
  Asian GPs in   43, 45, 48, 55
  proposals, in White Paper   37, 45
insulin
  dependency   133, 135
  religious restrictions affecting   119, 121,
    307
  therapy, compliance   135
interpreters   8, 38, 160, 173, 214, 277
  advocates, distinction between   67–8
  characteristics of   66
  checklist for interviewers using   66–7
  family members as   35–6, 66, 214, 277, 299,
    307
  need for, in general practice   35–6, 65
  problems, points to check   67
  in psychological and psychiatric
    disorders   299–300
  qualified   8, 65–6, 173, 299–300
  for terminally ill   307
interviewers, selection committees   46–7
intra-uterine contraceptive device (IUCD)   151
intra-uterine growth-retardation   180–1
iron-deficiency anaemia   125–6, 140–1
  in children   211, 231, 233
  in pregnancy   179, 219
iron supplements   25–6, 179, 231
Islam   10–11
  death and bereavement   214, 309, 311–15
  dietary restrictions   118–20
  see also Muslims

isolation of Asians 14, 290, 306
  women 159, 172, 216, 290, 306
isoniazid 142

Jainism 9, 121
jewellery, causing skin disease 283

karela 127, 142
Kaur 12, 13
keloids 284
ketoconazole 278
Koplick's spots 215
kushtays 105, 142

labour, care during 181–4
Labour Force Survey (LFS) 73–5
lactose malabsorption and intolerance 144
lacto-vegetarians 122
language 57
  appropriateness, culturally determined 61
  of Asians 4, 7–8, 164
  barrier 14, 61, 241, 277
    overcoming 63–9, 172–3
    to support of handicapped children 160
  development, assessment of progress 160
  distress for the dying patient and 307
  elderly Asians and 241–3
  English fluency/literacy 62–3, 150, 172,
    241–3, 307
  examination, for Asian doctors 34, 41, 48
  number spoken by Asian doctors 42
  problems,
    with diabetics 135
    in general practice 34–5
    in psychological and psychiatric
      disorders 299–300
  staff training 35–6, 69
  see also communication; interpreters
lead poisoning 142, 215, 284
learning difficulties 217
leishmaniasis 226–7, 275
leprosy 275
leucoderma, contact 279
lichen planus 276
lichen simplex 287
'life space', changes in 24
lifestyles 14–15
  dietary factors 117–24
link workers 68, 171, 173, 210
literacy 62–3, 150, 241–3
liver cirrhosis 141
lung cancer 136–7
lupus vulgaris 275

'Madura foot' 276
magic 107–8, 296
malaria 225–8, 234, 254–6
  diagnosis 254–5
  treatment and prevention 255–6
  vertical transmission 269
marriage
  arranged 14, 175, 217
  consanguineous, *see* consanguineous
    marriage
massage therapy 108–9
measles 215, 228, 262
  vaccine 262
Medical Act (1978) 48
medical records 36–7
medical school, discrimination in
    applications 46–7, 55
medical students 46–7, 211
medical sub-culture 19–20, 22
meditation 112–14
megaloblastic anaemia 139–41
melasma 277–8
Mendelian inherited disorders 193
meningitis 145
  tuberculous 145, 230, 234, 252
mental handicap 159–60
mental illness 22, 24–5
  rates 25, 293–4
  see also psychiatric disorders; psychological
    disorders
metabolic disorders, inherited 225
migration 23–5, 241, 291
  Asian doctors 41
  push-pull model 5–7, 24
  reasons for 5–7, 241, 291
  stress of 23–5, 292
  see also Asian population
milia 284
mineral clay 143
Mirpuris 5–7
miscarriage risk, prenatal diagnosis 201
molluscum contagiosum 284–5
Mongolian blue spot 218, 233, 277
monoamine oxidase inhibitors (MAOIs) 127,
    301
morbidity 85–7
mortality rates 85, 156, 308
Mosques 10
mourning 213–14, 313–16
multiple sclerosis (MS) 145
multi-racial approach, to health service
    provision 31
mumps 261–2
mumps-measles-rubella (MMR) vaccine 262
Muslims 4–5, 10–11, 62, 150
  attitude to termination of pregnancy 200–1,
    207
  belief in will of Allah, approach to 97, 100

birthweights of   182
consanguineous marriage   194–5, 223
contraceptive methods   151–2
dietary restrictions   118–20
names   13–14
perception of pain   306
place of death   309
skin diseases in   274
see also Islam
mycetoma   276

naming systems   10–14
  Hindu   11–12
  medical records and   12–13, 36–7
  Muslim   13–14
  Sikh   10, 12–13
nan bread   118, 123, 127
National Association of Health Authorities
      report (NAHA 1988)   48
National Health Service (NHS)
  Asian nurses in   49–54
  attitudes to   32, 34–5, 59–60
  doctors, *see* doctors, Asian, in NHS; general
      practitioner (GP)
  use of, by Asians   31–3, 84, 294
  see also health services
necropsies   213–14, 312
nephrotic syndrome, steroid-responsive   232
neural tube defects (NTDs)   203–6, 208
  prenatal screening and diagnosis   205
  recurrence risk   204
neurological disorders   145
neurosarcoid   145
New Commonwealth and Pakistan
      (NCWP)   73, 75, 81
nose-piercing   283
nurses, Asian, in NHS   49–54
  factors deterring   52–3
  numbers   52
  nursing curricula   51–4
  promotion prospects   50
  training   51–3
nutrition   117–29, 174–5, 219–20
nutritional disorders   124–6
  in children   124–5, 211, 231–2

obesity   135
obsessions   298–9
obstetrics   172–91
Office of Population Censuses and Surveys
      (OPCS)   73
oils, aromatherapy   95–6
oral tumours   136–7
organization of health-care   31–9
'oriental sore'   275
origins, of Asians in Britain   4–5

osteomalacia   124, 146, 180, 220
osteopathy   108–9, 116
over-the-counter medicine   109
ovo-lacto-vegetarians   120

paediatrics 210–36; *see also* children
pain   58, 180, 294
  perception, factors in   58, 305–6
  postnatal   187
  in pregnancy and labour   180, 183–4
Pakistanis   4–5, 63
  age-structure   76, 78
  population data   74–6
  year of entry into UK   76, 79
palmistry   109–10
paralinguistics   61
paranoia   295–6
paraphenylenediamine (PPD)   283
Parent Advisor   160
Pathans   5
peptic ulceration   143
perhaiz   122
periconceptional vitamin
      supplementation   205–6
perinatal mortality   80–3, 184–5, 220, 236
  causes   184–5, 220
  dietary and social factors   174
  rates (PMR)   81–3, 184–5, 220
  reactions to and communication on   188
  risk factors   82, 174–5, 186–7, 220
perinatal period   220–2
pernicious anaemia   139
pertussis   263–5
pertussis immunization   263–5
  neurological complications   265
  schedule   263, 266
'pesco-vegetarians'   120
phobias   298–9
physical abuse   217–18, 292
physical handicap   159–60
phytic acid and phytase   125
pigmentation disorders   273–4, 276–9
pityriasis alba   279
pityriasis capitis   280
pityriasis (tinea) versicolor   278
placental function monitoring   181, 183
polio vaccines   267
population, Asian *see* Asian population
pork and pork products   118–19, 121
'port medicine'   84
postgraduate training, Asian doctors   41, 43
post-inflammatory depigmentation   276
post-mortems   213–14, 312
postnatal care   187–8
postnatal rites and customs   157–8
practice nurses, female   47
prayer nodules   284
pre-eclampsia   180, 186

Preganvite Forte F   205–6
pregnancy   159
   antenatal complications   179–81
   care during   176–8
   care prior to   175–6
   diabetes in   175, 181
   dietary aspects   174–5, 219–20
   health education in   173, 176
   hepatitis Non-A Non-B (NANB) in   219
   perinatal mortality risk factors   174–5,
      186–7, 220
   risk factors in   174
   termination   175, 178–9, 200–2
      attitudes to   175, 200, 207
   working during   174, 186
prenatal diagnosis   200, 208, 218–19, 224
   neural tube defects (NTDs)   205
   thalassaemia   201–2, 218, 224
prenatal sex determination   153
pre-pregnancy counselling   175
prescription   215
primaquine   255
protozoal infections   225–7, 254–6
pruritus, generalized   282–3
psoriasis   276, 281, 286–7
psychiatric disorders   290–303
   conditions mistaken for, in children   234
   rates   293–4
   treatment   300–1
psychiatry   22, 34, 216, 296
psychological disorders   290–303
   background to, racism and   23–4, 291–2
   in children   216–290
   in parents, effects on child   216–17
   treatment   300–1
psychological responses to skin diseases   273–5
psychosis, acute reactive   297
psycho-social transitions   23–4, 26
psychosomatic disorders   216, 294, 297
   conditions mistaken for, in children   234
psychotherapy   101, 110, 112, 301
pulmonary tuberculosis, *see* tuberculosis
Punjabis   5, 52, 63
pustular skin disease   285
PUVA   279, 286
pyridoxine supplements   142
pyuria, sterile   135

rabies   234, 258–61
   diagnosis and immunization   234, 260–1
   'furious' and 'dumb'   259–60
   incubation period and presenting
      features   259
rabies human diploid cell strain (HDCS)
      vaccine   260
racial abuse and violence   43, 45, 292, 295
racism   291–2

Ramadan   11, 119, 274, 299
recruitment   36, 69, 173
   Asian doctors to UK, reasons   40–1
   Asian nurses   50–1
rectal examination   215
refugees   7, 296
reincarnation   9, 100, 120
religions   4–5, 8–11, 93, 95, 110
   attitudes to death and dying   212–14, 304
   contraceptive methods   151–2
   dietary restrictions   118–22, 212, 307–8
   obsessions and   299
   see also death and dying; *individual religions*
religious factors
   in pregnancy   174
   skin diseases and   274
religious leader, presence at death   309
religious rituals   101, 110–11
religious-therapist   100–1
renal disease   135–6
renal failure, chronic   135–6, 282
renal tuberculosis   135, 252
respiratory disease   138
resurrection doctrine   100
rheumatic conditions   111
rice   118, 127
rickets   124, 146, 211, 220
   adolescent   232, 234
   causes   221
   in children   124, 146, 231–2
   infantile   231–2
ringworm, scalp   280
roles, non-correspondence, and uncertainty   58
rose spots   256
rotavirus   227–8
roundworm   226, 230
Royal Colleges   47
rubella   218, 261–2
   vaccines   262

saand oil   95–6
Salmonella infections   227, 229, 256–7
salmonellosis, non-typhoid   227–8
'sanctity of life' doctrine   110, 120
sarcoidosis   139
scabies   285–6
scalp disorders   279–81
scented smoke, scented water   95–6
schizophrenia   101, 295–8
school problems   217
self-help groups   168–9
self-medication   109
self-poisoning   298
semen-losing syndrome   154, 295
sesame oil   96
sesame seeds   102
sexual dysfunction   154, 295

sheltered accommodation 246
Shia Muslims 10
shigellosis 227–8
sickle-cell disease 200, 22-.
Sikhs and Sikhism 4, 9–10, 62
  birthweights of 182
  contraceptive methods 151–2
  death and bereavement 213–14, 313–14
  dietary restrictions 121–2
  hair-removal and 274, 281
  names 10, 12–13
Singh 12
skin diseases 272–89
  altered prevalence 276–7
  cultural and psychological variations 273–5
  diagnosis, obscured in Asians 273, 276
  diagnosis and management, cultural factors
    affecting 272–3
  imported 272, 275–6
  management 277–87
  see also individual diseases
skin-lightening preparations 278
skin trauma 283–4
smells, cultural misunderstandings and 123,
  274
smoking 122, 132–3
social aspects, consanguineous marriage 195
social class, importance in general practice 34,
  84
social conventions 62
social factors, in pregnancy 159, 174
socio-economic factors
  elderly Asians and 161, 244
  influencing culture and ill-health 21–3
  perinatal mortality 174, 186
somatization of distress 58, 180, 216,
  294–5
spa therapy 111–12
sperm, importance of 153–4, 295
spina bifida 203
spinal meningitis 145
spine, tuberculosis of 252
spiritual medicine 100–1, 297, 309
staff training and development 35–6
Staphylococcus aureus 285–6
State enrolled nurse (SEN) 49–50
sterilization 153–4
steroid-responsive nephrotic syndrome 232
steroid therapy 139, 279, 287
stillbirths 213, 236
stress 112, 283, 290, 294
  of migration 23–5, 292
  reduction, overcoming language barrier 64
stress-induced psychosis 297
Strongyloides stercoralis 226
'stuck doctors' 43
subcaste names 12–13
sub-cultures 19–20, 22

medical 19–20, 22
  socio-economic factors influencing 21, 23
Sunni Muslims 10
support groups 168–9
surma 142, 215–16, 283–4
Swami Narayan sect 9

Takayasu's disease 145
Tamils 5, 7
tapeworms 226
tavees 296
terminal care 304–19
  alternative healers 97, 309–10
  information and literature on 317–18
  management of distress 307–8
  use of medical and social services 308
  see also death and dying
terminally ill, definition 305
tetanus 265–7
  immune globulin 266
tetanus toxoid vaccine 265–7
thalassaemia 140, 200–3, 208, 233
  beta- 140, 179, 201–3, 208, 218, 224
  carrier detection 202, 218
  iron therapy avoidance 126, 179
  prenatal diagnosis 201–2, 218, 224
Tibe-Unani 104–6, 247
tinea (pityriasis) versicolor 278
training 35–6
  Asian doctors, discrimination in 46–7, 55
  Asian nurses 51–4
  transcultural issues 69
transcendental meditation (TM) 112–13, 116
transplantation 312
trauma
  psychological effects 296
  skin response 284
travel, hazards of 250, 255, 257–8
Trichophyton violaceum 280
tricyclic antidepressants 300, 301
tuberculosis 138, 179, 251–3, 275
  abdominal 230, 252
  in children 230
  miliary 230, 251–2
  non-pulmonary 135, 230, 251–2
  pulmonary 138, 179, 230, 251
  reactivation 139, 251, 252
  renal 135, 252
  treatment and prevention 252–3
tuberculous meningitis 145, 230, 234, 252
typhoid fever 228–9, 256–7
typhoid vaccine 257

ulcerative colitis (UC) 143–4
ultrasound, in pregnancy 117, 179, 205
unhappiness 290

Urdu 7
urinotherapy 113

vaccine, *see* immunization; *individual vaccines*
vaginal bleeding 186
vaid 94, 98, 104, 247
varicella zoster virus 267–8
vegans 120–1
vegetarians 120–1, 126
  folate, vitamin B$_{12}$ deficiency 121, 126, 139,
    179, 219
  iron deficiency 125, 179, 219, 231
  pregnancy 174–5
  typical hospital menu 123–4
verbal communication 61
vertical transmission of infections 268–9
videotapes, health-education 155, 163, 243
viral skin infections 285
vitamin, periconceptional
    supplementation 205–6
vitamin B$_{12}$ deficiency 121, 126, 139–40,
    179
vitamin D
  binding protein 210–11
  deficiency 124, 146, 180, 220

  in children 124, 221, 231–2
    see also rickets
  supplements 125, 146, 180, 220, 232
vitiligo 273–4, 278–9
voluntary groups 168–9

weaning 158, 212, 222, 231
weight-gain, in pregnancy 186
whip-worm 226
White Paper *Promoting better health*
    (1987) 37, 45
whooping cough 263–5
women
  as carers 159–62, 174
  child rearing 157–9
  role of 14–15, 150, 163
women doctors 215
women's groups, addresses 191
women's health 150–71

xeroderma 282–3

yoga 114
yoghurt 102, 123, 127